ANNALS OF THE NEW YORK ACADEMY OF SCIENCES

VOLUME 151, ART. 2 PAGES 691–1001

July 31, 1968

Editor-in-Chief
TRUMAN L. HALL

Managing Editor
MARC KRAUSS

Associate Editor
KAREN SUSSELL

PHARMACOGENETICS*

Consulting Editors and Conference Cochairmen
BERT N. LA DU AND WERNER KALOW

CONTENTS

Introductory Remarks. *By* BERT N. LA DU 693

Part I. Drug Metabolism Enzymes

Pharmacogenetics in Animals and Man. *By* WERNER KALOW 694

Genetics of Esterases in Man. *By* NANCY E. SIMPSON 699

Properties of Plasma Cholinesterase Variants. *By* SANDRA W. CLARK, GEORGE A. GLAUBIGER AND BERT N. LA DU 710

Genetic Variations in the Acetylation of Isoniazid and Other Drugs. *By* DAVID A. PRICE EVANS 723

Purification and Properties of N-Acetyltransferase from Mammalian Liver. *By* WENDELL W. WEBER, SANFORD N. COHEN AND MICHAEL S. STEINBERG 734

Therapy of Prolonged Apnea after Suxamthonium with Purified Pseudocholinesterase: New Data on Kinetics of the Hydrolysis of Succinyldicholine and Succinylmonocholine and Further Data on N-Acetyltransferase-Polymorphism. *By* H. W. GOEDDE, K. ALTLAND AND W. SCHLOOT 742

Glucose-6-Phosphate Dehydrogenase Variants and Drug-Induced Hemolysis. *By* HENRY N. KIRKMAN 753

Hemolysis Due to Inherited Erythrocyte Enzyme Deficiencies. *By* PAUL E. CARSON 765

Effects of Drugs and Drug Metabolites on Erythrocytes from Normal and Glucose-6-Phosphate Dehydrogenase-Deficient Individuals. *By* IAN M. FRASER AND ELLIOT S. VESELL 777

Hereditary Methemoglobinemia, Toxic Methemoglobinemia and the Reduction of Methemoglobin. *By* ERNST R. JAFFÉ AND GERTRUDE NEUMANN 795

* This series of papers is the result of a conference entitled Pharmacogenetics, held by The New York Academy of Sciences on October 5, 6 and 7, 1967, and supported in part by grant no. GM 15487-01 from The National Institute of General Medical Sciences, National Institutes of Health, Bethesda, Md.

Drugs, Anesthesia and Abnormal Hemoglobins. *By* A. G. MOTULSKY AND G. STAMATOYANNOPOULOS ... 807

Acetophenetidin-Induced Methemoglobinemia. *By* N. T. SHAHIDI ... 822

Part II. Hereditary Diseases of Pharmacogenetic Interest

Pharmacologic and Genetic Determinants of Disordered Bilirubin Transport and Metabolism in the Liver. *By* LAWRENCE M. GARTNER AND IRWIN M. ARIAS ... 833

Experimental Hepatic Porphyria: Studies with Steroids of Physiological Origin in Man. *By* ATTALLAH KAPPAS AND S. GRANICK ... 842

Clinical Aspects of Drug Reactions in Hereditary Hepatic Porphyria. *By* DONALD P. TSCHUDY ... 850

Genetic Factors Related to Glaucoma. *By* MANSOUR F. ARMALY ... 861

Altered Drug Response in Familial Dysautonomia. *By* JOSEPH DANCIS ... 876

Inherited Forms of Diabetes Insipidus and Diagnostic Drug Applications. *By* RICHARD RELKIN ... 880

Part III. Genetic Variations that Modify Drug Response

Variations in Detoxication Enzymes During Mammalian Development. *By* SUMNER J. YAFFE, JOSEPH KRASNER AND CHARLOTTE S. CATZ ... 887

Genetic and Environmental Factors Affecting Hexobarbital Metabolism in Mice. *By* ELLIOT S. VESELL ... 900

Hereditary Resistance to Coumarin Anticoagulant Drugs in Man and Rat. *By* ROBERT A. O'REILLY, JUDITH G. POOL AND PAUL M. AGGELER ... 913

Variations in Metabolism of Coumarin Anticoagulant Drugs. *By* HARVEY M. SOLOMON 932

Atypical Human Liver Alcohol Dehydrogenase. *By* J. P. VON WARTBURG AND P. M. SCHÜRCH ... 936

Hyperrigidity and Hyperthermia Associated with Anesthesia. *By* B. A. BRITT AND W. KALOW ... 947

Part IV. Pharmacogenetics and Drug Toxicity

Variation of Drug Metabolism in Animals and the Prediction of Drug Action in Man. *By* J. J. BURNS ... 959

Pharmacogenetics in the Detection of the Hypersusceptible Worker. *By* H. E. STOKINGER, J. T. MOUNTAIN AND L. D. SCHEEL ... 968

Drug-Induced Chromosomal Aberrations. *By* KURT HIRSCHHORN ... 977

Genetic Factors in Hypersensitivity Reactions to Drugs. *By* BERNARD B. LEVINE ... 988

Teratology and Pharmacogenetics. *By* HAROLD KALTER ... 997

Concluding Remarks. *By* WERNER KALOW ... 1001

INTRODUCTORY REMARKS

B. N. La Du
Department of Pharmacology, New York University School of Medicine New York, N. Y.

The papers comprising this monograph were presented at the first international conference on pharmacogenetics and represent an introduction to this relatively new field of research and clinical investigation. Dr. Kalow and I intentionally did not restrict the papers to those areas which have been well developed or thoroughly explored. We sought to call attention to new examples, and in some cases, new possible examples of hereditary variations in drug metabolism or drug response.

The program emphasis has been on human pharmacogenetics but a number of papers on animal studies were included and we felt they were essential to balance the program. The relative value and applicability of animal studies in evaluating human hereditary variations in drug responses must still be determined and we do not know the answer today.

The plan to hold a conference on Pharmacogenetics came about by the stimulation and encouragement from the subcommittee of the Drug Research Board, National Academy of Sciences which is headed by Dr. John J. Burns, and is called the Committee on Applications of Biochemical Studies in Evaluating Drug Toxicity. We are pleased to acknowledge the cooperation and support of the New York Academy of Sciences and the financial support, which made the meeting possible, by the United States Public Health Service and the National Institute of General Medical Sciences.

PART I. DRUG METABOLISM ENZYMES

PHARMACOGENETICS IN ANIMALS AND MAN

W. Kalow

Department of Pharmacology
University of Toronto
Toronto, Canada

Different organisms respond differently to their environments because of different genetic endowments. Since drugs are part of the human environment, it is natural to encounter hereditary factors that affect the responsiveness of the human organism to drugs, and one should find these factors in all forms of life which are appropriately studied.[1]

In recent years, the discovery of antiviral agents was a major achievement, but it did not take long until mutant viruses appeared which were resistant to the antiviral drugs.[2,3] Hereditary resistance of bacteria to drugs was known for many years. The transfer of genetic material from one bacterial organism to the next by transformation and transduction were exciting discoveries, even when these processes were seen only under artificial conditions in vitro. Now it seems that under hospital conditions, bacterial genes conveying drug resistance have been transferred to bacterial strains which had been hitherto susceptible to antibiotics.[4,5] Until recently, plasmodia had not shown much hereditary resistance to antimalarial agents; now the existence of such altered strains are a major therapeutic problem.[6] One could cite many further examples concerning infectious organisms, but the problem is sufficiently well-known to make further elaboration unnecessary.

During recent years, concepts of pharmacogenetics have inspired much work on laboratory animals.[7] One way in which such animal studies were performed was by selecting rats or mice for a particular drug response and breeding them under continued selection.

For example, Nichols and Hsiao[8] selected and bred rats for susceptibility to morphine addiction. They first addicted the rats by injecting morphine, then maintained some addiction by intermittently adding it to drinking water, and finally withdrew morphine completely. After withdrawal, some rats preferred drinking water containing morphine, while others did not show this preference. By selecting, breeding and inbreeding these rats for a few generations, they obtained two strains which were distinctly different from each other by their preference for morphine. It turned out that the rats susceptible to morphine addiction could also be addicted to alcohol with greater ease than their morphine-declining counterparts.

In rats[9] and mice,[10] evidence for hereditary control of alcoholism has been known for many years. The inclination to take alcohol differs between strains;[9,10] that is, some animals refuse to drink water to which alcohol has been added, while others accept the addition avidly. Secondly, there are strains with differences of alcohol metabolism.[11] Thirdly, there are strains with different sensitivities to alcohol intoxication due to different sensitivities of brain cells.[12] Thus, there is evidence in animals for hereditary controls affecting intake and action of an addicting drug on three different levels.

I am not aware of any attempts to demonstrate a hereditary component in man for susceptibility to morphine addiction. However, there have been many attempts made to demonstrate genetic components in the propensity to becoming addicted to nicotine or alcohol. Various twin studies and family data which show a hereditary component in the propensity to become a cigarette smoker were summarized last year in a paper presented before this Academy.[13] Regarding alcohol addiction, many data do not support evidence for an hereditary predisposition in man.[14] However, there must be such a predisposition if the following experience is generally valid. Dr. Gordon Bell of Toronto told this story from his experience: Some decades ago a country doctor in Ontario performed tonsillectomies on several children in one family. In order to do so he anesthetized each child with ether, but he had a very difficult time getting one of the brothers to fall asleep. When this boy later, as an adult, became an alcoholic and thereby a patient, Dr. Bell heard of this childhood experience. Thereafter, Dr. Bell systematically enquired among alcoholics about their resistance to general anesthetics during childhood. On the basis of their answers, he suspects that the well-known resistance of alcoholics to general anesthetics is often not only due to acquired resistance, but also, in part, due to a personal trait present prior to alcohol intake. This makes sense if one believes that one factor predisposing to alcoholism is resistance to acute intoxication, so that a man tends to be stimulated by alcohol without getting sick. It may take years to prove or disprove by objective means this opinion of a keen observer. However, it will probably be worth the effort.

Among other attempts to find hereditary parameters affecting alcoholism in man, are those of Cruz-Coke and Varela in Chile,[15] whose starting point of investigation was the finding of a correlation between liver cirrhosis and color-blindness. At first sight this finding suggested a hereditary factor in alcoholic cirrhosis since color-blindness had been considered one of the best examples of a hereditary defect. It then appeared that color-blindness may occur as a consequence of severe liver damage.[16] However, Cruz-Coke extended his investigations, not limiting his efforts to cirrhosis. The circumstantial evidence shown by him last year[15] suggests that there is a connection between color-blindness and alcoholism, which is not due to the common factor of liver damage. The data imply that there might be a minor hereditary factor in alcoholism. Accordingly, a color-blind person is several times more likely to become an alcoholic than is one with normal vision, yet the great majority of alcoholics are not color-blind. It will be interesting to see whether these observations can be confirmed at other centers.

Some hereditary differences between animals have been a challenge to investigators, so that there are precise and extensive investigations of these differences, although there is no obvious utility of the data. I am thinking, for instance, of atropine esterase in rabbits.[17] More than 100 years ago, in 1852, the Viennese physician Schroff reported that rabbits do well on a diet of belladonna leaves.[17] This report initiated a number of studies which culminated in 1938 in the discovery by Bernheim and Bernheim[18] of an atropine esterase in liver and serum of some rabbits but absence of these enzymes in others. These studies were followed by the intensive genetic investigations of Sawin and Glick.[19] Since that time many pertinent reports have appeared in the literature. For instance, it has been shown that atropine esterase-deficient rabbits do not possess an immunologically related protein,[20] or, in other words, that the enzyme protein seems to be missing rather than changed into an inactive form. Despite all this progress, many observations are still lacking. We know that the presence and absence of atropine esterase strongly affect the response to injected atropine, and also atropine applied locally to the eye.[17] Whether it makes much difference to ingested atropine or ingested natural alkaloids has not been shown.[21] This would be a rather important piece of information for any theory on the role of atropine esterase in the process of natural selection. Furthermore, in individual rabbits esterases apparently different from atropine esterase may lack, e.g., a benzoylcholinesterase and a cocaine esterase.[22] A close investigation of the biochemical and genetic relationships between these enzymes may be very interesting.

A similar challenge has been the discovery of rats genetically resistant to the anaphylactoid reaction.[23] If a protein such as ovomucoid of egg white is injected, it normally causes a reaction that looks like an allergic reaction, yet it differs from an allergic reaction in that there is no previous sensitization required. In some rats the anaphylactoid reaction cannot be elicited. It is clear that these animals are homozygous for a recessive gene which conveys the lack of reactivity. These genes occur only in Wistar rats. Perhaps these studies will shed some light on the processes contributing to the anaphylactic reaction in man.

Another area of interest is presented by a number of investigations which one may classify under the term "comparative genetics." Many hereditary defects seem to occur in numerous species of animals and in man. Nachtsheim in 1959 published an extensive list of such defects, many of which were anatomical.[24] In addition, there are many examples of biochemical polymorphism.[7] For example, hemoglobin variants have been described in man,[25] cattle,[26] goats,[27] sheep,[28] and mice.[29] Enzymes variable in man and in other species are, for example, glucose-6-phosphate dehydrogenase,[27] catalase,[7] esterase,[30] phosphatase and others.[28] Hence there is more and more possibility of utilizing hereditary defects in animals for the study of similar hereditary defects in man. The study of Gunn rats who showed kernicterus and lack of glucuronidation similar to patients with the Crigler-Najjar syndrome is a prominent example.[1]

The more precisely one measures the effect of a drug in laboratory animals, the more likely one is to find differences between strains. There are numerous data showing differences of pharmacological response. Many of these differences are quite puzzling. It seems that males of all dark strains of mice are so susceptible to renal damage by chloroform[3] that one almost wonders whether one should develop a pesticide for mice on that basis.

An interesting strain difference became apparent by investigations of amphetamine toxicity on aggregated and isolated mice.[3] Amphetamine, dexedrine and stimulants of similar nature are about eight times as toxic to mice which are in group cages than to those caged singly. This difference is so regular and well-established that it has been used to test new chemicals for similarity of action with amphetamine. Further, this observation has stimulated many studies of the causes of reduced fertility in crowded populations of different kinds of animals. Yet this difference of susceptibility between isolated and aggregated mice was not there for DBA/2 or BDF mice. Would Nature control the rate of reproduction in these strains differently from those of other strains of mice?

Some authors tried to correlate differences of behavior with different susceptibilities to drug effect, and both or either to amine levels in brain. Thus there are strain differences of serotonin content of the limbic system. Bourgault *et al.*[33] have shown that C57BL mice have higher levels of brain serotonin and brain epinephrine than SC-I mice. In behavior, the C57BL mice are the more active, but they are also more susceptible to chlorpromazine, reserpine, phenobarbital and also to pentylenetetrazol. The former are tranquillizers or sedatives, while the last named is a convulsant. This may be surprising but it has also been suggested that humans tolerant to excitant drugs are also tolerant to sedative agents. Perhaps, such studies will lead to a new understanding of drug effects on the brain.

The diversity of these examples shows that hereditary variation may affect all kinds of responses to all kinds of drugs. If one were to neglect pharmacogenetics in the study of animals one would miss some very stimulating research experiences. I thought this should be stated at the beginning of a monograph mostly devoted to the study of man.

References

1. KALOW, W. 1962. Pharmacogenetics. Heredity and the Response to Drugs. W. B. Saunders, Phila., Pa.
2. RENIS, H. E. & D. A. BUTHOLA. 1965. Development of resistance to antiviral drugs. Ann. N. Y. Acad. Sci. **130:** 343.
3. EGGERS, H. J., N. IKEGAMI & I TAMM. 1965. Comparative studies with selective inhibitors of picornavirus reproduction. Ann. N. Y. Acad. Sci. **130:** 267.
4. KABINS, S. A. & S. COHEN. 1966. Resistance-transfer factor in enterobacteriaceae. New Engl. J. Med. **275:** 248.
5. WATANABE, T. 1966. Infectious drug resistance in enteric bacteria. New Engl. J. Med. **275:** 888.
6. SCHNITZER, R. J. 1966. Drug resistance of pathogenic protozoa. Trans. N. Y. Acad. Sci. **28:** 923.
7. MEIER, H. 1963. Experimental Pharmacogenetics. Physiopathology of Heredity and Pharmacologic Responses. Academic Press, N. Y.
8. NICHOLS, J. R. & S. HSIAO. 1967. Addiction liability of albino rats: breeding for quantitative differences in morphinen drinking. Science **157:** 561.
9. REED, J. 1951. A study of the alcoholic consumption and amino acid excretion patterns of rats of different inbred strains. Univ. Texas Pub. 5109: 144.
10. MCCLEARN, G. E. & D. A. RODGERS. 1961. Genetic factors in alcohol preference of laboratory mice. J. Comp. Physiol. **54:** 116.
11. BENNETT, E. L. & M. HEBERT. 1960. Univ. Calif. Radiat. Lab. Quart. Rept. No. 9208, April, quoted in "Brain sensitivity to alcohol in inbred mouse strains," Kakihana, R. *et al.*, 1966. Science **154:** 1574.
12. KAKIHANA, R., D. R. BROWN, G. E. MCCLEARN & I. R. TABERSHAW. 1966. Brain sensitivity alcohol in inbred mouse strains. Science **154:** 1574.
13. SELTZER, C. C. 1967. Constitution and heredity in relation to tobacco smoking. Ann. N. Y. Acad. Sci. **142:** 322.
14. GREGORY, I. 1960. Family data concerning the hypothesis of hereditary predisposition toward alcoholism. J. Ment. Sci. **106:** 1068.
15. CRUZ-COKE, R. & A. VARELA. 1966. Inheritance of alcoholism. Lancet **II:** 1282.
16. FIALKOW, P. J., H. C. THULINE & L. F. FENSTER. 1966. Lack of association between cirrhosis and the common types of color blindness. New Engl. J. Med. **275:** 584.
17. WERNER, G. 1965. Fermentdefekte als Ursache Unterschiedlicher Mydriatischer Wirksamkeit von Atropin und Cocain bei Kaninchen. Arch. Exp. Path. **251:** 320.
18. BERNHEIM, F. & M. L. C. BERNHEIM. 1938. The hydrolysis of homatropine and atropine by various tissues. J. Pharmac. Exp. Ther. **64:** 209.
19. SAWIN, P. B. & D. GLICK. 1943. Atropinesterase, a genetically determined enzyme in the rabbit. Proc. Natn. Acad. Sci. **29:** 55.
20. MARGOLIS, F. & P. FEIGELSON. 1964. Genetic expression and developmental studies with rabbit serum atropinesterase. Biochim. Biophys. Acta **90:** 117.
21. HARRIS, H. 1967. Personal communication.
22. ELLIS, S. 1948. Enzymic hydrolysis of morphine esters. J. Pharmac. Exp. Ther. **94:** 130.
23. WEST, G. B. & J. M. HARRIS. 1964. Pharmacogenetics. A fresh approach to the problem of allergy. Ann. N. Y. Acad. Sci. **118:** 439.
24. NACHTSHEIM, H. 1959. Probleme vergleichender Genetik bei Saugern. Naturwissenschaften **46:** 565.
25. BEALE, D. & H. LEHMANN. 1965. Abnormal haemoglobins and the genetic code. Nature **207:** 259.
26. SHREFFLER, D. C. & G. W. SALISBURY. 1959. Distribution and inheritance of hemoglobin variants in American cattle. J. Diary Sci. **42:** 1147.

27. Khanolkar, V. R., S. N. Naik, A. J. Baxi & H. M. Bhatia. 1963. Studies on haemoglobin variants and glucose-6-phosphate dehydrogenase in Indian sheep and goats. Experimentia **19:** 472.
28. Evans, J. V., H. Harris & F. L. Warren. 1958. The distribution of haemoglobin and blood potassium types in British breeds of sheep. Proc. R. Soc., B, **148:** 249.
29. Gluecksohn-Waelsch, S., H. Ranney & B. F. Sosken. 1957. The hereditary transmission of hemoglobin differences in mice. J. Clin. Invest. **36:** 753.
30. Augustinsson, K.-B. 1961. Multiple forms of esterase in vertebrate blood plasma. Ann. N. Y. Acad. Sci. **94:** 844.
31. Bennet, R. A. & A. Whigham. 1964. Chloroform sensitivity of mice. Nature **204:** 1328.
32. Weaver, L. C. & T. L. Kerley. 1962. Strain difference in response of mice to d-amphetamine. J. Pharmacol. Exp. Ther. **135:** 240.
33. Bourgault, P. C., A. G. Karczmar & C. L. Scudder. 1963. Contrasting behavioral, pharmacological, neurophysiological, and biochemical profiles of C57 B1/6 and SC-1 strains of mice. Life Sciences **8:** 533.

GENETICS OF ESTERASES IN MAN

Nancy E. Simpson
Departments of Biology and Pediatrics
Queen's University
Kingston, Ontario, Canada

INTRODUCTION

Most of the known genetic enzyme deficiencies and variants in man are rare and have been recognized through the study of metabolic diseases. Harris (1966) has demonstrated that genetic control of enzyme variation in normal people, however, can be rapidly discovered by mass screening methods, and knowledge of inherited enzyme diversity in apparently normal people may soon supersede that in the diseased. An additional approach to discovery of inherited enzyme variation has been pharmacogenetics. Like disease, an unusual pharmacological response selects individuals for study who are more likely to have a genetic variant when an enzyme is known to metabolize the drug in question. Conscious pursuit of enzyme diversity may, in time, make it possible to describe an "enzyme profile" of an individual as distinctive as his finger prints or blood group. The genetics of esterases in man to be described has been studied by both the "mass screening" and the "unusual pharmacological response" methods.

TISSUE ESTERASES

Soluble Esterases in Tissues

Extensive studies have been made of classification and comparison of esterases in tissue homogenates of man (Paul & Fottrell, 1961; Blanco & Zinkham, 1966; Ecobichon & Kalow, 1961, 1962, 1963, 1964 & 1965; Ecobichon, 1966). Esterases in these studies were characterized by their substrate specificities and inhibition properties. Their molecular variation was shown in zymograms; a technique using the starch-gel electrophoresis of Smithies (1955) coupled with conventional histochemical stains introduced by Hunter and Markert (1957) to localize the enzyme activity.

These studies have shown that in man most forms of esterase isozymes are common to all organ tissues but a few forms are organ-specific. The esterase zones of activity from human organs were, however, markedly different from those in human serum. Genetic control of esterases in organs seems likely because their isozymes are species-specific (Paul & Fottrell, 1961).

Observations of intra-species variation of the middle of three groups of isozymes in human liver (Ecobichon & Kalow, 1961; Blanco & Zinkham, 1966) also suggest genetic control, although proof of genetic transmission in man is not practical. Ecobichon and Kalow (1961) suggested that the variation in mobility of the middle group is continuous. From the study by Blanco and Zinkham (1966) it is not clear if the variation in the middle group was descretely dichotomous or continuous. Both data suggest that the variation of the same group of isozymes occurs commonly, but it is not possible to postulate a single gene controlling this group of isozymes as has been shown for a group of esterase isozymes in the protazoan *Tetrahymena* by Allen (1961).

The middle group of isozymes in liver appears later in development than the slow and fast groups when studied from fetal life to three years of age, and its activity increases faster during development than the other two groups (Blanco & Zinkham, 1966), suggesting that there is control of the isozymes by regulator genes. Increase in esterase activity in the small intestine of man was not evident during the 7–22 postconceptual weeks (Pelichova *et al.*, 1966). Complex control of esterases by regulator genes as well as structural genes has been demonstrated in maize (Schwarz, 1963), but we are a long way from showing similar complexity of genetic control of tissue esterases in man.

Esterases in Cell Cultures

The same pattern of esterase isozymes has been retained in cells from human tissue, including liver cells, when cultured in heterologous media containing calf serum (Paul & Fottrell, 1961), which suggests that they are not adaptive enzymes. Study of esterase isozyme variation in more readily available cultured skin fibroblasts, if the enzymes are present in these cells, would seem to be a likely method of studying their genetic control in man. Komma (1963) has carefully classified esterases from cultured cells grown from various epithelial tissues such as cervical carcinoma, normal amnion and normal cervix and found no differences in mobility of the isozymes on starch-gels. He did observe, however, variability in amounts of cholinesterase which he suggests may be due to contamination by serum used in the growth medium. His study provides a base line from which variation could be sought, although, again, genetic control in man is somewhat impractical. Such methods as the sib-pair analysis used by Robson and Harris (1965) to study the genetics of placental alkaline phosphatase from dizygotic twin births could be applied, however, to studies of amniotic cell lines.

Drug Metabolizing Esterase in Liver

Variable rates of the biotransformation of demerol hydrochloride (1-methyl-4-phenylisonipecotic acid) in man have been described by Burns, Berger, Lief, Wollack, Papper and Brodie (1955). Bernheim and Bernheim (1945) have demonstrated hydrolysis of demerol hydrochloride in human liver. The drug is also demethylated in the liver (Plotnikoff, 1951) by N-demethylase in the microsomes (Clouet, 1964). Way, Swanson and Gimble (1947) observed only slight hydrolysis by liver from two persons and more active hydrolysis from a third person which suggests that amounts of esterase are variable in different people. Species differences in hydrolysis of the drug are evident from studies by Bernheim and Bernheim (1945) and Burns *et al.* (1955) which again suggests genetic control of the enzyme. Ammon and Takeo (1966) have described an activator of demerol esterase in human plasma. The relative contributions to differences in rates of biotransformation of the drug by variation in the liver esterase, the serum activator and the demethylase are not known.

Erythrocyte Esterases

Carboxylesterases

Enzymes in blood rather than in tissues are much better candidates for genetic studies in man and a number of esterase variants in both erythrocytes and serum have been documented. Tashian and Shaw (1962) have described a genetic variant of carboxylesterase in erythrocytes. The variant was seen as two extra bands in two different groups of isozymes (A_1 and A_3) which had greater mobility than the more usual bands during starch-gel electrophoresis using α napthylacetate as substrate. The variant was first described for sera from monozygotic twins; data from three generations of the family suggested two codominant autosomal alleles for an A and B gene. The heterozygote was named AB type; one occurred in 2600 Caucasians (Tashian & Shaw, 1962) and one in 600 American Negroes (Tashian, 1965). Homozygotes of the rare B gene have not been observed. In addition, Tashian (1965) reported a variant among the 600 Negroes with extra bands of slower mobility than the usual bands of the A_2 and A_3 groups of isozymes known as AC type, but study of the family was not possible. Since the two variants showed variation in the three esterase zones, each of which had distinct biochemical properties, Tashian suggested that they share a common polypeptide unit with the same genetic control. Neither of the variants were observed in 360 American Indians, 500 Micronesians (Tashian, 1965), or in 186 Xavante Indians (Tashian *et al.*, 1967).

Carbonic Anhydrases

Three genetic variants of carbonic anhydrase (CA-I) with esterase activity produced by three alleles (b, c and d) of a common gene (a) have been reported (Shaw *et al.*, 1962; Tashian *et al.*, 1963; & Tashian, 1965). The enzyme variants were seen by starch gel electrophoresis; showed a preference for β over α napthylacetate as substrate, and were visible with conventional protein stain as well. Sera from all persons tested had one band of activity which migrated towards the anode; most sera had this band only and were designated as CA-Ia type. The variant types had cathodic zones of carbonic anhydrase activity with varying mobilities in addition to the band which migrates towards the anode. The first variant, known as CA-Ib, was observed in serum from a mongol of the 21-trisomic type. It was found during a survey of mentally retarded children and was shown to be inherited by a single autosomal gene. Persons with the variant were heterozygotes. Association of the variant with 21-trisomy was excluded (Shaw *et al.*, 1962).

The second variant CA-Ic was observed in sera from four persons in a survey of 500 Micronesians by Tashian *et al.* (1963), and analysis of pedigrees again suggested that the variant was controlled by an autosomal codominant gene. Recently, Tashian, Riggs and Yu (1966) have presented evidence that the CA-Ic type differs from the CA-Ia type by a single amino-acid substitution which probably involves only one change of base pairs in DNA. Tashian *et al.* (1966) also observed disproportional synthesis of the two enzymes produced by the two alleles in heterozygotes; the ratio being 0.56: 1 of amounts of CA-Ia: CA-Ic respectively. Two probable CA-Ic variants were observed in 120 Filipinos (Eng, 1967).

The third variant which Tashian (1965) has designated as CA-Id was observed in one woman and her daughter from the sample of 600 American Negroes and he suggests it is another heterozygote with the CA-Ia gene.

None of the variants of carbonic anhydrase are particularly common and they have not been observed in their homozygous forms.

Acetylcholinesterase

Johns (1962) has reported a reduction of acetylcholinesterase activity (acetylcholine hydrolase E.C. 3.1.1.7) in erythrocytes in a family of Lithuanian Jewish extraction. The propositus was ascertained during a routine measurement of the enzyme because he was engaged in the manufacture of organophosphates. Levels of his erythrocyte acetylcholinesterase were about one-third of normal on repeated determinations. There was no evidence of organophosphate inhibition of his acetylcholinesterase, and his levels of serum cholinesterase were normal. He was not suffering from paroxysmal nocturnal hemoglobinuria, a condition known to have reduced activity of the enzyme. Family data suggest a dominant gene for reduction of enzyme activity, although it is not possible to state whether the gene is on an autosome or the X-chromosome. Members of the family with reduced levels of the enzyme were apparently healthy.

Serum Esterases

Cholinesterase

More is known about genetic variants of cholinesterase (acylcholine acylhydrolase E.C. 3.1.1.8) than other esterases even though they are uncommon because three of the variants have been selected for study through unusual pharmacological response; prolonged apnea after a standard dose of succinylcholine and of course, variants in sera are easy to study in man.

In 1957 Kalow and Staron showed that two cholinesterase types were controlled by two codominant alleles E_1^u for usual and E_1^a for atypical enzyme. The atypical enzyme was recognized by its resistance to dibucaine inhibition (DN) and heterozygotes for the two alleles had an intermediate DN. Persons with only the atypical enzyme had prolonged apnea after succinylcholine and one occurred in about 2000 persons (Kalow & Gunn, 1959). The frequency of the atypical gene is more variable than was first thought (see reviews by Kalow, 1964; Walter *et al.*, 1965; Szeinberg *et al.*, 1966a). The frequency of heterozygotes is 2–4% in many populations but is high (7%) in Czechoslovakians (Goedde & Altand, 1963); 6% in Israeli Jews (Szeinberg, *et al.*, 1963); 10% in Iraqi and Irani (Szeinberg *et al.*, 1966a) and low (1%) in North Africans (Szeinberg *et al.*, 1966a) and 1% in Australian aborigines (Horsfall *et al.*, 1963). Heterozygotes were not observed in 250 Japanese (Omoto & Goedde, 1965); 285 Xavante Indians (Tashian *et al.*, 1967) 500 Easter Islanders and 500 Thais (Simpson, unpublished).

Irwin and Hein (1966) suggest that there are more than one kind of atypical enzyme with low dibucaine inhibition. Cholinesterase in sera from two male sibs who were heterozygous for the atypical gene had different kinetics when acetylcholine was used as substrate. The mother, whose serum had the atypical enzyme, may have transmitted two different atypical genes to her sons. Serum from one atypical out of eight tested in our laboratory showed no activity with acetylcholine as substrate although the serum had the expected level of activity with benzoylcholine for atypical type.

Harris and Whittaker (1961 & 1962) described a second variant recognized by its resistance to sodium fluoride inhibition (E_1^f) and suggested that the gene was allelic to the E_1^u and E_1^a genes. Observation of predicted homozygotes for the E_1^f gene soon followed and additional family data fitted the allelic hypothesis (Liddell *et al.*, 1963; Whittaker, 1964; Griffiths *et al.*, 1966; Simpson & Kalow, 1965). Moderate apnea has been observed in some individuals with only the fluoride-resistant enzyme (Lehmann *et al.*, 1963; Simpson, 1967). The frequency of heterozygotes for the fluoride-resistant gene (E_1^u E_1^f) was 1.5% in a sample of 800 southwest German parents (Goedde *et al.*, 1964); about 1% in 216 Brazilian parents (Simpson & Kalow, 1965) and one in 41 unrelated Canadian Caucasians (Simpson, unpublished). 1967.

The third variant is a gene for little or no activity of cholinesterase. The first homozygote for the "silent" gene ($E_1{}^s$) was observed in a succinylcholine-sensitive patient by Liddell, Lehmann and Silk (1962). Data for the dose of succinylcholine and length of apnea in homozygotes for the silent gene (TABLE 1) suggest that the duration of apnea is probably similar to that for those who have the atypical enzyme. Simpson and Kalow (1964) suggested that the silent gene was allelic to the $E_1{}^u$ and $E_1{}^a$ genes, and probably not due to a gene which suppressed activity. Heterozygotes for the $E_1{}^s$ allele with the $E_1{}^u$ or $E_1{}^a$ alleles can only be recognized by family data (Simpson & Kalow, 1964). The silent gene is the rarest of the variants; heterozygotes ($E_1{}^u$ $E_1{}^s$) are estimated to occur in one in 200 Canadians (Simpson & Kalow, 1964). The remarkably high frequency of homozygotes for the silent gene of 1.5% in 379 Alaskan Eskimos of one isolated group has been reported recently by Gutsche, Scott and Wright (1967) which suggests a frequency of 21% for heterozygotes. The above authors did not observe homozygotes for the silent gene in another group of 122 Eskimos, 141 Athabascan Indians or 58 Aleuts.

Some homozygotes for the silent gene have been reported as having no activity of cholinesterase (Liddell *et al.*, 1962; Hodgkin *et al.*, 1965; Szeinberg *et al.*, 1966b). Hodgkin and his colleagues could not demonstrate presence of enzyme in serum of their patient by reaction with a cholinesterase antiserum. Goedde, Gehring and Hofmann (1965) on the other hand, reported minimal amounts of activity in homozygotes and cross reaction with cholinesterase antiserum. One in five Canadian families studied had four homozygotes for the silent gene whose sera showed minimal activity towards benzoylcholine, and two homozygotes whose sera had no detectable activity. Since there was consanguinity in this family, the silent genes are likely to be the same mutant (Simpson, unpublished). Eight persons showed minimal activity and nine did not in Eskimos from the same isolate studied by Gutsche *et al.* (1967); again, it probably was the same mutant allele.

The predicted $E_1{}^f$ $E_1{}^s$ heterozygote has only recently been observed in two individuals (Whittaker, 1967; Simpson, 1967) providing confirmation of allelism for the four E_1 genes. Inhibition data for the two heterozygotes ($E_1{}^f$ $E_1{}^s$) were similar to and levels of activity somewhat lower than for homozygotes of the $E_1{}^f$ gene, as would be expected. The E_1 locus for the four alleles is linked to that which controls types of serum transferrins with a recombination fraction of about 0.16 (Robson *et al.*, 1966).

TABLE 1

LENGTH OF APNEA AFTER SUCCINYLCHOLINE IN SIX PERSONS WITH NO CHOLINESTERASE ACTIVITY

Age (yr)	Dose of Drug (mg)	Duration of Apnea (min)
53	50	25
	10	30
40*	70	300
60*	80	300
2	26	300
28	40	60
7	20	60

* Members of the same family.

There is another locus (E_2) which controls a variant of cholinesterase in human serum recognized by a zone with reduced mobility in addition to the zone usually observed on starch-gel electrophoresis with α naphylacetate as substrate (Harris *et al.*, 1962; Harris *et al.*, 1963). Persons with the extra zone are said to be C5+ phenotype and heterozygous for the E_2^- and E_2^+ genes; the latter gene is for C5+.

Harris *et al.* (1963) observed that the E_2^+ gene increased the activity of the usual enzyme about 30% which is a similar increase to that observed for the usual type of sera in members of Canadian families (TABLE 2). Data for the atypical C5+ type are insufficient to suggest that the E_2^+ gene increases activity of the atypical enzyme. The frequency of the C5+ phenotype is about 8% in usual, intermediate and atypical phenotypes (TABLE 2) suggesting that there is no association between the two loci. The lack of observed C5+ phenotypes in the 44 heterozygotes for the fluoride-resistant gene (UF) is probably not significant; the heterozygotes were found in only eight families. There is no evidence for linkage between the E_1 and E_2 loci (Ashton & Simpson, 1966).

The frequency of the C5+ gene in different populations (TABLE 3) appears to be more variable than that of the atypical gene; the frequency of heterozygotes ranges from 29% in one Greek village to none at all in 64 Iraqi Jews (Robson & Harris, 1966); none in 285 Xavante Indians (Tashian *et al.*, 1967) or in 500 Easter Islanders (Simpson, unpublished).

The presence of the C5+ gene in persons with only the atypical enzyme does not protect against apnea as suggested by Price (1967); six of the nine AC5+ phenotypes were individuals with apnea after the drug (TABLE 4).

Neitlich (1966) has described another electrophoretic variant which greatly increased cholinesterase activity; it appeared to be controlled by a dominant gene and occurred in one of 1,000 American males who were screened.

There is evidence for genetic control of cholinesterase activity from twin and family studies in addition to the established single genes (Wetstone *et al.*, 1965; Schloot *et al.*, 1966; Simpson, 1966). Whether the basis of the control is additional unrecognized single genes or a result of effects of additive genes is not established.

Recently, preliminary observations (FIGURE 1) suggest variation in another plasma esterase during starch-gel electrophoresis at pH 5.3 with the discontinu-

TABLE 2

MEAN ACTIVITY OF CHOLINESTERASE BY PHENOTYPES IN 100 CANADIAN FAMILIES

Phenotype	Mean Activity*	Standard Error	Number
U C5+	268	14.9	19
U C5−	208	4.0	261
I C5+	208	11.3	24
I C5−	175	2.6	269
A C5+	115	16.8	9
A C5−	107	3.8	93
UF C5−	191	2.7	44
IF C5−	147	15.5	6
F C5−†	92		1
Total			726

* Units for usual type represent micromoles of acetylcholine hydrolyzed by one ml of serum at 37° C during one hour.

† F was heterozygous for E_1^f and E_1^s genes.

TABLE 3

FREQUENCY OF C5+ PHENOTYPE FOR CHOLINESTERASE IN DIFFERENT POPULATIONS

Population	Percent C5+	Number of Tested	Reference
British*	10	1941	
Greek {Village A†	9	138	
Greek {Village B†	29	100	
Negro (Seattle)*	2	100	Robson & Harris (1966)
Iraqi Jews*	0	64	
Icelandic*	16	25	
Tristan da Cunha‡	17	214	
Canadians§	7	726	
Brazilians§	8	6500	Ashton & Simpson (1966)
Negro (Seattle)*	5	317	
Polish*	6	445	Trela (1966)
Xavante Indians*	0	285	Tashian, Brewer, Lehmann, Davies & Rucknagel (1967)
Easter Islanders‡	0	497	
Thais§	14	81	Simpson (unpublished)
Cree Indians*	14	589	

* Random population, unselected for C5+
† Parents, unselected for C5+
‡ Almost whole population
§ In family groups

TABLE 4

COMPARISON OF FREQUENCY OF A C5+ PHENOTYPES FOR SERUM CHOLINESTERASE AMONG SUCCINYLCHOLINE SENSITIVE PATIENTS AND FAMILY MEMBERS

Ascertainment	Phenotype A C5+	A C5—	Percent
Apneic	6	82	7
Family member	3	34	8
Total	9	116	

ous buffer system of Poulick (1957). The esterase showed a preference for phenylacetate as substrate over α and β napthylacetates and Fast Black was used as a dye-coupler (Stern & Lewis, 1962). The esterase appears to migrate with the albumin fraction. The faster moving zone of activity occurred together with the more usual zone in 4% of 589 Cree Indians from the Canadian province of Saskatchewan and was not seen in 350 Canadian Caucasians. The extra zone appeared as a distinct band about one hour after incubation with substrate; it was neither eserine nor EDTA sensitive. It has been observed in two sibs, and family studies are now in progress.

The significance of esterase variation is not known. The genetic variants of esterases which have been discussed occur in healthy people. The gene frequencies are for the most part rare, which does not suggest any major selective advantage in the recent past and there is no known disadvantage. Even those individuals with no cholinesterase activity are apparently healthy, and reduced erythrocyte acetylcholinesterase is compatible with health.

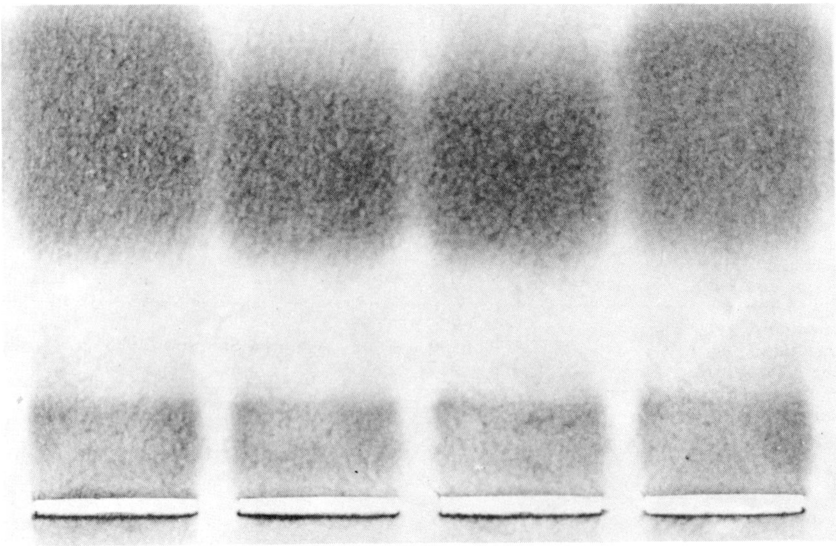

FIGURE 1. Starch gel electrophoresis at pH 5.3 of sera from four Cree Indians. Two samples in the middle are type usually observed and the two on the extreme right and left with faster migratory zone occur in 4% of Cree Indians. The esterase variant can be seen with phenylacetate as substrate coupled with Fast Black or with protein stain (Amido Black). The sample slot is at the bottom; the proteins have migrated towards the top of the photograph i.e., the anode.

The atypical variant of cholinesterase is less inhibited by solanine in potatoes (Harris & Whittaker, 1962) but it is not clear whether the toxic effects of solanine can be attributed to cholinesterase inhibition. Since persons with no cholinesterase activity are healthy, it seems unlikely that the rare cholinesterase types have been selected for in the past because they were less inhibited than the usual type by some other naturally occurring inhibitors.

[Note added in proof: The esterase variant described in Cree Indians which was thought to be an esterase which hydrolyzed phenylacetate (FIGURE 1) has now been shown to be identical to that of the albumin variant described by Melartin and Blumberg (1966) in Naskapi Indians.]

REFERENCES

ALLEN, S. L. 1961. Ann. N. Y. Acad. Sci. **94:** 753–773.
AMMON, R. & K. TAKEO. 1966. Enzymologia **30:** 69–79.
ASHTON, G. C. & N. E. SIMPSON. 1966. Amer. J. Hum. Genet. **18:** 438–477.
BERNHEIM, F. & M. L. C. BERNHEIM. 1945. J. Pharmacol. Exp. Ther. **85:** 74–77.
BLANCO, A. & W. H. ZINKHAM. 1966. Bull. Hopkins Hosp. **118:** 27–39.
BURNS, J. J., B. L. BERGER, P. A. LIEF, A. WOLLACK, E. M. PAPPER & B. B. BRODIE. 1955. J. Pharmacol. Exp. Ther. **114:** 289–298.
CLOUET, D. H. 1964. J. Pharmacol. Exp. Ther. **144:** 354–361.
ECOBICHON, D. J. 1966. Canad. J. Physiol. Pharmacol. **44:** 225–232.
ECOBICHON, D. J. & W. KALOW. 1961. Canad. J. Biochem. Physiol. **39:** 1329–1332.
ECOBICHON, D. J. & W. KALOW. 1962. Biochem. Pharmacol. **11:** 573–583.
ECOBICHON, D. J. & W. KALOW. 1963. Canad. J. Biochem. Physiol. **41:** 1537–1546.
ECOBICHON, D. J. & W. KALOW. 1964. Canad. J. Biochem. **42:** 277–286.
ECOBICHON, D. J. & W. KALOW. 1965. Canad. J. Biochem. **43:** 73–79.
ENG, L. L. 1967. Amer. J. Hum. Genet. **19:** 130–132.

GOEDDE, H. W. & K. ALTLAND. 1963. Nature **198:** 1203–1204.
GOEDDE, H. W., D. GEHRING & R. A. HOFMANN. 1965. Humangenetik **1:** 607–620.
GOEDDE, H. W., K. OMOTO, H. RITTER & H. BAITSCH. 1964. Humangenetik **1:** 1–13.
GRIFFITHS, P. D., D. DAVIES & H. LEHMANN. 1966. Brit. Med. J. **2:** 215–216.
GUTSCHE, R. B., E. M. SCOTT & R. C. WRIGHT. 1967. Nature **215:** 322–323.
HARRIS, H. 1966. Proc. Roy. Soc. B. **164:** 298–310.
HARRIS, H., D. A. HOPKINSON & E. B. ROBSON. 1962. Nature **196:** 1296–1298.
HARRIS, H., D. A. HOPKINSON, E. B. ROBSON & M. WHITTAKER. 1963. Ann. Hum. Genet. **26:** 359–382.
HARRIS, H. & M. WHITTAKER. 1961. Nature **191:** 496–498.
HARRIS, H. & M. WHITTAKER. 1962. Ann. Hum. Genet. **26:** 59–72.
HARRIS, H. & M. WHITTAKER. 1962. Ann. Hum. Genet. **26:** 73–76.
HODGKIN, W. E., E. R. GIBLETT, H. LEVINE, W. BAUER & A. G. MOTULSKY. 1965. J. Clin. Invest. **44:** 486–492.
HORSFALL, W. R., H. LEHMANN & D. DAVIES. 1963. Nature **199:** 1115.
HUNTER, R. L. & C. L. MARKERT. 1957. Science **125:** 1294–1295.
IRWIN, R. L. & M. M. HEIN. 1966. Biochem. Pharmacol. **15:** 145–154.
JOHNS, R. J. 1962. New Eng. J. Med. **267:** 1344–1348.
KALOW, W. 1964. Anesthesiology **25:** 377–387.
KALOW, W. & D. R. GUNN. 1959. Ann. Hum. Genet. **23:** 239–250.
KALOW, W. & N. STARON. 1957. Canad. J. Biochem. Physiol. **35:** 1306–1320.
KOMMA, D. J. 1963. J. Histochem. Cytochem. **11:** 619–623.
LEHMANN, H., J. LIDDELL, B. BLACKWELL, D. C. J. O'CONNOR & A. V. DAWS. 1963. Brit. Med. J. **1:** 1116–1118.
LIDDELL, J., H. LEHMANN & D. DAVIES. 1963. Acta Genet. (Basel) **13:** 95–108.
LIDDELL, J., H. LEHMANN & E. SILK. 1962. Nature **193:** 561–562.
MELARTIN, L. & B. S. BLUMBERG. 1966. Science **153:** 1664–1665.
NEITLICH, H. W. 1966. J. Clin. Invest. **45:** 380–387.
OMOTO, K. & H. W. GOEDDE. 1965. Nature **205:** 726–727.
PAUL, J. & P. FOTTRELL. 1961. Biochem. J. **78:** 418–424.
PELICHOVA, H., O. KOLDOVSKY, J. UHER, J. KRAML, A. HERINGOVA & V. JIRSOVA. 1966. Biol. Neonat. **10:** 281–287.
PLOTNIKOFF, N. P. 1951. J. Pharmacol. Exp. Ther. **101:** 31.
POULICK, M. D. 1957. Nature **180:** 1477–1479.
PRICE, J. 1967. J. Med. Genet. **4:** 44–67.
ROBSON, E. B. & H. HARRIS. 1965. Nature **207:** 1257–1259.
ROBSON, E. B. & H. HARRIS. 1966. Ann. Hum. Genet. **29:** 403–408.
ROBSON, E. B., I. SUTHERLAND & H. HARRIS. 1966. Ann. Hum. Genet. **29:** 325–332.
SCHWARTZ, D. 1963. Erwin-Baur-Gedachtnisvorlesungen **III:** 201–203.
SCHLOOT, W., J. MURKEN & H. W. GOEDDE. 1966. Humangenetik **2:** 36–41.
SHAW, C. R., F. N. SYNER & R. E. TASHIAN. 1962. Science **138:** 31–32.
SIMPSON, N. E. & W. KALOW. 1964. Amer. J. Hum. Genet. **16:** 180–188.
SIMPSON, N. E. & W. KALOW. 1965. Amer. J. Hum. Genet. **17:** 156–162.
SIMPSON, N. E. 1966. Amer. J. Hum. Genet. **18:** 243–252.
SIMPSON, N. E. 1967. J. Med. Genet. **4:** 264–267.
SMITHIES, O. 1955. Biochem. J. **61:** 629–641.
STERN, J. & W. H. P. LEWIS. 1962. J. Ment. Defic. Res. **6:** 13–21.
SZEINBERG, A., M. MEYER, Z. EISENBERG, E. OSTFELD, R. BAR-OR & R. EZRA. 1963. Israel Med. J. **22:** 137–146.
SZEINBERG, A., S. PIPANO & E. OSTFELD. 1966a. Acta Anaesth. Scand. Supp. **24:** 199–205.
SZEINBERG, A., S. PIPANO, E. OSTFELD & L. EVIATAR. 1966b. J. Med. Genet. **3:** 190–193.
TASHIAN, R. E. 1965. Amer. J. Hum. Genet. **17:** 257-272.
TASHIAN, R. E., G. J. BREWER, H. LEHMANN, D. A. DAVIES & D. L. RUCKNAGEL. 1967. Amer. J. Hum. Genet. **19:** 524–531.
TASHIAN, R. E., C. C. PLATO & T. B. SHOWS. 1963. Science **140:** 53–54.
TASHIAN, R. E., S. K. RIGGS & Y. L. YU. 1966. Arch. Biochem. Biophys. **117:** 320–327.
TASHIAN, R. E. & M. W. SHAW. 1962. Amer. J. Hum. Genet. **14:** 295–300.
TRELA, F. 1966. Med. Dosw. Mikrobiol. **18:** 293–296.
WALTER, H., S. NEUMANN, R. BACKHAUSZ & J. NEMESKERI. 1965. Humangenetik **1:** 651–657.
WAY, E. L., R. SWANSON & A. I. GIMBLE. 1947. J. Pharmacol. Exp. Ther. **91:** 178–184.
WETSTONE, H. J., M. S. HONEYMAN & R. B. MCCOMB. 1965. JAMA **192:** 1007–1009.
WHITTAKER, M. 1964. Acta Genet. (Basel) **14:** 281–285.
WHITTAKER, M. 1967. Acta Genet. (Basel) **17:** 1–12.

DISCUSSIONS OF THE PAPER

DR. EARL USDIN (*Atlantic Research Corp., Alexandria, Va.*): In your talk, you mentioned that cholinesterase isozymes could be detected in tissues grown in culture. Considering the known tendency of tissue culture lines to de-differentiate on passage, I wonder if the isozyme pattern remains stable from passage to passage?

DR. SIMPSON: Apparently they are stable. However these are not cholinesterase isozymes, but other types of esterases. Cholinesterases may be found in these cells but variations have not been described.

DR. USDIN: Do you have any indication that pseudocholinesterase variant individuals are lacking one or more of the isozymes found in normals, or even have isozymes with different mobilities than normal, or are the low pseudocholinesterase values obtained in the case of the variants a resultant of an approximately proportional amount of each of the isozymes?

DR. SIMPSON: The isozymes are the same regardless of the type of esterase, we can't tell atypical or fluoride-resistant esterase types from normal by the isozyme technique. The identification depends upon differences in response to the particular inhibitors.

DR. USDIN: In normal serum you can show a very nice picture of a major component C_4 and minor components (C_1, C_2 and C_3) by the zymogram technique.

DR. SIMPSON: Yes, and you find the same pattern if you use serum from individuals with normal, intermediate or atypical plasma cholinesterase.

DR. H. W. GOEDDE (*Institute of Human Genetics, University of Hamburg*): I have two comments to make about Dr. Simpson's paper. From population genetic studies on the polymorphism of the E_1 locus of pseudocholinesterases (frequency of the atypical allele E_1^a) it can be concluded that there are roughly three levels of frequency: one group with a frequency $>$ 0.014, one with almost

High ($>$ 0,014)	Intermediate (0,005-0,01)	Low (0-0,002)
North African (0,0142)	Oriental pop. mostly Japanese (0,0047)	Thais (0)
Brazilian (0,0149)	Australian (0,0051)	Japanese (0)
Greek (0,0162)	Seattle-Negro (0,0053)	Eskimo (0)
German (0,0162)	Indian (Mexican) Tribes (0,0093)	3 South Amer. Indian pop. (0)
Cauc. Americans (0,0163)	Maroccan Jewish (0,0098)	Congolese Negro (0,0009)
Portuguese (0,0168)		Formosan Chinese (0,0015)
Berber (0,0182)		Filipino (0,0024)
Canadian (0,0188)		
British (0,0192)		
Israeli (0,0312)		

none (0 — 0.002) and a third one with an intermediate frequency (0.005 — 0.01).*

Investigations on the so-called "silent gene" phenotype of the pseudocholinesterase polymorphism have furnished evidence for both qualitative and quantitative differences. In addition to those cases without any pseudocholinesterase activity or cross reacting material (crm), we found some with enzyme activity of about 1% of normal with high quantities of crm and others with enzyme activity of about 3%, but with small amounts of crm.

Comparative studies in collaboration with Altland, Dietz and Jenkins on 15 sera of the so-called phenotype S will be published elsewhere.

* Altland, K. *et al.* 1967. Humangenetik 4: 129.

PROPERTIES OF PLASMA CHOLINESTERASE VARIANTS

Sandra W. Clark, George A. Glaubiger* and Bert N. La Du
Department of Pharmacology
New York University School of Medicine
New York, N. Y.

INTRODUCTION

Genetic variants of plasma cholinesterase have been described by Kalow and Staron[1] and by others,[2-5] and the basis for classification of these variants, i.e., differential inhibition by dibucaine, fluoride and other compounds, has been reviewed by Kalow in his book *Pharmacogenetics*.[6] The nature of the structural alterations in the variant enzymes which still possess esterase activity has not been determined. We have undertaken a series of experiments on the kinetic properties of the esterases as well as effects of stimulators, inhibitors, pH effects and the effect of changing ionic strength, and it is expected that these studies will aid in the elucidation of the structural differences of the variant enzymes. In this paper, we will confine our discussion to a comparison of the usual and atypical (dibucaine-resistant) esterases.

MATERIALS AND METHODS

Benzoylcholine Hydrolysis

All experiments involving inhibitors and activators were performed with benzoylcholine at the concentration of 5×10^{-5} M unless indicated otherwise in the figures. Esterase activity was measured spectrophotometrically at 240 mμ according to the method of Kalow and Lindsay,[7] using absorption cells of 10 mm light path. Some reactions were read directly, but most were recorded automatically by a Gilford Multiple Sample Absorbance Recorder.

The cholinesterase variants were classified by dibucaine numbers and fluoride numbers according to the criteria of Kalow and Genest[8] and Harris and Whittaker.[2]

Phosphorylation Followed by Reactivation with Paraoxon

The procedure used was a modification of that developed by Heilbronn[9] with serum as the source of enzyme. Diethyl-p-nitrophenylphosphate (paraoxon, E-600) was added to the serum to yield a final concentration of 1×10^{-6} M. The treated sera stood at room temperature for at least 30 minutes and then were dialyzed in the cold room (4°) overnight against 0.15 M NaCl, to remove excess paraoxon. The extent of phosphorylation of the esterase was determined before dialysis and on the following day, prior to the reactivation studies. Control sera, not treated with paraoxon, were dialyzed and tested similarly.

For standard reactivation studies, NaF in phosphate buffer was added to the dialyzed sera (both control and phosphorylated to give a final concentration of 5×10^{-3} M NaF in 0.1 M phosphate buffer pH 6.0. Aliquots were removed at various time intervals, diluted 1:50 with M/15 phosphate buffer pH 7.4 and mixed with an equal volume of benzoylcholine 10×10^{-5} M in the same buffer. Spectrophotometric assays were made immediately to determine the amount of dephosphorylated (reactivated) enzyme.

* Predoctoral trainee, U. S. Public Health Service Training Grant 5T05GM16–68.

Enzyme Sources and Partial Purification

For some studies, whole serum was used, but Cohn fraction IV-4 was also employed for some of the stimulation studies of the usual enzyme. It was found that the latter preparation showed no substantial differences in behavior from serum.

Partial purification of the esterase from usual and atypical sera was achieved by fractionation with ammonium sulfate followed by filtration through G-200 Sephadex. The resulting enzymes were purified about 600-fold.[10] Purified enzymes were used in experiments over a range of pH values so that sufficiently high activity would be available at low pH to give accurate results.

Results

Stimulation and Inhibition Studies

We reported some time ago[11] that in low ionic strength buffer (M/1500 tris), the activity of the usual esterase could be greatly enhanced by increasing amounts of sodium chloride (FIGURE 1B). The highest activity obtained, with salt present as 0.2 M NaCl, was approximately three times that obtained without added salt.

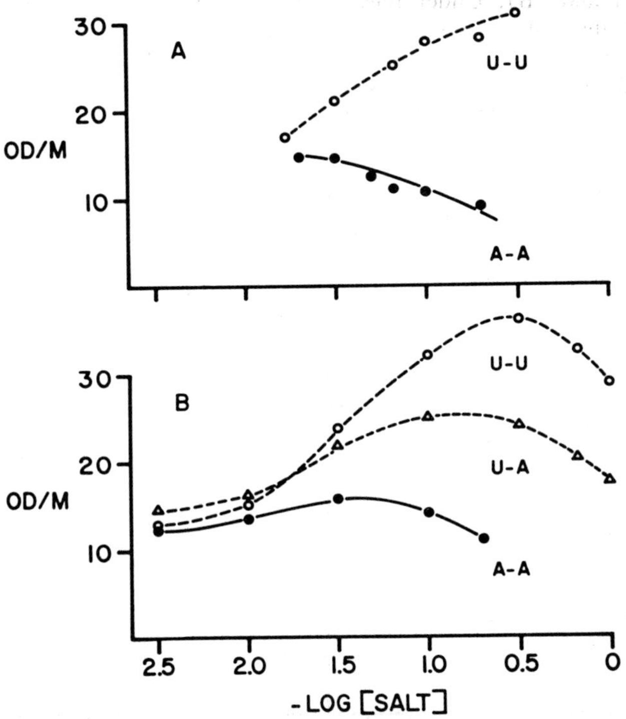

FIGURE 1A. Effect of increasing concentrations of KCl on the rate of hydrolysis of benzoylcholine, measured spectrophotometrically.[7] FIGURE 1B, effect of increasing concentrations of NaCl in M/1500 tris buffer, pH 7.3.

UU = serum from individual homozygous for usual allele.
UA = serum from individual heterozygous for usual and atypical alleles.
AA = serum from individual homozygous for atypical allele.

In contrast, the activity of the atypical enzyme was not affected except for inhibition at high salt concentrations. Enzyme from an individual heterozygous for the atypical trait was enhanced one half as much as the enzyme from a person with the usual esterase. Other salts tested were NaBr, Na_2SO_4 and KCl (FIGURE 1A). The results obtained with these salts were essentially the same as those with NaCl, indicating that the stimulatory effect was a general one with increasing ionic strength.

When higher concentrations of tris buffer itself were tested, it was found that much lower concentrations (about one-tenth of the concentration of NaCl) stimulated not only the usual, but also the atypical enzyme. However, the atypical enzyme was stimulated to a lesser degree, only about one-half as much as the usual enzyme. The effects of tris at a series of relatively low concentrations were studied using a range of substrate (benzoylcholine) concentrations, and the results are shown in plots of 1/v against 1/s (FIGURES 2A and 2B). Although stimulation of the usual esterase is apparent, the kinetics of the stimulation are complex, and these complications are well illustrated by the data presented in FIGURE 2A. The stimulation of the atypical esterase (FIGURE 2B), on the other hand, seems to be a clear-cut example of uncompetitive stimulation. Testing with higher concentrations of tris in the same manner results in a different set of curves (FIGURES 3A and 3B). Under these circumstances tris acts as a competitive inhibitor for the usual enzyme, although the V_{max} progressively increases. In contrast, higher concentrations of tris do not stimulate the atypical enzyme and the small amount of inhibition observed is not competitive.

Other compounds known to be competitive inhibitors of the enzyme were also

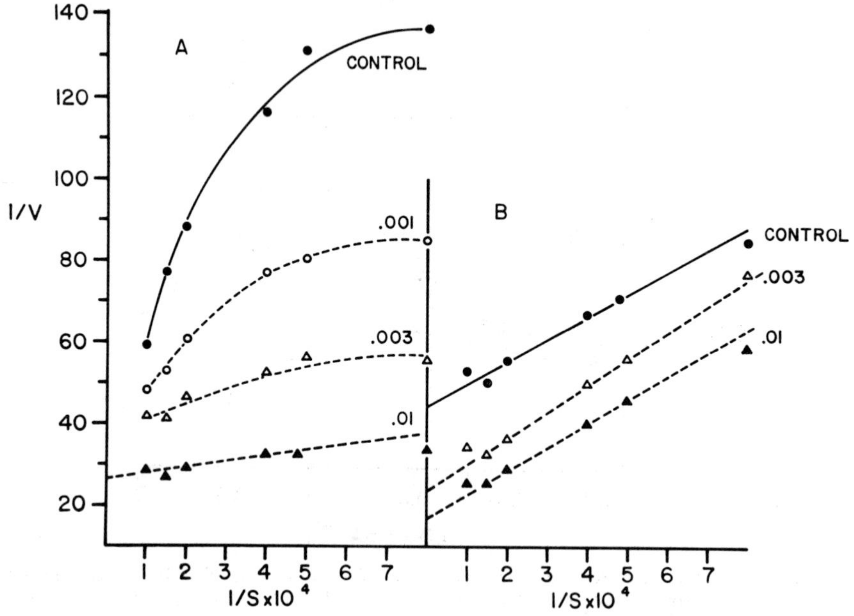

FIGURE 2A. Effect of various concentrations of tris on the kinetics of benzoylcholine hydrolysis by usual esterase. FIGURE 2B, effect of tris buffer benzoylcholine hydrolysis by atypical esterase.

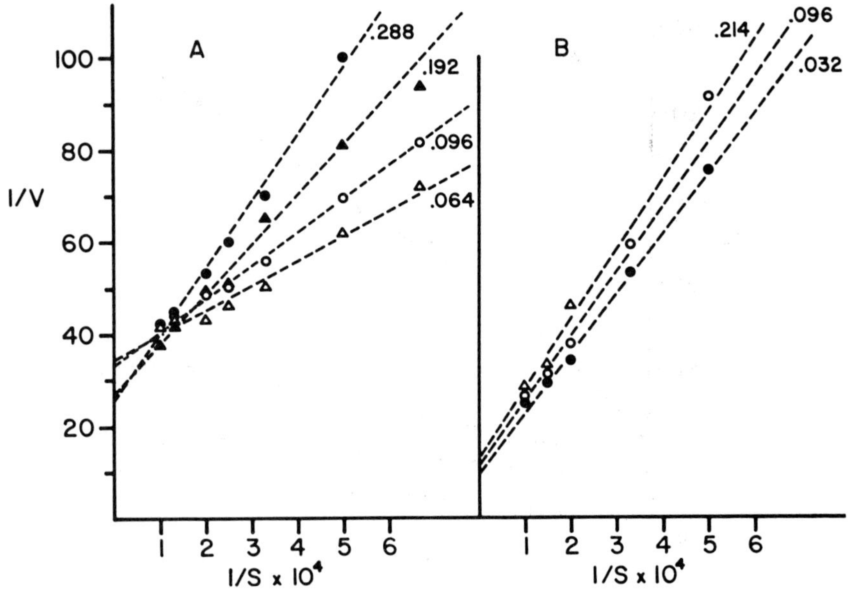

FIGURE 3. Effects of higher concentrations of tris buffer on the hydrolysis of benzoylcholine. 3A, usual esterase; 3B atypical esterase.

tested to see if they had a stimulatory effect at low concentrations in low ionic strength buffer. Inhibitors such as dibucaine and decamethonium did not stimulate under these conditions. However, choline and tetramethylammonium (TMA) stimulated the usual enzyme but not the atypical enzyme. Other workers have noted that these and other quaternary ammonium compounds[12] and some alkaloids[13,14] stimulate usual esterase activity but no detailed study of this effect was made in low ionic strength buffer. TMA and choline react in much the same manner and can be considered interchangeable in the studies to be reported here. Using TMA for example, the effect of low levels of either compound on the usual enzyme is shown in FIGURE 4A. The lines, except for the control, approach being parallel, again suggesting uncompetitive stimulation. There was no effect on atypical esterase.

With higher concentrations of TMA or choline there was competitive inhibition with both the usual and atypical enzymes. FIGURES 4B and 4C illustrate these effects with choline. From these results it can be seen that the higher concentrations of choline have two opposing effects on the usual enzyme; one, a stimulatory effect and two, as a competitive inhibitor. With the atypical enzyme (FIGURE 4C) the stimulatory effect is much less. In order to analyze the nature of the stimulatory effect of choline it is necessary to correct for the competitive inhibition effects by suitable kinetic analysis. To make this type of analysis possible, a higher buffer concentration was used so that the points of the control curve formed a straight line and a Km and Vmax could be calculated (FIGURE 5A). In M/15 phosphate, the lines reflecting choline inhibition look essentially the same as in M/1500 phosphate, but there is a marked difference in the two control lines. The extent of stimulation by choline though drastically reduced at the high ionic strength (FIGURE 5A), is still present and can be determined.

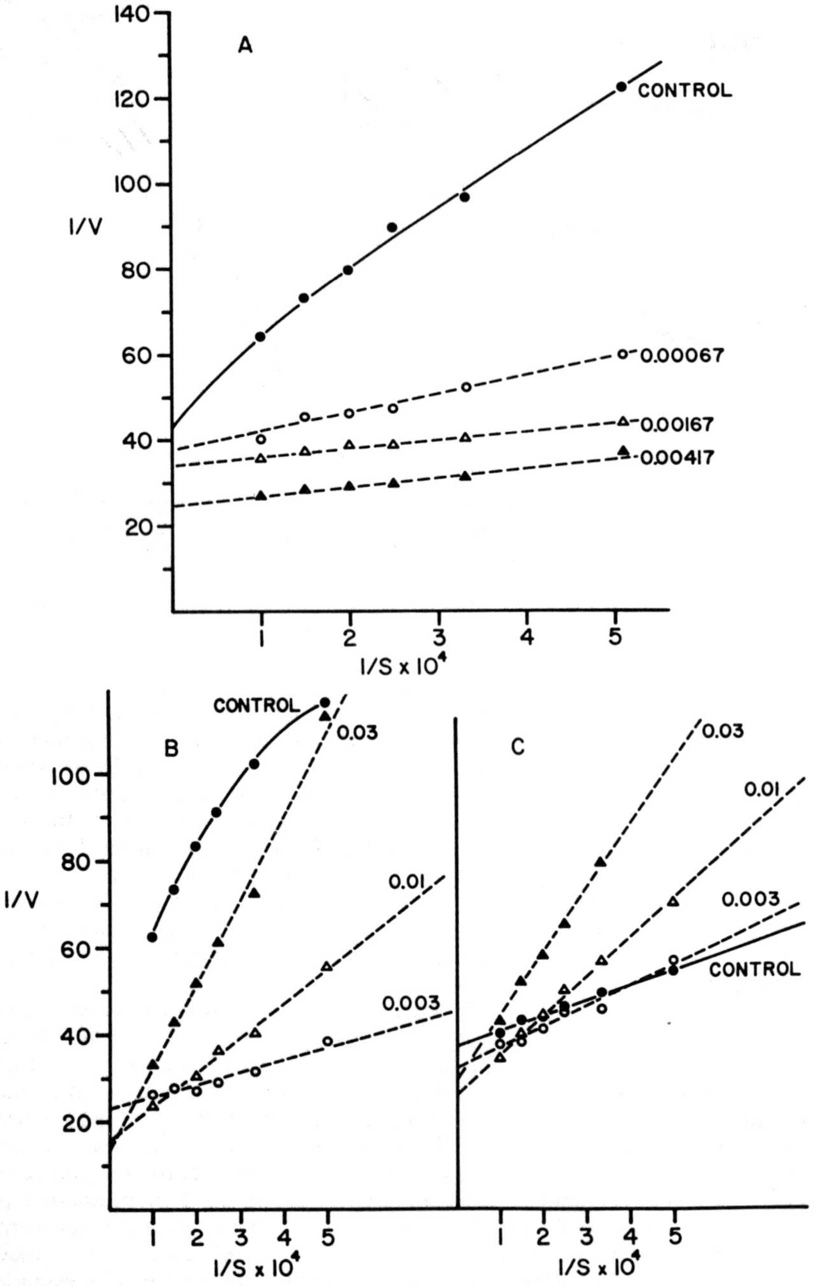

FIGURE 4A. Effects of low concentrations of tetramethylammonium (TMA) on the hydrolysis of benzoylcholine by usual esterase in M/1500 phosphate buffer, pH 7.3. FIGURES 4B and 4C, effects of higher concentrations of choline on the hydrolysis of benzoylcholine by usual (4B) and atypical (4C) esterases.

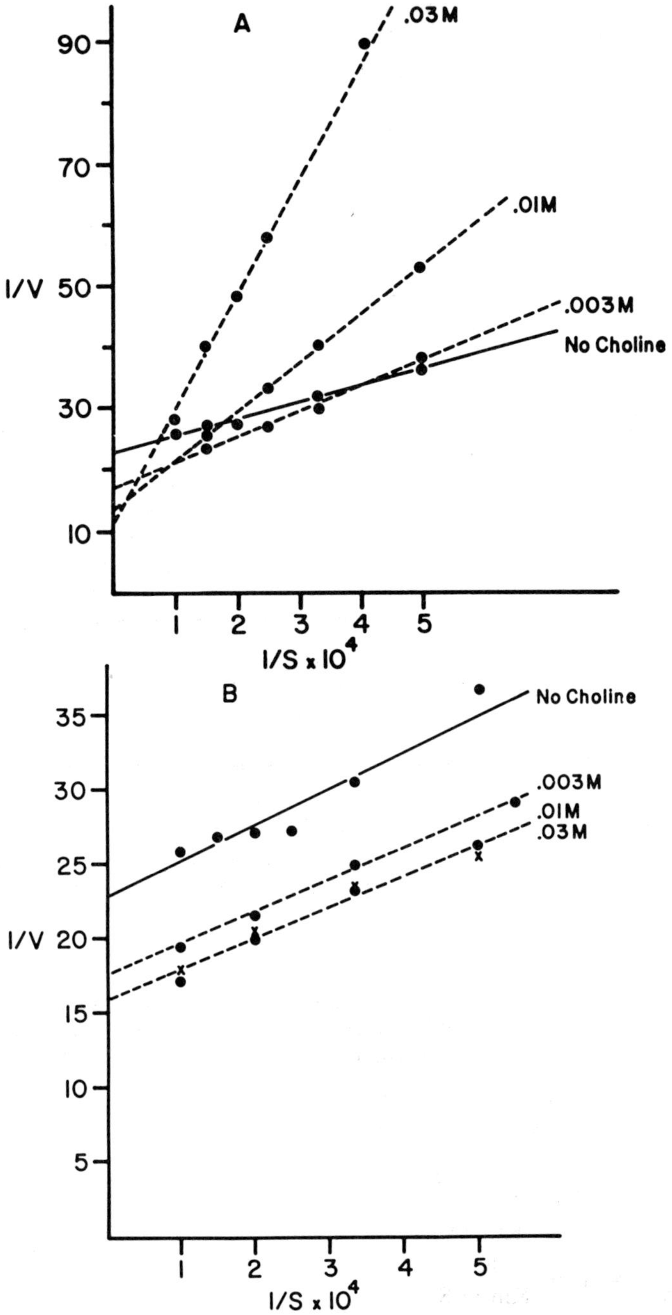

FIGURE 5A. Effects of higher concentrations of choline on the hydrolysis of benzoylcholine by usual esterase in M/15 phosphate buffer, pH 7.3. FIGURE 5B, uncompetitive stimulation by choline of benzoylcholine hydrolysis by usual esterase. Calculations are corrected for the competitive inhibition by choline, as explained in the text.

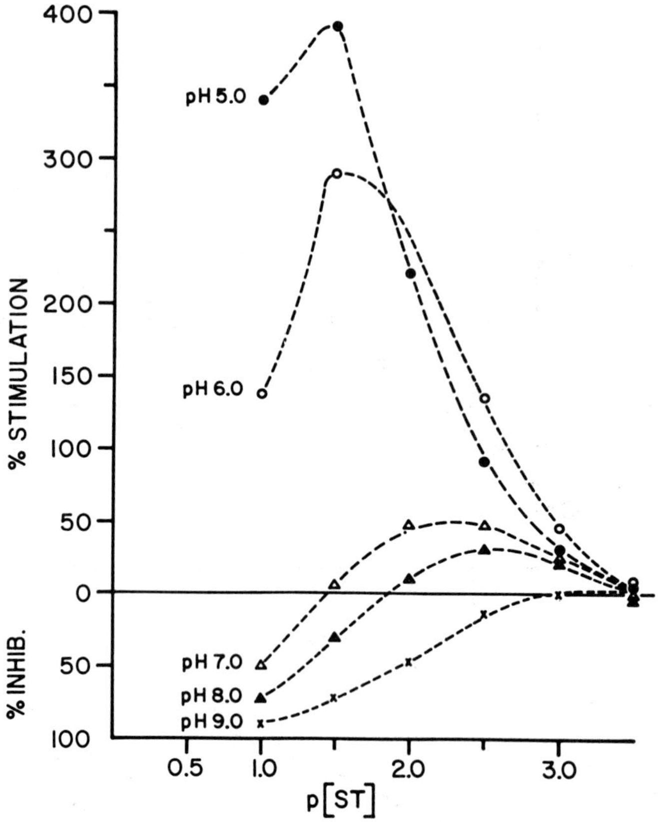

FIGURE 6. Effects of choline on the hydrolysis of benzoylcholine by usual esterase at various pH values. Buffer (0.01M) was phosphate except at pH 9, which was borate. Benzoylcholine concentration, 5×10^{-5}M.

An expression can be derived which makes it possible to calculate the *uninhibited velocities* (Vo) at various inhibitor and substrate concentrations and thus "correct" the lines in FIGURE 5A for the competitive inhibition by choline.

$$\frac{1}{Vo} = \frac{Km}{Vmax} \cdot \frac{1}{S} + \frac{1}{Vmax} \quad (1)$$

$$\frac{1}{V_i} = \frac{Km}{Vmax}\left(1 + \frac{(I)}{K_I}\right) \cdot \frac{1}{S} + \frac{1}{Vmax} \quad (2)$$

$$\frac{Vo}{Vi} = 1 + \frac{\frac{Km(I)}{K_I}}{Km + S} \quad (3)$$

Equation 2 for competitive inhibition, divided by Equation 1 results in an Equation 3 from which V_{max}, and thus, the stimulatory effect, has been eliminated. The Km is calculated in the usual manner from the straight control line,

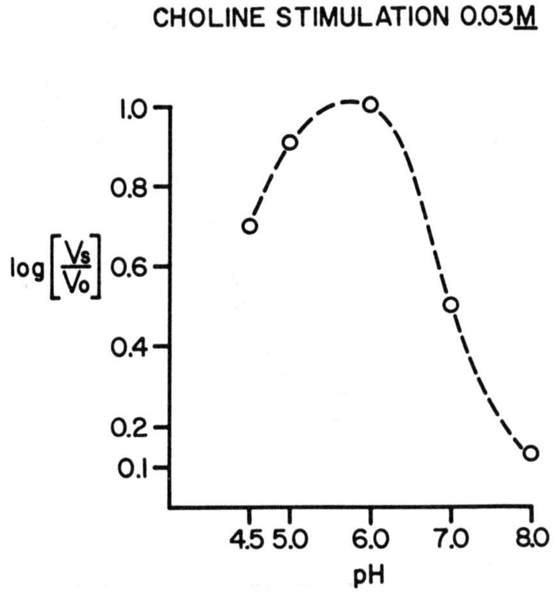

FIGURE 7. pH Dependence of the stimulatory effect of choline on benzoylcholine hydrolysis by usual esterase.

Ordinate: $\log \frac{\text{maximum velocity of stimulated reaction}}{\text{maximum velocity of unstimulated reaction}}$

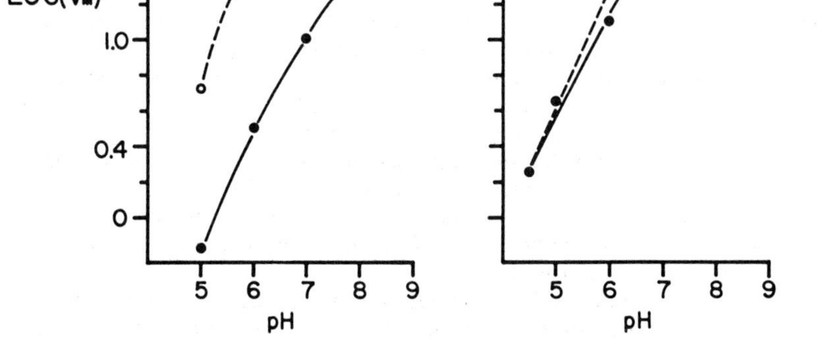

FIGURE 8. The log of the maximum velocities versus pH in the presence of 0.03 M choline and without choline of the usual esterase (8A) and atypical esterase (8B).

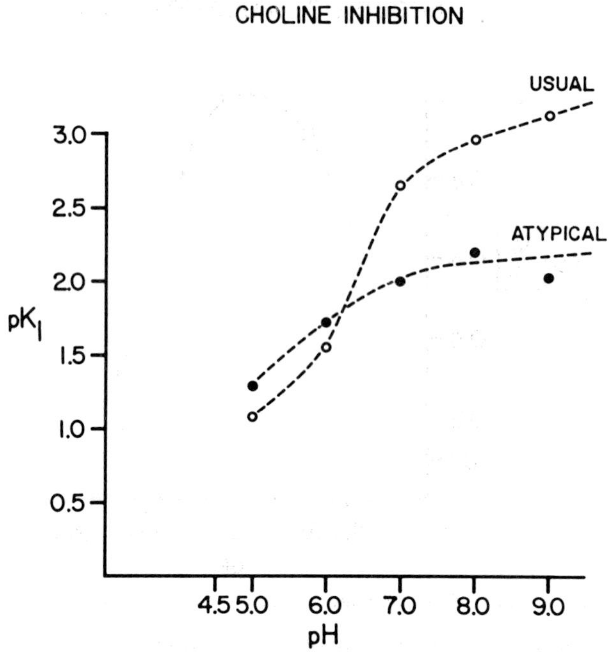

FIGURE 9. The changes in the pK_I for choline at various pH values with usual and atypical esterase.

and K_I is calculated from the following equation, derived by plotting the slopes the inhibited lines against the choline (inhibitor) concentrations:

$$\frac{\text{Slope}}{\text{(Inhibited line)}} = \frac{Km}{Vmax} + \frac{Km}{Vmax} \cdot \frac{(I)}{K_I}$$

Recalculation of the velocities by this method resulted in a set of parallel lines (FIGURE 5B). This is expected if the stimulation by choline is uncompetitive and similar to that seen at lower concentrations of TMA (FIGURE 4A) and tris (FIGURE 2B).

The stimulatory effect of choline was investigated over a range of pH values. Several choline concentrations were tested at each pH (FIGURE 6). The atypical enzyme, tested in a similar manner, was not stimulated at all. At the higher choline concentrations, the inhibitory effect predominates over the stimulatory effect with the usual enzyme and a true maximum pH for stimulation cannot be determined. Maximum velocities were calculated by testing the choline effect over several substrate levels, using reciprocal plots and eliminating the inhibitory effect. By plotting the ratios of the stimulated maximum velocities to the control velocities at various pH values, the pH for maximum stimulation was found to be approximately 6.0 (FIGURE 7).

This data can also be used to calculate the pK of the enzyme and the effect of choline upon this value by plotting the log of the maximum velocities versus pH (FIGURE 8A). The pK of atypical enzyme was determined in the same manner (FIGURE 8B). The pK of the usual enzyme was around pH 7.7, and the value was shifted to pH 6.0 by 0.03 M choline. The pK of the atypical enzyme, on the other hand, was somewhat lower, around pH 7.0, and it was not affected by choline. Since we assume that the pK of the enzyme represents the ionization of an amino acid at (or near) the anionic site, choline probably alters the ionization of this site in the usual, but not in the atypical esterase.

From these data, it was also possible to calculate the K_I's for choline at all the pH values for both types of esterase. If the assumption is made that the ionization of a single group in the protein is essential for the binding of cationic inhibitors, then a plot of the negative log of the K_I's against pH should show a change in slope corresponding to the pK of that group. Plotting the negative log of K_I versus pH for choline inhibition of both esterases (FIGURE 9) shows a change in slope at pH 7.7 for the usual enzyme at pH 7.0 for the atypical enzyme. Since these values are the same as the pK calculations above, it is probable that these cationic inhibitors are bound by the essential group undergoing ionization in the active center of the enzyme.

Reactivation of Phosphorylated Esterases

It was pointed out above, that stimulation of esterase activity by choline and other quaternary ammonium compounds is of an uncompetitive nature. This finding implies that the action of choline should be to enhance the rate of enzyme-substrate complex breakdown and not an earlier step concerned with the formation of the enzyme-substrate complex. The series of reactions believed to represent the hydrolysis of ester substrates is as follows:

$$E + S \underset{k_2}{\overset{k_1}{\rightleftarrows}} ES \qquad (1)$$

$$ES \xrightarrow{k_3} ES' + ROH \qquad (2)$$

$$ES' \xrightarrow{k_4} E + ROOH \qquad (3)$$

TABLE 1

REACTIVATION OF CHOLINESTERASE VARIANTS BY 5×10^{-3} M NaF

Type of Esterase*	Genotype	Percent Recovery† after			
		1 hr	2 hr	3 hr	4 hr
Atypical (4)	AA	46.5	67.7	77.2	82.0
Intermediate (4)	AU	31.2	48.5	57.0	64.5
Usual (17)	UU	18.5	33.5	43.0	50.7
Fluoride-resistant (4) (heterozygous)‡	UF	10.5	21.3	29.7	41.0
Fluoride-resistant-silent (heterozygous) (1)‡	FS	11.0	15.0	18.0	16.0

* The number in parenthesis is the number of individuals tested. Each individual was tested several times except the fluoride-resistant-silent heterozygous individual, who was tested once.

† The relative activity of the dephosphorylated enzyme to control enzyme.

‡ We are indebted to Dr. Nancy E. Simpson for providing us with serum samples of the fluoride-resistant types for these studies.

TABLE 2

POTENTIATION OF NaF REACTIVATION BY CHOLINE IN THE USUAL ENZYME

NaF → / Choline ↓	Percent Reactivation at 2 hr: 0	5×10^{-4} M	1.5×10^{-3} M	5×10^{-3} M
0	0	4.3	10.2	27.0
0.033 M	0	9.6	19.2	49.1
0.11 M	2.3	15.0	30.8	67.5
0.33 M	2.3	25.3	50.2	84.5

In this scheme, choline might increase the rate of formation of the acyl-enzyme (ES′) with release of the alcohol moiety (step 2), or catalyze the rate of cleavage of the acyl-enzyme complex itself (step 3).

A means to study the rate of cleavage of the acyl-enzyme complex is provided by using diethyl-p-nitrophenylphosphate (paraoxon). This organophosphate compound can be considered both an inhibitor and a very poor substrate for the esterase since it reacts with the enzyme but the spontaneous rate of hydrolysis of the enzyme-phosphate ester (step 3) is very slow.

Cleavage of the phosphorylated enzyme to restore active esterase can be accelerated by a number of agents, including fluoride ion.[9] The rate of dephosphorylation of the inhibited enzyme by NaF under standard conditions (see Methods) can be used to evaluate the influence of choline on this process and whether the reactivation step differs according to the genetic type of esterase.

The rates of reactivation of usual atypical and fluoride resistant choline esterases are given in TABLE 1. The atypical esterase was reactivated faster than the usual type of esterase, suggesting that the acyl- or phosphoryl-enzyme complex is more labile in the atypical enzyme. On the other hand, the reactivation rate of the phosphorylated fluoride-resistant esterase is slower than the usual enzyme, and the acyl bond may be more stable in the fluoride-resistant type of esterase. However, these findings are preliminary results and further studies will be needed to confirm this hypothesis.

The effect of choline on the rate of reactivation was also studied. Choline alone did not reactivate the phosphorylated esterases, but in combination with NaF, it potentiated the rate of reactivation (TABLE 2). When a concentration of 5×10^{-3} M NaF was used, the rate of reactivation of the usual esterase was increased approximately 3-fold by 0.33 M choline. Furthermore, when 5×10^{-4} M NaF (which produces essentially no reactivation alone) was used, the addition of 0.33 M choline caused a very significant rate of reactivation.

In contrast to the above results, choline had very little influence on the rate of reactivation of phosphorylated atypical esterase. However, it should be noted that the rate of reactivation by NaF of the usual esterase without choline is much slower than that of the atypical esterase, and the addition of choline seems to increase the rate of reactivation of the usual esterase to approximately the same value as that of the atypical enzyme with NaF alone. The particular experimental conditions selected may also be those which happen to favor stimulation of the usual esterase and not atypical esterase. The studies with choline do indicate that the rate of acyl-enzyme cleavage (step 3) of the usual esterase is accelerated by choline and this is not found with atypical esterase. A difference in functional activity at the esteratic site of the usual and atypical esterases is thus clearly indicated.

Discussion

Since choline has a positively charged nitrogen it is presumed that choline interacts with the anionic site of the esterase, just as the cationic portion of substrate molecules. The inhibitory effect of choline should be competitive with substrate for this reason. A comparison of the usual and atypical esterases as far as choline inhibition has shown a lower apparent affinity for the atypical enzyme since the pK_I of choline for this enzyme is higher above pH 6.0 and is less affected by increases in pH. Thus, there is convincing evidence for an alteration at the anionic site of the atypical esterase. In addition, since the pK of the atypical enzyme is lower than that of the usual enzyme, one would expect a different ionizable group at the binding site, presumably the anionic site. The fact that choline alters the pK of this group in the usual enzyme but not in the atypical lends further support to this hypothesis.

The stimulatory effect of choline, however, is more complex. The uncompetitive nature of the stimulation was confirmed by the dephosphorylation studies, but these studies also helped to characterize additional differences in the usual and atypical esterases. The stimulation by choline of the dephosphorylation step of the usual enzyme but not the atypical enzyme, and the difference in rates of dephosphorylation by NaF alone, are very significant for these differences imply that the *esteratic* site must be different in the two enzymes.

The evidence presented above might at first appear to require alterations in the primary structure of the atypical esterase at both the anionic and esteratic sites, to account for these functional changes. To propose a double alteration in the primary enzyme structure would be inconsistent with the well-documented mode of inheritance of the serum esterases.

Consequently, in view of all the known facts, it would be more logical to propose that there is a single alteration in the primary structure of the atypical esterase which modifies the properties of both the anionic and esteratic sites.

References

1. Kalow, W. & N. Staron. 1957. On distribution and inheritance of atypical forms of human serum cholinesterase, as indicated by dibucaine numbers. Can. J. Biochem. Physiol. **35:** 1305.
2. Harris, H. & M. Whittaker. 1961. Differential inhibition of human serum cholinesterase with fluoride: recognition of two new phenotypes. Nature **191:** 496.
3. Harris, H. & M. Whittaker. 1962. The serum cholinesterase variants. A study of twenty-two families selected via the 'intermediate' phenotype. Ann. Human. Genet. Lond. **26:** 59.
4. Liddell, J., H. Lehmann & E. Silk. 1962. A "silent" pseudocholinesterase gene. Nature **193:** 561.
5. Lehmann, H., J. Liddell, B. Blackwell, D. C. O'Connor & A. V. Daws. 1963. Two further serum pseudocholinesterase phenotypes as causes of suxamethonium apnoea. Brit. Med. J. **1:** 1116.
6. Kalow, W. 1962. Pharmacogenetics. Heredity and response to drugs : 69. W. B. Saunders Co. Phila. & Lond.
7. Kalow, W. & H. A. Lindsay. 1955. A comparison of optical and manometric methods for the assay of human serum cholinesterase. Can. J. Biochem. **33:** 568.
8. Kalow, W. & K. Genest. 1957. A method for the detection of atypical forms of human serum cholinesterase. Determination of dibucaine numbers. Can. J. Biochem. Physiol. **35:** 339.
9. Heilbronn, E. 1965. Action of fluoride on cholinesterase – II. *In vitro* reactivation of cholinesterases inhibited by organophosphorous compounds. Biochem. Pharm. **14:** 1363.
10. Glaubiger, G. Unpublished observations.
11. Callahan, S. & B. N. La Du. 1965. Effect of ionic strength on normal and atypical plasma pseudocholinesterase activity. Fed. Proc. **24:** 610.

12. ERDOS, E. G., F. F. FOLDES, E. K. ZSIGMOND, N. BAART & J. A. ZWARTZ. 1958. Acceleration of plasma cholinesterase activity by quaternary ammonium salts. Science **128:** 92.
13. ERDOS, E. G., F. F. FOLDES, N. BAART & E. K. ZSIGMOND. 1957. Activation of enzymatic hydrolysis of benzoylcholine by tryptamine. Science **126:** 1176.
14. ERDOS, E. G., F. F. FOLDES, N. BAART, E. K. ZSIGMOND & J. ZWARTZ. 1959. The accelerating effect of narcotic analgesics on the hydrolysis of aromatic substrates by human plasma cholinesterase. Biochem. Pharm. **2:** 97.

DISCUSSIONS OF THE PAPER

DR. EARL USDIN (*Atlantic Research Corp., Alexandria, Va.*): Couldn't some of your data, particularly the data on inhibition and enhancement of cholinesterase activity, be interpreted as implying the presence of more than one enzyme? In the case of the normal individuals, the plots were obviously curved and did not conform to classical kinetics for a single enzyme. Main (personal communication) has indicated to me that he has preliminary results which seem to indicate that the concentration of pseudocholinesterase isozymes can calculated by resolution of similar inhibition curves into components. Furthermore, from the facts that the data from your variants is much closer to linear, couldn't one guess that this might imply that the variants have less enzymes, i.e., isozymes, than the normals?

DR. S. CLARK: It is difficult to understand how the minor components (C_1, C_2 and C_3) which together account for less than 10 percent of the total activity could influence the overall kinetics very much. Besides, Mr. Glaubiger has been purifying the enzyme and during the purification most of the minor components are lost, so we have really purified C_4. Kinetic studies with purified C_4 show even a more pronounced curve than we found when serum was used.

DR. F. F. FOLDES (*Montefiore Hospital, Bronx, N. Y.*): I would like to compliment Drs. Clark and La Du for their interesting kinetic studies on the NN and DD variants of plasma butyrylcholinesterase. We have also observed several years ago that the hydrolyses of aromatic substrates (e.g. benzoylcholine, procaine) by plasma butyrylcholinesterase can be markedly accelerated by narcotic analgesics.* None of these compounds accelerated the hydrolysis of aliphatic substrates (e.g. acetylcholine) by this enzyme. I wonder whether the activators employed by Drs. Clark and La Du were only effective with aromatic substrates, or they also increased the hydrolysis rates of aliphatic substrates?

DR. S. CLARK: We have tested phenylacetate and found that there was some stimulation but it required about ten times as much salt to show it as when bezoylcholine was used as the substrate. We found no stimulation using acetylthiocholine or butyrylthiocholine as the substrate, however. There are reports that acetylcholinesterase activity is stimulated by various cations. For example, Krupka found tetraethylammonium ions to increase the velocity of acetylcholine hydrolysis.†

* Erdos, *et al.* 1959. Biochem. Pharmacol. **2:** 97.
† Krupka, R. M. 1966. Biochemistry **5:** 1988.

GENETIC VARIATIONS IN THE ACETYLATION OF ISONIAZID AND OTHER DRUGS

David A. Price Evans
Department of Medicine, University of Liverpool
Liverpool, U. K.

Preliminary Observations

Isoniazid (1-isonicotinyl hydrazine) was first synthesized by Meyer and Mally in 1912 but its chemotherapeutic value was not discovered until forty years later. Grunberg and Schnitzer (1952) and Grunberg, Leiwant, D'Ascension and Schnitzer (1952) showed that the compound had bacteriostatic action against *Mycobacterium tuberculosis* strain H37Rv *in vitro* and that it protected mice from developing tuberculosis when they were given i.v. injections of tubercle bacilli. Robitzek, Selikoff and Ornstein (1952) and Selikoff and Robitzek (1952) then showed that the compound was effective in the treatment of tuberculosis in man.

A considerable amount of work has been carried out on the metabolism of isoniazid both in animals and in man. These studies have shown that there is rapid and complete absorption of the drug giving an initial high blood level. As this falls the greater part of the isoniazid appears in the urine either unchanged or enzymatically biotransformed into metabolites, within 24 hours of oral administration (Elmendorf *et al.*, 1952; Barclay *et al.*, 1953).

A large variation in the metabolism of isoniazid was found to exist among human beings by Bönicke and Reif (1953); Hughes (1953); Hughes, Biehl, Jones and Schmidt (1954) and Hughes, Schmidt and Biehl (1955). The latter workers studied the products excreted in the urine after isoniazid was given to human beings and found that: (1) all the drug given could be accounted for; (2) isoniazid was found in the urine as free unchanged drug, as acetyl isoniazid, as isonicotinic acid and in small quantities in the form of other metabolic products; (3) there was an inverse relationship between the percentage of the given dose which is recovered as free drug and that recovered as acetylated derivative. The percentage recovered as acetyl isoniazid varied from 14 to 70 percent of the dose given, and (4) the pattern of excretion for a given subject remained constant even when the drug was given daily for months.

Distribution histograms of the percentage of the administered isoniazid excreted in the free unchanged form in the urine were given by Biehl (1956, 1957). These were bimodal suggesting that subjects might belong to one of two classes—either rapid or slow inactivators.

Genetics

A twin study was carried out by Bönicke and Lisboa (1957) in which they estimated the free isoniazid excreted in the urine during 24 hours as a percentage of the dose administered. The results showed that there was a remarkable similarity between monozygous twins, but that dizygous twins differed from each other to a much greater degree.

Mitchell, Riemensnider, Harsch and Bell (1958) thought that this polymorphism for isoniazid metabolism in man might be genetically determined. Support for this view was afforded by their finding that the proportion of rapid inactivators in groups of Japanese subjects was much larger than in groups of Caucasian subjects (Harris *et al.*, 1958). To test the genetic hypothesis a study of twenty families was carried out by Knight, Selin and Harris (1959). They showed that it was probable that slow inactivators of isoniazid (who have high blood levels of the free compound and excrete a high proportion of the free drug in the urine) had a trait recessive to rapid inactivation and moreover that the genes concerned were autosomal.

Evans, Manley and McKusick (1960) determined plasma isoniazid concentrations six hours after subjects had swallowed a dose of 10 mg isoniazid per kg body weight. The distribution histogram of these values is bimodal allowing the phenotype of a subject to be expressed as either a rapid inactivator with a low plasma isoniazid concentration, or a slow inactivator of the drug. In this study 267 members of 53 Caucasian two-generation family units were phenotyped. Examination of the pedigrees proved that slow inactivation of isoniazid is an autosomal recessive trait. In addition, the mean six-hour plasma isoniazid concentration in recognizable heterozygotes is higher than that for other rapid inactivators in the pedigrees. This indicates that dominant homozygotes have lower values than the heterozygotes (though they did not form a separate mode). In other words, a dosage effect is shown for the character (Evans *et al.*, 1960).

Further work using a precise microbiological technique has shown that the genotype of a person can be determined directly from a trimodal distribution curve in both Japanese and Caucasian subjects (Sunahara *et al.*, 1963b; Sunahara *et al.*, 1963a; Dufour *et al.*, 1964). A similar trimodal distribution curve in Japanese subjects, determined by a chemical estimation technique, each mode of which probably represents a genotype has recently been published by Nakagawa and Sunahara (1967).

Minor Genes Controlling Acetylation

It is generally agreed that a single major gene controlling a polymorphic character functions against a background provided by a number of other genes. There may be alleles of these other genes also and hence the background against which the major gene operates can vary between individuals. The background genes should vary less within families than between families and so siblings who are of the same character as determined by the major genes should tend to be similar to each other.

The following are two pieces of evidence for the existence of such minor genes controlling acetylation in man:

(1) The percentage of urinary sulfamethazine which appears in the acetylated form after a standard oral dose of the drug shows significantly greater variability between individuals of a given acetylator phenotype than within repeat tests in the same individual (White & Evans, 1968).

(2) The plasma isoniazid concentrations in the data of Evans, Manley and McKusick (1960) have a significant positive regression on body weight (see also Evans *et al.*, 1961). A value has been computed for plasma isoniazid concentration which has been corrected for body weight. When families consisting entirely of slow acetylators are considered there is a significantly greater variability of this corrected plasma isoniazid concentration between sibships than within sibships (TABLE 1). A regression of mean-offspring value on mid-parent value just fails to attain significance at the $p = 0.05$ level (FIGURE 1).

TABLE 1.

ANALYSIS OF VARIANCE OF PLASMA ISONIAZID CONCENTRATION (μg/ml) CORRECTED FOR BODY WEIGHT IN SIBSHIPS CONSISTING ENTIRELY OF SLOW ACETYLATOR SUBJECTS*

Total Number of Offspring	Number of Sibships	Within Sibships Mean Square = W	Between Sibships Mean Square = B	$\frac{B}{W} = F$	p
47	13	0.5397	2.4849	4.6	<0.001

* Data of Evans, Manley & McKusick, 1960.

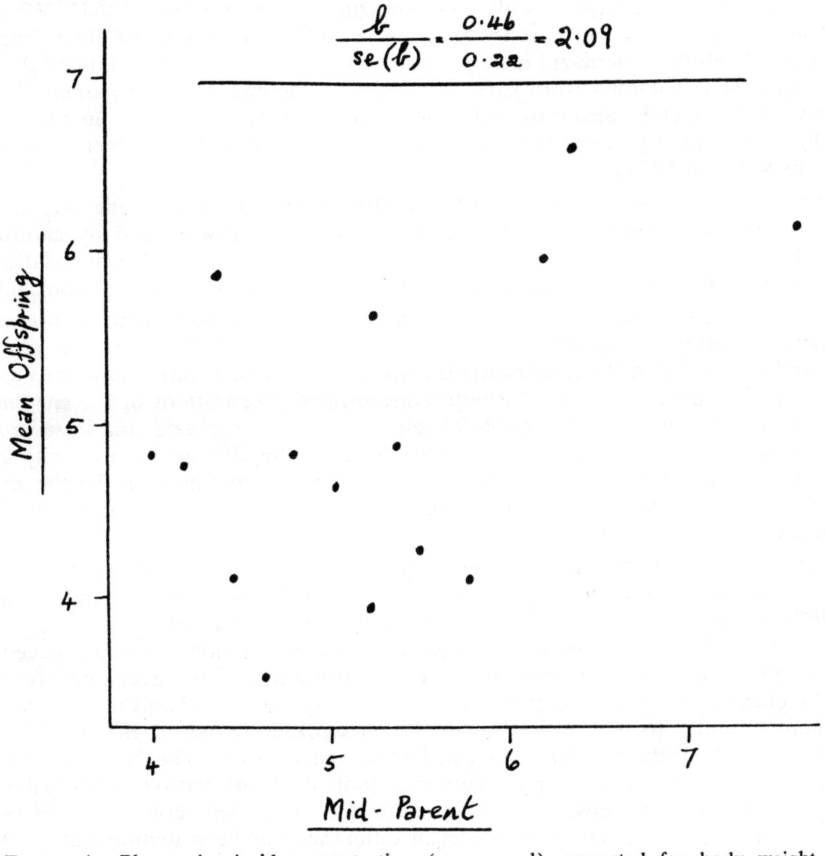

FIGURE 1. Plasma isoniazid concentration (μg per ml) corrected for body weight, in families which consist entirely of slow acetylators. b = regression coefficient, se (b) = standard error of b. (Data of Evans, Manley and McKusick, 1960).

Biochemical Basis for the Polymorphism

Intestinal absorption factors are not responsible for the difference between the two phenotypes since Jenne, MacDonald and Mendoza (1961) measuring the plasma half-life have shown that the rapid and slow inactivator phenotypes are recognizable when isoniazid is given intravenously. The same investigators have also shown that renal glomerular clearance and renal tubular reabsorption of the drug are the same in both phenotypes. These facts strongly suggested that a metabolic difference existed between the two phenotypes and in view of the observations of Hughes, Biehl, Jones and Schmidt (1954) and of Hughes, Schmidt and Biehl (1955) mentioned above, it was likely that this difference consisted of different speeds of acetylation.

Evans (1962) studying the metabolism of sulfamethazine (syn. sulfadimidine) has produced evidence to support this hypothesis. The acetylation of sulfamethazine in human volunteer subjects is polymorphic, and rapid inactivators of isoniazid are extensive acetylators of sulfamethazine (Evans & White, 1964). When supplied with ATP, acetate and coenzyme A biopsy specimens of liver from rapid inactivators of isoniazid have greater acetylating powers for isoniazid than liver specimens obtained from slow inactivators. One enzymic step namely that catalyzed by acetyl-transferase was shown to be polymorphic by incubating healthy liver biopsy specimens with sulfamethazine and acetyl coenzyme A (Evans & White, 1964).

Peters, Gordon and Brown (1965) confirmed that sulfamethazine and isoniazid were both polymorphically acetylated in the same way, and by careful analytical techniques Peters, Miller and Brown (1965) showed that acetylation was the primary metabolic reaction determining inactivator status for isoniazid.

Jenne (1963) found that jejunal mucosa as well as liver homogenates showed *in vitro* polymorphic capacity to acetylate isoniazid. Jenne (1965) partially purified and concentrated the liver acetyl-transferase 300-fold. From livers representative of the "rapid" and "slow" groups concentrated preparations of the enzyme showed no differences in apparent Michaelis constant for isoniazid, and in several other respects the enzymes behave identically. Thus the differences in activity of these phenotypes do not appear to result from differences in affinity of the enzyme for isoniazid but may be due to differences in amount of an identical enzyme molecule.

Further work on N-acetyltransferase purified from human and rabbit liver by a procedure similar to that of Jenne (1965) has been reported by Weber (1967), Cohen and Steinberg (1967) and Weber and Cohen (1967). An analysis of the enzyme's kinetic properties suggests that the acetylation reaction proceeds by a "ping-pong Bi-Bi" mechanism with the formation of the acetylated form of the enzyme as the first step in the over-all acetylation mechanism. This conclusion is similar to that arrived at by earlier workers (Jenne & Boyer, 1963) studying an N-acetyltransferase purified from pigeon liver. The N-acetyltransferase preparations from rapid acetylator individuals of various mammalian species differ in their substrate requirements (Cohen & Steinberg, 1967). However, to date, no clear cut enzymological difference has been demonstrated between the slow and rapid acetylator phenotypes.

The enzyme responsible for acetylating isoniazid in human liver has been shown to be "non-inducible" by Levi and Walker (1966), and this is in keeping with the observation of Sunahara, Urano and Kawait (1963) who showed that acetylating enzymes in animals were mostly located in liver cell supernatant fractions (inducible enzymes are generally microsomal).

Skin and white blood cells have been shown to be devoid of the capacity to acetylate sulfamethazine *in vitro* (Evans & White, Unpublished observations). Red cells similarly lack the capacity to acetylate isoniazid (Motulsky & Steinmann, 1962).

Other Drugs for Which There Is Evidence for Polymorphic Acetylation

McIsaac and Kanda (1964) had demonstrated in rabbits that 25 to 30% of C^{14}-1-hydrazinophthalazine (hydralazine) given either intragastrically or intraperitoneally appeared in the urine as N-acetyl-l-hydrazinophthalazine.

Evidence has been obtained to show that hydrallazine is most probably a substrate for polymorphic acetylation in man. Evans and White (1964) showed by *in vitro* incubation of liver homogenates containing acetyl coenzyme A and hydrallazine that more unconjugated drug was present at the end of incubation in slow than in rapid acetylator livers (as determined by previous testing with sulfamethazine). Jenne (1965) showed competitive inhibition by hydralazine of isoniazid acetylation by partially purified liver preparations. Weber (1967) and also Cohen and Steinberg (1967) showed that purified N-acetyltransferase preparations from rapid acetylator human livers were able to acetylate hydralazine *in vitro*.

It is probable that some other sulphonamides as well as sulfamethazine will undergo polymorphic acetylation in man. Suggestive evidence for this process was obtained at the I.C.I. laboratories some years ago. Persons who acetylate sulfamethazine to a considerable extent also deal with sulphamaprine in the combination tablet "Bimez" in a similar way (Spinks, 1962, Personal communication.) White and Evans (1968) have shown that the serum concentration of unconjugated sulfamethoxypyridazine 30 hours following drug ingestion is not different in the two acetylator phenotypes. The percentage of sulfamethoxypyridazine appearing in the urine in the acetylated form was, however, slightly though significantly greater in rapid than in slow acetylators.

Toxicological Aspects

Early studies by Hughes, Biehl, Jones and Schmidt (1954) and Biehl (1957) had suggested that slow inactivators of isoniazid were more susceptible to develop peripheral neuropathy than rapid inactivators of the drug. This was amply confirmed by Devadatta, Gangadharam, Andrews, Fox, Ramakrishnan, Selkon and Velu (1960) in a much bigger survey in Madras.

It is probable that the acetylation polymorphism also underlies the observation of Smirnov and Kozulitzina (1962) that toxic effects of the hydrazide drug, phtivazid, were noted relatively seldom in patients excreting large amounts of the drug in the acetylated form.

The very bizarre effects of hydralazine which include a systemic lupus erythematosus-like syndrome and peripheral neuropathy (see Meyler 1960) are more common in slow acetylators of the drug. (Perry *et al.* 1967).

Phenelzine, the antidepressive drug (Nardil) which is a substituted hydrazine, from its molecular configuration, should be a substrate for polymorphic acetylation. Evans, Davison and Pratt (1965) in a double-blind investigation found that the severe side-effects of phenelzine occurred only in slow acetylator subjects.

An unexpected toxicological aspect of the acetylator polymorphism has been found in patients receiving treatment for epilepsy with diphenylhydantoin, and also simultaneously for tuberculosis with a regimen including isoniazid. Toxic effects of diphenylhydantoin were found in slow acetylators and not in rapid acetylators. (Brennan *et al.*, 1968).

Observations on Possible Natural Substrates

Polymorphisms like the acetylator polymorphism are presumably maintained by natural selection. However, the chemical basis of the maintaining environmental factors ("environmental pressure") is unknown. There is very little information available concerning naturally occurring hydrazine compounds. Peters, Miller and Brown (1965) estimated values of di-methyl-amino-benzaldehyde reacting substances in the urines of persons who had not taken drugs. These values were estimated after hydrolysis and so should include all hydrazines; they gave a value below 0.8 mg total hydrazine equivalents per 12 hours. This would suggest that the body does not deal with a great weight of naturally occurring hydrazines but this fact may not, of course, correlate with their biochemical importance.

White and Evans (1967a) estimated urinary total hexosamine and urinary free N-acetyl hemosamine in subjects of known acetylator phenotype. The results show no significant difference in the acetylation of excreted urinary endogenous hexosamine between the two phenotypes.

White and Evans (1967b) administered 5 gram oral L-tryptophan loads to subjects who had received a sulfamethazine (SM) phenotyping test. Kynurenine (K) and 3-hydroxy-kynurenine (OH-K) were estimated by elution from two-way paper chromatograms in both the unconjugated and the acetylated forms. There was no correlation between the percentage acetylation of urinary (K + OH − K) and the percentage acetylation of urinary SM.

These two pieces of work suggest, therefore, that hexosamine and tryptophan metabolites are unlikely to be natural substrates for the human acetylation polymorphism.

Substances Which Are Monomorphically Acetylated

The likelihood that para-aminosalicylic acid (PAS) and para-aminobenzoic acid (PABA) are monomorphically acetylated in human populations is suggested by the following observations.

Jenne, MacDonald and Mendoza (1961) found that the fall-off of serum PAS concentrations was the same in rapid and slow acetylator subjects. Motulsky and Steinmann (1962) found that the acetylation of PAS by red cell homogenates was unimodally distributed amongst 131 subjects. Evans (1963) gave PAS orally to 52 healthy subjects and showed that the ratio of free to total drug (both determined chemically) in the urine was an unimodally distributed character. Evans (1964) showed that the PABA acetylating properties of human jejunal mucosa *in vitro* were not correlated with the power of liver biopsy tissue from the same persons to acetylate sulfamethazine. Finally Jenne (1965) gave 300 mg doses of PAS to human subjects and then separated urinary PAS and acetyl PAS chromatographically and showed that the ratio of the latter to the former was not different in rapid and slow acetylators of isoniazid.

Evans and White (1964) found that liver biopsy specimens when homogenized with acetate, ATP and coenzyme A would acetylate isoniazid and sulfamethazine but not sulphanilamide. In contrast, rat liver which was used in preliminary work was able to acetylate sulphanilamide in the same system. This latter observation was confirmed by Hartiala and Terho (1965) who showed that many rat and guinea pig tissues were able to acetylate sulphanilamide. Peters, Gordon and Brown (1965) estimating the acetylation of excreted sulphanilamide, sulfamethazine and isoniazid in the same human subjects demonstrated that the acetylation of sulphanilamide was closely similar in both slow and rapid acetylators of the other two drugs.

The evidence therefore points to the existence of two acetylating systems in man – one polymorphic and the other monomorphic. Although it seems likely that steric factors or the molecular electronics (Perault & Pullman, 1963) of substrates determine by which system they are dealt with in the body, this is an area in which comparatively little work has been done.

Acetylator Phenotypes and Disease Processes

Since rapid acetylators have lower plasma isoniazid levels than slow acetylators it might be expected that tuberculous rapid acetylators might respond less well to treatment.

This idea has been very thoroughly tested by Harris (1961) who studied 744 patients with pulmonary tuberculosis on standardized treatment schedules. There was a tendency for cavity closure and sputum conversion (i.e. disappearance of tubercle bacilli) to occur earlier in slow acetylators, but the eventual outcome after six months treatment was the same in both phenotypes.

Gow and Evans (1964) similarly found that neither acetylator phenotype was associated with reversion (i.e. reappearance of tubercle bacilli in the urine), following a course of therapy for genito-urinary tuberculosis.

As anticipated by McDermott (1960) the acetylator polymorphism does not seem to influence the outcome of tuberculosis treated by standard schedules including isoniazid as used in so-called developed countries.

The polymorphism turns out, however, to be of great importance when intermittent dosage regimens are employed as recent results (British Medical Journal, 1967) testify (TABLE 2). The patients were fresh cases with drug sensitive organisms on admission, studied in the Tuberculosis Chemotherapy Centre. Madras. Treatment was given for one year. Patients with bacteriologically quiescent disease at the end of the year are said to have a favorable response if they had negative cultures at 10, 11 and 12 months, or only one positive culture out of

TABLE 2

RESULTS OF INTERMITTENT DOSAGE REGIMENS IN TUBERCULOSIS PATIENTS OF DIFFERENT ACETYLATOR PHENOTYPES*

Dosage Regimen				Numbers of Patients	
Abbreviations	Drugs Administered	Frequency of Drug Administration	Acetylator Phenotype	Favorable Response	Poor Response
SHTW	Streptomycin (1.00 or 0.75 g; 27 or 20 mg per kg) and isoniazid 15.5 mg per kg (scaled according to body weight)	Twice Weekly	Slow	75	7
			Rapid	33	3
SHOW	As above	Once Weekly	Slow	49	11
			Rapid	33	22
SH/SHOW	One month of streptomycin 1.00 or 0.75 g and isoniazid 10 mg per kg	Daily	Slow	61	3
	then followed by dosage as above	Once Weekly	Rapid	28	9
SZHOW	Dosage of streptomycin and isoniazid as above plus pyrazinamide 89 mg per kg	Once Weekly	Slow	58	9
			Rapid	18	16

* Data from the Madras Tuberculosis Chemotherapy Centre published by kind permission of Dr. D. A. Mitchison.

about 9 set up during these months. Patients with an unfavorable response may have remained positive during treatment or had a relapse or may have deteriorated and had their treatment changed; they included a few deaths from tuberculosis.

In the SHTW regimen acetylator phenotype did not influence the response to treatment. In all of the once-weekly regimens the response in the rapid acetylators was much worse than in the slow acetylators. (Mitchison, Personal communication, 1967)

There is no association between the acetylator phenotypes and the development of isoniazid resistant tubercle bacilli (Biehl, 1957; Harris 1961).

Pantothenate deficient rats are unable to synthesize coenzyme A and hence suffer from an inability to acetylate, thus simulating the metabolic situation in human slow acetylators. The reports of Berg (1959), Seronde (1963) and Zucker, Seronde and Zucker (1955) that pantothenate deficient rats develop duodenal ulcer led to speculation concerning possible association between human acetylator phenotype and duodenal ulcer. Evans (1967) therefore subjected 56 patients with typical uncomplicated duodenal ulcers to a sulfamethazine test, and of these 27 were rapid acetylators. There is thus no overwhelming susceptibility to duodenal ulcer in slow acetylators since the phenotype incidences in this disorder are very similar to those found in healthy persons in the same population.

In the study of Evans, Davison and Pratt (1965) it was noted that slow acetylator depressives tended to be heavier than rapid acetylators, and also that the mean age at presentation of the slow acetylator endogenous depression category tended to be higher than the mean ages at presentation of the other clinical categories. Evans and Davison (Unpublished observations, 1967) have now examined a new series of depressed patients and again a similar pattern emerges particularly among females (TABLES 3 and 4). One difficulty in the interpretation of these body weight data at the present time is the lack of a

TABLE 3

BODY WEIGHTS OF DEPRESSED FEMALE PATIENTS

Type of Depression	Acetylator Phenotype	Number	Body Weight (lbs) Mean ± SE
Neurotic	Slow	14	139.07 ± 4.77
	Rapid	13	120.00 ± 4.73
Endogenous	Slow	13	138.23 ± 6.91
	Rapid	11	123.18 ± 2.83
All	Slow	27	138.67 ± 4.06
	Rapid	24	121.46 ± 2.83

TABLE 4

AGES OF PRESENTATION OF FEMALE DEPRESSED PATIENTS

Type of Depression	Acetylator Phenotype	Number	Age (years) Mean ± SE
Neurotic	Slow	14	37.64 ± 3.04
	Rapid	13	41.46 ± 4.52
Endogenous	Slow	13	52.61 ± 4.16
	Rapid	11	45.36 ± 3.17

suitable large control population of phenotyped healthy middle-aged females whose weights have been recorded.

Racial Distribution of Acetylator Phenotypes

Using the precise microbiological technique referred to earlier, the serum isoniazid concentration can be very accurately determined. This method, when applied to serum 6 hours after an oral dose of 4 mg isoniazid per kg body weight, allows genotypes to be directly determined from a trimodal frequency distribution curve. Caucasian, Negro and Japanese populations have been studied in the same laboratory in this way by Dufour, Knight and Harris (1964). In Negro and Caucasian populations the "slow" allele is approximately three times more frequent than the rapid allele, but among the Japanese exactly the reverse proportions are found.

Impressive evidence for a "cline" of increasing frequency of the slow alleles from the Ainu in the North to the Thai in the South has been produced by Sunahara, Urano, Ogawa, Yoshida, Mukoyama and Kawai (1963) and by Sunahara, Urano, Lin, Cheg and Jarumilinda (1963) by studying populations along the coast of Asia and in the islands of Japan. This fits with an earlier observation by Armstrong and Peart (1960) that Eskimo populations contain only a very low percentage (about 5%) of slow inactivators of isoniazid.

The implication of this work would seem to be that there is some correlation between the "set" of the polymorphism and latitude – more rapid acetylators towards the Arctic circle and more slow acetylators towards the Equator. This simple hypothesis is not sustained, however, by the similarity in acetylator phenotype distributions between the populations of Northern Europe and Africa. Meaningful ecological interpretations must probably await the recognition of the natural substrate.

References

ARMSTRONG, H. R. & H. E. PEART. 1960. A comparison between the behavior of Eskimos and Non-Eskimos to the administration of isoniazid. The Amer. Rev. Resp. Dis. **81**: 588.

BARCLAY, W. R., R. H. EBERT, G. V. LEROY, R. W. MANTHEI & L. J. ROTH. 1953. Distribution and excretion of radioactive isoniazid in tuberculous patients. J.A.M.A. **151**: 1384.

BERG, B. N. 1959. Duodenitis and duodenal ulcer produced in rats by pantothenic acid deficiency. Brit. J. Exp. Path. **40**: 371.

BIEHL, J. 1956. The role of the dose and the metabolic fate of isoniazid in the emergence of isoniazid resistance. Trans. Conf. Chemotherapy of Tuber. 15th Conf. : 279.

BIEHL, J. 1957. Emergence of drug resistance as related to the dosage and metabolism of isoniazid. Trans. Conf. Chemotherapy of Tuber. 16th Conf. : 108.

BÖNICKE, R. & B. P. LISBOA. 1957. Uber die Erbbedingtheir der intraindividuellen Konstanz der Isoniazidausscheidung. Naturwissenschaften **44**: 314.

BÖNICKE, R. & W. REIF. 1953. Enzymatische Inaktivierung von Isonicotinsaure-hydrazid im menschlichen und tierischen Organismus. Arch. exper. Path. u. Pharmakol. **220**: 321.

BRENNAN, R. W., H. DEHEJIA, H. KUTT AND F. MCDOWELL. 1968. Diphenylhydantoin intoxication attendant to slow inactivation of INH. Neurology **18**: 283.

BRIT. MED. J. 1967. Chemotherapy of Tuberculosis in Developing Countries. Brit. Med. J. **4**: 230.

COHEN, S. M. & M. S. STEINBERG. 1967. Variation in substrate specificity of N-Acetyl-Transferase from mammalian liver. Fed. Proc. **26**: 683.

DEVADATTA, S., P. R. J. GANGADHARAM, R. H. ANDREWS, W. FOX, C. V. RAMAKRISHNAN, J. B. SELKON & S. VELU. 1960. Peripheral neuritis due to isoniazid. Bull. World Health Org. **23**: 587.

DUFOUR, A. P., R. A. KNIGHT & H. W. HARRIS. 1964. Genetics of isoniazid metabolism in Caucasian, Negro and Japanese populations. Science **145**: 391.

ELMENDORF, D. F., W. U. CAWTHON, C. MUNSCHENHEIM & W. MCDERMOTT. 1952. The absorption, distribution, excretion and short-term toxicity of isonicotinic acid hydrazide (Nydrazid) in man. Am. Rev. Tuberc. **65**: 429.

EVANS, D. A. P. 1962. Pharmacogenetique. Medecine et Hygiene **20**: 905.

EVANS, D. A. P. 1963. Pharmacogenetics. Amer. J. Med. **34**: 639.

EVANS, D. A. P. 1964. Acetylation polymorphisms. Proc. R. S. M. **57**: 508.

EVANS, D. A. P. 1967. The acetylator phenotypes of duodenal ulcer patients. Scand. J. Gastroenterol. **2**: 289.

EVANS, D. A. P., K. DAVISON, R. T. C. PRATT. 1965. The influence of acetylator phenotype on the effects of treating depression with phenelzine. Clin. Pharmacol. & Therap. **6**: 430.

EVANS, D. A. P., K. MANLEY & V. A. MCKUSICK. 1960. Genetic control of isoniazid metabolism in man. Brit. Med. J. **II**: 485.

EVANS, D. A. P., P. B. STOREY & V. A. MCKUSICK. 1961. Observations on the determination of the isoniazid inactivator phenotype. Bull. Johns Hopkins Hosp. **108**: 60.

EVANS, D. A. P. & T. A. WHITE. 1964. Human acetylation polymorphism. J. Lab. Clin. Med. **63**: 387.

GOW, J. G. & D. A. P. EVANS. 1964. A study of the influence of the isoniazid inactivator phenotype on reversion in genito-urinary tuberculosis. Tubercle. **45**: 136.

GRUNBERG, E. & R. J. SCHNITZER. 1952. Studies on the activity of hydrazine derivatives of isonicotinic acid in the experimental tuberculosis of mice. Quarterly Bulletin, Sea View Hospital **13**: 3.

GRUNBERG, E., B. LEIWANT, I-L. D'ASCENSION & R. J. SCHNITZER. 1952. On the lasting protective effect of hydrazine derivatives of isonicotinic acid in the experimental tuberculosis infection of mice. Diseases of the Chest **21**: 369.

HARRIS, H. W., A. KNIGHT & M. J. SELIN. 1958. Comparison of isoniazid concentrations in the blood of people of Japanese and European Descent – Therapeutic and genetic implications. The Amer. Review of Tuberc. & Pulm. Dis. **78**: 944.

HARRIS, H. W. 1961. High-dose isoniazid compared with standard-dose isoniazid with PAS, in the treatment of previously untreated cavitary pulmonary tuberculosis. Trans. Conf. Chemotherapy of Tuber., 20th Conf. : 39.

HARTIALA, K. J. W. & T. TERHO. 1965. Metabolic acetylation by the mucosal membrane of the gastro-intestinal tract. Nature **205**: 809.

HUGHES, H. B. 1953. On the metabolic fate of isoniazid. J. of Pharmacology & Exper. Therapeutics **109**: 444.

HUGHES, H. B., J. BIEHL, A. P. JONES & L. H. SCHMIDT. 1954. Metabolism of isoniazid in man as related to the occurrence of peripheral neuritis. The Amer. Rev. of Tuberculosis **70**: 266.

HUGHES, H. B., H. SCHMIDT & J. BIEHL. 1955. The metabolism of isoniazid: its implications in therapeutic use. Trans. Conf. Chemotherapy of Tuberc. 14th Conf. : 217.

JENNE, J. W. 1963. Isoniazid acetylation by human liver and intestinal mucosa. Fed. Procs. **22**: 540.

JENNE, J. W. 1965. Partial purification and properties of the isoniazid trans-acetylase in human liver. Its relationship to the acetylation of p-aminosalicylic acid. J. Clin. Invest. **44**: 1992.

JENNE, J. W. & P. D. BOYER. 1963. Kinetic characteristics of the acetylation of isoniazid and p-aminosalicylic acid by a liver-enzyme preparation. Biochim. et Biophys. Acta **65**: 121.

JENNE, J. W., F. M. MACDONALD & E. MENDOZA. 1961. A study of the renal clearances, metabolic inactivation rates, and serum fall-off interaction of isoniazid and para-aminosalicylic acid in Man. The Amer. Rev. of Resp. Dis. **84**: 371.

KNIGHT, R. A., J. SELIN & H. W. HARRIS. 1959. Genetic factors influencing isoniazid blood levels in humans. Trans. Conf. Chemotherapy of Tuber. 18th Conf. : 52.

LEVI, A. J. & D. M. WALKER. 1966. Drug metabolism and liver disease. Gut **7**: 105.

MCDERMOTT, W. 1960. Antimicrobial therapy of pulmonary tuberculosis. Bull. World Health Org. **23**: 427.

MCISAAC, W. M. & M. KANDA. 1964. The metabolism of I-hydrazinophthalazine. J. Pharmacol. and Exp. Therap. **143**: 7.

MEYER, H. & J. MALLY. 1912. Uber Hydrazinderivate der Pyridincarbonsauren. Monatsh. Chem. **33**: 393.

MEYLER, L. 1960. Side effects of drugs. Excerpta Medica Fdn: Amsterdam.

MITCHELL, S., D. K. RIEMENSNIDER, J. R. HARSCH & J. CARROLL BELL. 1958. New information on the clinical implications of individual variations in the metabolic handling of antituberculous drugs, particularly isoniazid. Trans. Conf. Chemotherapy of Tuber. 17th Conf. : 77.

MOTULSKY, A. G. & L. STEINMANN. 1962. Aryl amine acetylation in human red cells. J. Clin. Invest. **41**: 1387.

NAKAGAWA, H. & S. SUNAHARA. 1967. Studies on metabolism of isoniazid by a new chemical determination of isoniazid. Kekkaku **42**: 203.

PERAULT, A-M. & B. PULLMAN. 1963. Electronic aspects of enzymic acetyl-transfer reactions. Biochim. Biophys. Acta **66**: 86.

PERRY JR. H. M., A. SAKAMOTO & E. M. TAN. 1967. Relationship of acetylating enzyme to hydralazine toxicity. Proc. Central Soc. for Clin. Res. **40**: 81.

PETERS, J. H., G. R. GORDON & P. BROWN. 1965. Studies on the metabolism of isoniazid in sub-human primates. Proc. of the Society for Exper. Biol. & Med. **120**: 575.

PETERS, J. H., K. S. MILLER & P. BROWN. 1965. The determination of isoniazid and its metabolites in human urine. Analyt. Biochem. **12**: 379.

ROBITZEK, E. H., I. J. SELIKOFF & G. G. ORNSTEIN. 1952. Chemotherapy of human tuberculosis with hydrazine derivatives of isonicotinic acid. Quarterly Bull., Sea View Hospital **13**: 27.

SELIKOFF, I. J. & E. H. ROBITZEK. 1952. Tuberculosis chemotherapy with hydrazine derivatives of isonicotinic acid. Diseases of the Chest **21**: 385.

SERONDE, J. 1963. The pathogenesis of duodenal ulcer in the pantothenate-deficient rat. Yale, J. Biol. & Med. **36**: 141.

SMIRNOV, G. A. & T. I. KOZULITZINA. 1962. Interrelation between toxic effect and metabolic patterns of phtivazid. Vop. Med. Khim. **8**: 401.

SUNAHARA, S., M. URANO & K. KAWAIT. 1963. Biochemical and genetical studies on isoniazid metabolism. Tokyo Nat. Chest Hosp. Annual Report.

SUNAHARA, S., M. URANO, H. T. LIN, T. J. CHEG & A. JARUMILINDA. 1963a. Further observations on trimodality of frequency distribution curve of biologically active isoniazid blood levels and 'cline' in frequencies of alleles controlling isoniazid inactivation. Acta Tuberc. Pneumol. Scand. **43**: 181.

SUNAHARA, S., M. URANO, M. OGAWA, S. YOSHIDA, H. MUKOYAMA & K. KAWAI. 1963b. Genetical aspect of isoniazid metabolism. Jap. J. Human Genetics **8**: 93.

WEBER, W. W. 1967. Purification and properties of human liver N-Acetyl-transferase. Fed. Proc. **26**: 683.

WEBER, W. W. & S. N. COHEN. 1967. N-Acetylation of drugs: isolation and properties of an N-Acetyltransferase from rabbit liver. Molecular Pharmacology **3**: 266.

WHITE, T. A. & D. A. P. EVANS. 1968. The acetylation of sulfamethazine and sulfamethoxypyridazine by human subjects. Clin. Pharmacol. & Therap. **9**: 80.

WHITE, T. A. & D. A. P. EVANS. 1967a. Urinary hexosamine and Acetyl-hexosamine excretion in human acetylator phenotypes. Clin. Chim. Acta. **18**: 161.

WHITE, T. A. & D. A. P. EVANS. 1967b. The acetylation of tryptophan metabolites by rapid and slow acetylators of sulfamethazine. Experientia, Basel. **23**: 959.

ZUCKER, L. M., J. SERONDE, JR. & T. G. ZUCKER. 1955. Acetylating activity in the rat in relation to other signs of pantothenic acid deficiency. Arch. Biochem. **55**: 9.

PURIFICATION AND PROPERTIES OF N-ACETYLTRANSFERASE FROM MAMMALIAN LIVER

Wendell W. Weber,* Sanford N. Cohen† and Michael S. Steinberg‡

Department of Pharmacology
New York University School of Medicine
New York, N. Y.

Introduction

Acetylation is a major route for the metabolism of aromatic amines in many different species (Williams, 1959). Early *in vitro* studies of acetylation of sulfanilamide by rabbit liver slices were reported by Klein and Harris (1938). Acetylation of sulfanilamide by rabbit and pigeon liver homogenates was reported by Lipmann who used the acetylating enzyme system as an analytical tool in the investigations which led to the identification of coenzyme A (Lipmann, 1948). This system was also used by Lynen (1952) in his work on the isolation and identification of acetyl coenzyme A.

Early studies of the properties of the acetylating enzyme itself indicated that the enzyme from pigeon liver catalyzes the acetylation of isoniazid (INH) (Johnson, 1954) as well as sulfanilamide. Jenne and Boyer (1962) reported on the kinetic characteristics of the acetylation of INH by a pigeon liver extract. In their studies, the acetyl coenzyme A generating system, which had been used in earlier studies, was replaced by purified acetyl coenzyme A. They suggested that an acetyl-enzyme was formed in the acetylation of INH and they proposed a mechanism for this reaction.

The properties of the acetylating enzyme system from human liver were reported by Evans (1962; Evans & White, 1964) from studies in which INH and various other substrates were utilized in investigations of the human acetylation polymorphism. He showed that there is a correlation between the rate of acetylation of INH *in vivo* and the level of activity of the liver acetylating enzyme system.

Frymoyer and Jacox (1963; 1963a) reported that a polymorphism in the rate of acetylation of INH exists in the rabbit. They found a correlation between the rate of acetylation *in vivo* and the level of activity in liver homogenates which was similar to the correlation found in man.

Studies of partially purified human N-acetyltransferase prepared from liver of rapid and of slow inactivators of INH were reported by Jenne (1965). The purified enzyme preparations from the liver of slow inactivators of INH had less N-acetyltransferase activity than those from the liver of rapid inactivators. He found that the enzyme obtained from slow inactivators had kinetic and temperature stability characteristics similar to the enzyme obtained from rapid inactivators. He suggested that the difference between slow and rapid inactivator phenotypes "may be due to differences in amount of an identical enzyme molecule."

This report summarizes our studies of partially purified N-acetyl-transferase from 4 mammalian species—rabbit, human, monkey and rat—and from the slow INH-inactivator rabbit (Weber & Cohen, 1967, 1967a; Cohen & Steinberg, 1967; Weber *et al.*, 1967).

* Recipient of Career Scientist Award of the Health Research Council of the City of New York under contract I–441.

† Special Fellow, NICHD, 1965–1967. John and Mary R. Markle Scholar in Academic Medicine.

‡ Predoctoral trainee, U.S. Public Health Service Training Grant, 5TO5GM16–68.

Results

N-acetyltransferase from various species. The 100,000 g supernatant of liver homogenates contained all of the N-acetyltransferase activity. Purification of this fraction is shown in TABLE 1. This procedure consistently yielded 300–500-fold purification of the enzyme from rabbit liver and could also be used to prepare the enzyme from human, monkey, and rat liver to the same level of purification. Compounds found to be substrates for the purified enzyme from all species include those listed in TABLE 2. Each of these compounds has either a primary amino group attached to an unsaturated ring or a hydrazino group attached, either directly or via a carbonyl group, to an unsaturated ring. In general, we have found that drugs and other foreign compounds which have these structural features are substrates for liver N-acetyltransferase.

Families of parallel lines were obtained for the acetylation of INH with N-acetyltransferase from each species studied when reciprocal initial velocity was plotted against reciprocal substrate concentration. Initial velocity data obtained with rabbit and with human N-acetyltransferase, plotted in this way, are shown in FIGURES 1 and 2. These studies, together with product inhibition studies on rabbit liver N-acetyltransferase, led us to propose that the acetylation of INH takes place according to a "ping-pong" mechanism in which two substrates react and two products are formed (Weber & Cohen, 1967). Thus, in the acetylation of INH, acetyl coenzyme A (AcCoA) reacts with N-acetyltransferase, and the first product, coenzyme A (CoA), is released before INH enters the reaction. The reaction may be written in the following way:

$$\begin{array}{ccccccc} & \text{AcCoA} & \text{CoA} & & \text{INH} & \text{AcINH} & \\ & \downarrow & \uparrow & & \downarrow & \uparrow & \\ \hline \text{E} & & & \text{E-Ac} & & & \text{E} \rightarrow \end{array}$$

The initial steady state rate equation for the reaction is:

$$\frac{1}{v_o} = \frac{1}{V} + \frac{K_{m},AcCoA}{V} \cdot \frac{1}{(AcCoA)} + \frac{K_m\ INH}{V} \cdot \frac{1}{(INH)}$$

where v_o is the initial velocity, V is the maximum velocity of the reaction when both substrates are at infinite concentration, and K_m for each substrate is the limiting Michaelis constant, i.e., the concentration which half saturates the enzyme in the presence of an infinite concentration of the other substrate. Limiting values of the Michaelis constants for each substrate were calculated from initial rates determined with enzyme from each species (TABLE 3). Since there was a

TABLE 1

PURIFICATION OF N-ACETYLTRANSFERASE FROM RABBIT LIVER

Step	Activity* (units/ml)	Protein Concentration	Specific Activity (units/mg)	Fold Purification
Supernatant fraction (100,000 g)	0.014	30.6	0.00046	1
Ammonium sulfate fraction (0.45–0.60)	0.032	25.6	0.0012	2.6
Sephadex G–100 (peak fraction)	0.010	1.1	0.0091	20
DEAE-cellulose (peak fraction)	0.021	0.14	0.16	350

* The enzyme was assayed with INH at pH 9.0 (Weber & Cohen, 1967). One unit of activity represents 1 μM of 2-acetyl INH formed per min per ml of enzyme fraction.

3-fold variation in the limiting values between two preparations of human N-acetyltransferase, both obtained from rapid inactivators of INH, the differences between the species seen in TABLE 3 are probably not significant.

A K_m value can be determined from each line in FIGURES 1 and 2. The approach of these apparent K_m values for INH to the limiting K_m value for INH, determined with rabbit and with human liver N-acetyltransferase, is shown in FIGURE 3. The apparent $K_{m,INH}$ of human enzyme approaches its limiting value at a different rate than that of the rabbit enzyme and more acetyl coenzyme A

TABLE 2

SUBSTRATES OF LIVER N-ACETYLTRANSFERASE

Aniline	Isoniazid
p-Aminobenzoic acid	p-Phenetidin
p-Aminosalicylic acid	Sulfamethazine
Hydralazine	Sulfanilamide

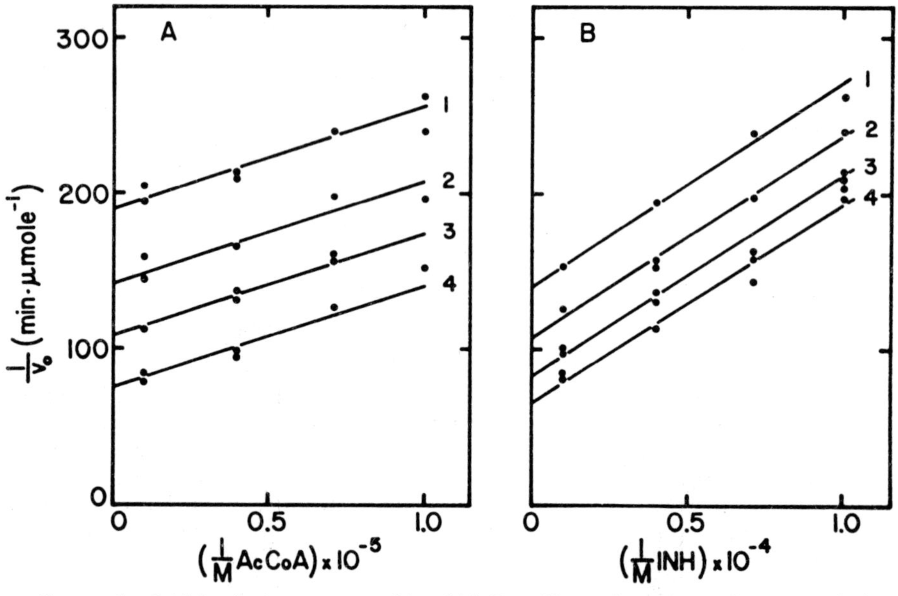

FIGURE 1. Initial velocity patterns with rabbit liver N-acetyltransferase from a rapid inactivator of INH. **A**. Acetyl coenzyme A as the varied substrate. INH concentration: line 1, 0.10 mM; line 2, 0.14 mM; line 3, 0.25 mM and line 4, 1.0 mM. **B**. INH as the varied substrate. Acetyl coenzyme A concentration: line 1, 0.01 mM; line 2, 0.014 mM; line 3, 0.025 mM and line 4, 0.10 mM. The enzyme preparation was the DEAE-cellulose fraction. The rate of the reaction was determined by following the appearance of sulfhydryl groups from acetyl coenzyme A in an automatic recording spectrophotometer at 412 mµ and 27° by a procedure utilizing 5,5′-dithiobis-(2-dinitrobenzoic acid) (Ellman, 1959). These experiments were carried out in a 2.0 ml reaction mixture in 0.1 M borate buffer, pH 8.0. INH, acetyl coenzyme A and 0.12 µmole of 5,5′-dithiobis-(2-dinitrobenzoic acid) were added to each cuvette (1.0 cm. light path) and the reaction was started by the addition of 0.1 ml of enzyme with an adder-mixer (Boyer & Segal, 1952). Initial velocities were determined by extrapolating the recorded curve to the time of addition of the enzyme and measuring the slope of the tangent to the curve at that point.

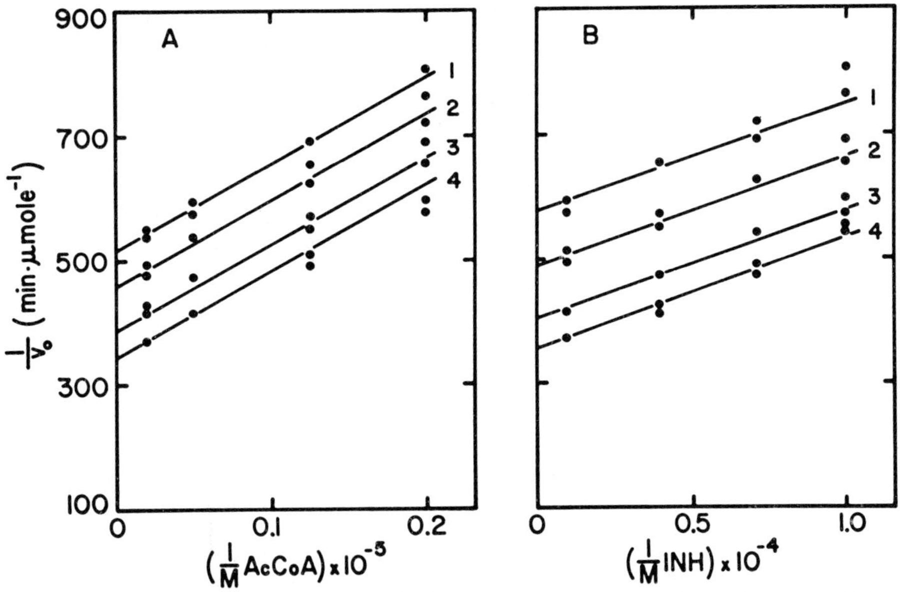

FIGURE 2. Initial velocity patterns with human liver N-acetyltransferase from a rapid inactivator of INH. **A**. Acetyl coenzyme A as the varied substrate. INH concentration: line 1, 0.1 mM; line 2, 0.14 mM; line 3, 0.25 mM; and line 4, 1.0 mM. **B**. INH as the varied substrate. Acetyl coenzyme A concentration: line 1, 0.05 mM; line 2, 0.08 mM; line 3, 0.20 mM and line 4, 0.50 mM. The enzyme preparation was the DEAE-cellulose fraction. The conditions for assay were the same as those described in FIGURE 1.

TABLE 3

LIMITING VALUES OF THE APPARENT $K_{M, AcCoA}$ AND $K_{M, INH}$ DETERMINED WITH N-ACETYLTRANSFERASE FROM 4 MAMMALIAN SPECIES*

Species	$K_{M, AcCoA}$ (M) × 10^5	$K_{M, INH}$ (M) × 10^5
Human†	3.9	5.8
Monkey	2.7	10.4
Rabbit†	2.0	18.2
Rat†	2.2	6.0

* K_M for each substrate at infinite concentration of the other substrate. The experimental conditions are described in FIGURE 1.

† Computed with aid of PING PONG program (Cleland, 1963).

is required to achieve the same fraction of the limiting $K_{m,INH}$ with the human enzyme than with the rabbit enzyme.

The catalytic activity of N-acetyltransferase from these species was also studied with substrates other than INH. The value of the apparent K_m for several substrates for rabbit liver N-acetyltransferase varies widely between 8.9 × 10^{-4} M for INH and 0.009 × 10^{-4} M for p-phenetidin (TABLE 4). The ratio of the apparent K_m value for each substrate to that for INH was determined for each species (TABLE 5). There are species-related differences in this ratio, and these differences are most pronounced with sulfamethazine, p-amino salicylic acid and p-phenetidin. On the basis of the differences in this ratio for these three sub-

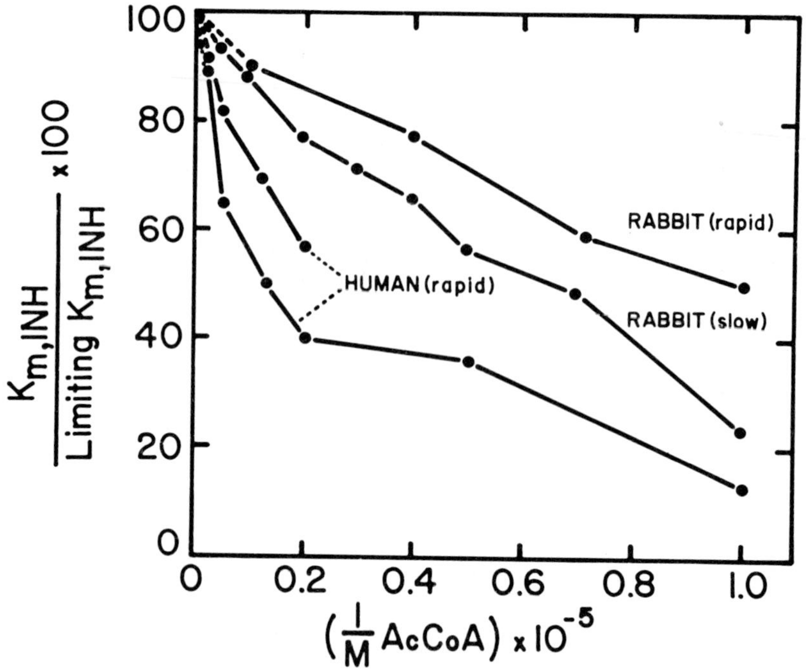

FIGURE 3. The approach of $K_{m, INH}$ to its limiting value for liver N-acetyltransferase. Note that data for enzyme obtained from two humans are included.

TABLE 4

APPARENT $K_{M, Substrate}$ DETERMINED WITH N-ACETYLTRANSFERASE FROM RABBIT LIVER*

Substrate	$K_{M, Substrate}$† ($M \times 10^4$)
INH	8.9
Hydralazine	3.6
p-NH_2 benzoic acid	0.55
Sulfamethazine	0.42
p-NH_2 salicylic acid	0.38
Aniline	0.28
p-Phenetidin	0.009

*K_M determined with (AcCoA) $= 2 \times 10^{-4}$ M. The experimental conditions were the same as those described in FIGURE 1.

† K_M computed with aid of HYPER program (Cleland, 1963).

strates, these species may be divided into two groups—human-monkey and rabbit-rat. The difference between the properties of N-acetyltransferase from these two groups was much more obvious when the acetylation of p-aminobenzoic acid and sulfanilamide was studied. Both of these substrates produced marked inhibition of the enzyme from human and monkey liver at concentrations which did not inhibit the enzyme from both rabbit and rat. For example, p-aminobenzoic acid markedly inhibited the enzyme from human and monkey liver at concentrations above 0.14mM while the enzyme from the other species was not inhibited at 1.0m

TABLE 5

$\frac{K_{M,\,Substrate}}{K_{M,\,INH}}$ DETERMINED WITH N-ACETYLTRANSFERASE FROM 4 DIFFERENT SPECIES*

Substrate	Human	Monkey	Rabbit	Rat
INH	1.0	1.0	1.0	1.0
Hydralazine	0.50	0.34	0.41	0.11
Aniline	0.04	0.02	0.03	0.11
Sulfamethazine	1.5	0.59	0.048	0.12
p-Aminosalicylic acid	6.3	4.3	0.042	0.039
p-Phenetidin	0.15	0.18	0.001	0.0008

* K_M determined when (AcCoA) = 2×10^{-4} M. The experimental conditions were the same as those described in FIGURE 1.

M concentration. It may be significant that all of the substrates which differentiate the human and monkey enzymes from the rabbit and rat enzymes have a substitution para to the group which is acetylated.

Slow vs. rapid N-acetyltransferase. Recently, we have studied the acetylation of INH with liver N-acetyltransferase from a single slow inactivator rabbit, purified according to the procedure in TABLE 1. Initial velocity determinations with this enzyme preparation yielded families of parallel lines (FIGURE 4) indicating that the acetylation of INH probably proceeds by the same mechanism in the slow as in the rapid inactivator rabbit. Limiting values of the K_m for acetyl coenzyme A and for INH were the same in the slow as in the rapid inactivator

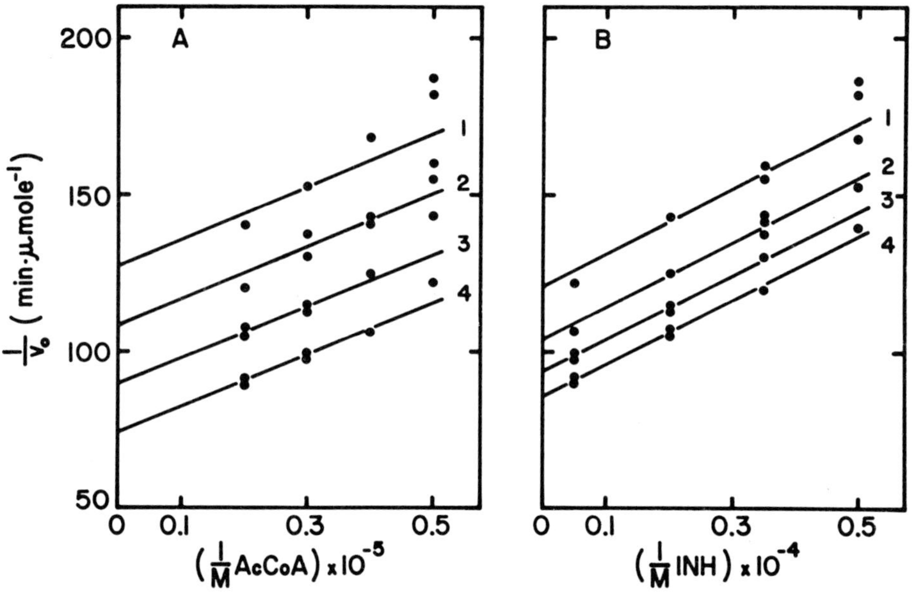

FIGURE 4. Initial velocity patterns with rabbit liver N-acetyltransferase from a slow inactivator of INH. **A**. Acetyl coenzyme A as the varied substrate. INH concentration: line 1, 0.20 mM; line 2, 0.28 mM; line 3, 0.50 mM and line 4, 2.0 mM. **B**. INH as the varied substrate. Acetyl coenzyme A concentration: line 1, 0.020 mM; line 2, 0.025 mM; line 3, 0.033 mM and line 4, 0.050 mM. The conditions for assay were the same as those described in FIGURE 1. The enzyme preparation was the DEAE-cellulose fraction.

TABLE 6

LIMITING VALUES OF THE APPARENT $K_{M, AcCoA}$ AND $K_{M, INH}$ DETERMINED WITH N-ACETYLTRANSFERASE FROM RAPID AND SLOW ACETYLATOR RABBITS*

Phenotype	$K_{M, AcCoA}$† (M) × 10^5	$K_{M, INH}$† (M) × 10^5
Rapid	2.0	18.2
Slow	2.9	17.8

* K_M determined when (AcCoA) = 2 × 10^{-4} M. The experimental conditions were the conditions were the same as those described in FIGURE 1.

† Computed with aid of PING PING program (Cleland, 1963).

rabbit (TABLE 6). However, the approach of the K_m for INH of the slow inactivator enzyme to its limiting value differs from that of the rapid inactivator enzyme (FIGURE 3).

Summary

1) N-acetyltransferase has been purified from liver of the human, monkey, rat and both rapid and slow inactivator rabbits.

2) N-acetyltransferase from all of these sources catalyzes the acetylation of INH by the same mechanism (ping-pong). The limiting values of the Michaelis constants for acetyl coenzyme A and for INH obtained with enzyme from each of these sources do not differ significantly.

3) Studies with substrates other than INH show that the catalytic properties of enzyme from rapid inactivator rabbits and from rats differ from the properties of enzyme from rapid inactivator humans and from monkeys.

4) Further examination of the kinetic data on the acetylation of INH shows that the catalytic properties of enzyme from rapid inactivator rabbits differ from the properties of rapid inactivator human enzyme.

5) Examination of the kinetic data on the acetylation of INH by the enzyme from slow inactivator rabbits shows that it may differ from the enzyme from rapid inactivator rabbits.

Conclusions

The results presented in this report show that the catalytic center of N-acetyltransferase from rapid inactivator rabbit liver differs from that of the enzyme from human liver. In addition, the data suggest that there are differences in the catalytic properties of N-acetyltransferase from rapid and slow inactivator rabbits.

Acknowledgments

We thank D. J. Hearse, University College of South Wales and Monmouthshire, Cardiff, Wales, for carrying out the studies on rat liver N-acetyltransferase as a visiting scientist in our laboratory, Dr. D. Marsh of the Department of Physiology for assistance in modifying the Fortran computer program, Dr. H. Siegel of the Department of Forensic Medicine for providing the human liver samples and Mrs. R. Szabadi for technical assistance. This work was supported in part by National Institutes of Health grants AM 08577, GM 15064 and by computer grant FR–00331–01A1.

References

WILLIAMS, R. T. 1959. Detoxication Mechanisms. John Wiley & Sons. N. Y., N. Y.

KLEIN, J. R. & J. S. HARRIS. 1938. The acetylation of sulfanilamide *in vitro*. J. Biol. Chem. **124:** 613–626.

LIPMANN, F. 1948–1949. Biosynthetic mechanisms. The Harvey Lectures. Charles C. Thomas. Springfield, Ill.
LYNEN, F. 1952–1953. Acetyl coenzyme A and the "fatty acid cycle." The Harvey Lectures. Charles C. Thomas. Springfield, Ill.
JOHNSON, W. J. 1954. Biological acetylation of isoniazid. Nature **174**: 744–745.
JENNE, J. W. & P. D. BOYER. 1962. Kinetic characteristics of the acetylation of isoniazid and p-aminosalicylic acid by a liver-enzyme preparation. Biochim. Biophys. Acta **65**: 121–127.
EVANS, D. A. P. 1962. Pharmacogenetique. Medecine et Hygiene **20**: 905.
EVANS, D. A. P. & T. A. WHITE. 1964. Human acetylation polymorphism. J. Lab. & Clin. Med. **63**: 394–403.
FRYMOYER, J. W. & R. F. JACOX. 1963. Investigation of the genetic control of sulfadiazine and isoniazid metabolism in the rabbit. J. Lab. & Clin. Med. **62**: 891–904.
FRYMOYER, J. W. & R. F. JACOX. 1963a. Studies of genetically controlled sulfadiazine acetylation in rabbit livers: Possible identification of the heterozygous trait. J. Lab. & Clin. Med. **62**: 905–909.
JENNE, J. W. 1965. Partial purification and properties of the isoniazid transacetylase in human liver. Its relationship to the acetylation of p-aminosalicylic acid. J. Clin. Invest. **44**: 1992–2002.
WEBER, W. W. & S. N. COHEN. 1967. N-acetylation of drugs: Isolation and properties of an N-acetyltransferase from rabbit liver. Mol. Pharm. **3**: 266–273.
WEBER, W. W. & S. N. COHEN. 1967a. The mechanism of isoniazid acetylation by human N-acetyltransferase. Biochim. Biophys. Acta. **151**: 276–278.
COHEN, S. N. & M. S. STEINBERG. 1967. Variation in substrate specificity of N-acetyltransferase from mammalian liver. Fed. Proc. **26**: 683.
WEBER, W. W., S. N. COHEN & M. S. STEINBERG. 1967. Species differences in the kinetic properties of the INH-acetylating enzyme. Pharmacologist **9**: 190.
ELLMAN, G. L. 1959. Tissue sulfhydryl groups. Arch. Biochem. Biophys. **82**: 70–77.
BOYER, P. D. & H. L. SEGAL. 1952. *In* Mechanism of Enzyme Action. W. D. McElroy and B. Glass, Eds. Johns Hopkins Press. Baltimore, Md. p. 523.
CLELAND, W. W. 1963. Computer programmes for processing enzyme kinetic data. Nature **198**: 463–465.

THERAPY OF PROLONGED APNEA AFTER SUXAMTHONIUM WITH PURIFIED PSEUDOCHOLINESTERASE: NEW DATA ON KINETICS OF THE HYDROLYSIS OF SUCCINYLDICHOLINE AND SUCCINYLMONOCHOLINE AND FURTHER DATA ON N-ACETYLTRANSFERASE-POLYMORPHISM

H. W. Goedde, K. Altland and W. Schloot

Institute of Human Genetics, University of Hamburg and Department of Biochemical Genetics, Institute of Human Genetics and Anthropology, University of Freiburg, Germany

Introduction

In recent years many authors have tried to characterize different cholinesterases in human serum. If one remembers the many esterase zones of a starch gel electrophoretic pattern of human serum, one really likes to assume the existence of more than one enzyme. However, looking at the esterase patterns of the serum with the ineffective "silent" pseudocholinesterase (phenotype S), there is nothing to be seen, but a faint coloration in the albumin region.

But, what is the situation with the enzymatic activities on various substrates such as acetylcholine, benzoylcholine, succinyldicholine, succinylmonocholine and others? Are they metabolized by the same enzyme or not? And what is the situation with the different enzymes Berry[1] postulated from saturation curves with benzoylcholine and acetylcholine, and the different inhibition of these activities by dibucaine? If, for example, the hydrolysis of benzoylcholine at high substrate concentration with the V_{max} at 10^{-2} M is due to an enzyme different from pseudocholinesterase, one would expect that it is not controlled by the alleles at the E_1-locus.

Tests with sera from homozygotes for the so-called "silent gene" are very appropriate to study such questions. As I demonstrated last year[2] analyzing five of these cases, and as Dietz[3] found in another case of a "silent gene," neither benzoylcholine nor acetylcholine are hydrolyzed at high as well as low concentration for more than 3% of normal rate. The same results are to be found with succinyldicholine.

Kinetic Data on the Conversion of Succinyldicholine and Succinylmonocholine

We have tried to get more kinetic data on the breakdown of succinyldicholine, and especially on its split product, the monocholine ester, using C^{14}-labeled substrates.[4] After incubation, substrate and split products are separated by high voltage electrophoresis on paper, which is then cut into small pieces and analyzed by means of a liquid scintillation counter. The method has the advantage that the hydrolysis can be estimated at concentrations of substrate as low as 10^{-6} M. The test is particularly accurate and sensitive for the monocholine ester.

The pH-optimum for the enzymatic breakdown of succinyldicholine in serum of phenotype U is about 8. The relatively rapid spontaneous hydrolysis of succinyldicholine at physiological and alkaline pH renders exact measurements of very small enzymatic activities impossible. In terms of an assay, the situation is rather more favorable if we look at the serum activity for the hydrolysis of succinylmonocholine. As one would not expect, the pH-optimum is between 5 and 6 for the catalytic activity of sera with both phenotypes U and A. This low

Substrate	Succinyldicholine			Succinylmonocholine		
Phenotype	U	A	Ratio A/U	U	A	Ratio A/U
pH-optimum	8 - 9	—	—	5 - 6	5 - 6	—
K_M	$4,2 \times 10^{-5}$ (pH 7,4)	—	—	$8,3 \times 10^{-3}$ (pH 5,7)	$1,7 \times 10^{-1}$ (pH 5,7)	21
K_I substrate: benzoylcholine (pH 7,4)	$2,2 \times 10^{-5}$	$3,1 \times 10^{-3}$	141	$4,4 \times 10^{-3}$	—	—
pI_{50}	4,1 (4,01*) 5×10^{-5}M	2,1 (2,02*) benzoylcholine	$I_{50}(A)/I_{50}(U) = 99$	1,88 2×10^{-5}M	1,0 benzoylcholine	$I_{50}(A)/I_{50}(U) = 7,6$

*) data from KALOW

FIGURE 1. Comparison of kinetic data of the enzymic hydrolysis of succinyldicholine and succinylmonocholine.

pH-optimum is strikingly different from that for the other known choline esters, which are metabolized by human serum. One might think that an enzyme different from that converting succinyldicholine is responsible for this activity. However, this seems to be unlikely for the following reasons. Investigating 15 sera of the very rare phenotype S with little or no activity towards succinyldicholine, we found that also succinylmonocholine was hydrolyzed at rates below 1% of normal. By contrast, controls and control assays with a 5000-fold purified pseudocholinesterase from serum of phenotype U showed high catalytic activity towards succinylmonocholine.

Comparison data for the hydrolysis of succinyldicholine and succinylmonocholine are shown in FIGURE 1. The differences of affinity for the phenotypes U and A as reflected by the K_M- and K_I-values of the dicholine and monocholine esters, as well as the different V_{max}-values are striking.

Therapy of Prolonged Apnea in Persons with Atypical Pseudocholinesterase

As previously described by Kalow,[5] Thompson and Whittaker[6] two-thirds of those people suffering from prolonged apnea after injection of succinyldicholine, have atypical pseudocholinesterases in their serum.

FIGURE 2 shows that individuals of the phenotypes A and S as well as heterozygotes for two atypical alleles are unable to convert succinyldicholine. A comparison of the conversion of ^{14}C-succinyldicholine and benzoylcholine shows a good correlation between both substrates in one phenotype. "Silent gene" sera show no activity with both substrates; the phenotypes A and AS no activity with succinyldicholine.

Therapeutic possibilities of shortening prolonged apnea have often been discussed. An effective therapy against prolonged apnea in persons with atypical pseudocholinesterases as well as in persons having normal pseudocholinesterase,

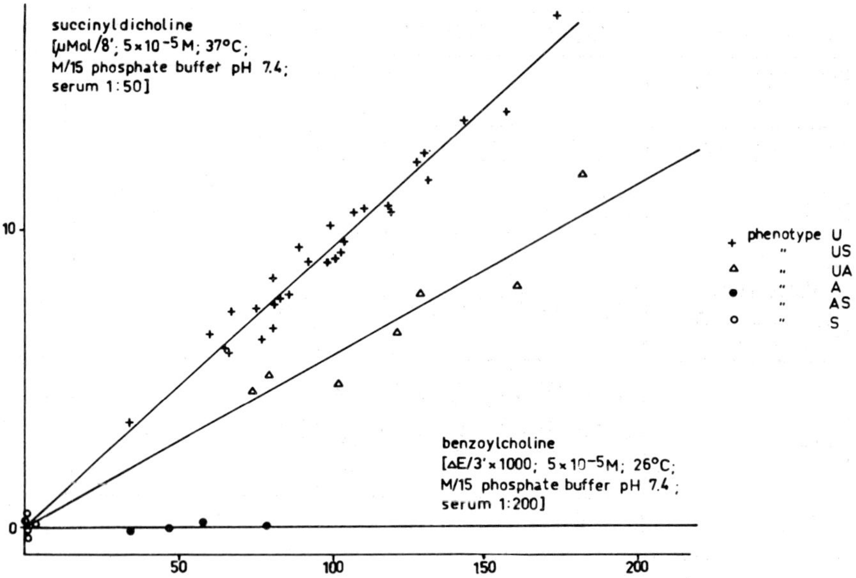

FIGURE 2. Correlation of the enzymic hydrolysis of succinyldicholine and benzoylcholine in sera of different pseudocholinesterase phenotypes.

has not yet been reported. The infusion of fresh plasma is recommended by some authors, but a convincing positive effect has not been described. Borders *et al.*[7] reported shortening the duration of apnea by injecting cholase (concentrated human pseudocholinesterase) before the application of succinyldicholine. Injection of cholase during relaxation showed no abbreviation of apnea.

Experiments, performed together with Dr. Scholler[8] from the Department of Anesthesiology, show that effective therapy of prolonged apnea in persons with atypical pseudocholinesterases is possible by injection of normal purified pseudocholinesterase before and after injection of succinyldicholine. This is a practical example of overcoming a genetic enzyme defect by normalizing the metabolic disorder with application of the missing normal enzyme.

FIGURE 3 shows the segregation of the atypical alleles in the six probands' families. Three persons became known by showing prolonged apnea during operations, the others, were detected in a routine study of the sera of 8,000 blood donors. None of the six persons had ever suffered from a disease which might cause a decrease in pseudocholinesterase activity. These were the subjects.

The narcoses were started with a short-time acting barbiturate, N_20 and 1 mg/kg bodyweight of suxamethonium. Sixteen minutes later – twice the time of normal relaxation after this dosage – the whole plasma activity of pseudocholinesterase, calculated from individual plasma volume and normal enzyme level, was injected. A 1300-fold purified enzyme preparation from human plasma was used. First, before the experiments, and 10 minutes after the application of pseudocholinesterase, blood was taken for measurements of pseudocholinesterase activity.

In three persons 20 hours after the first narcosis with injection of pseudocholinesterase, a second narcosis with 1 mg succinyldicholine per kg bodyweight was performed, but this time without application of pseudocholinesterase. The duration of apnea lasted a bit longer than that of the day before, but was far shorter than during the control narcosis without any normal pseudocholinesterase activity (FIGURE 4). In the three persons, who were found by the routine investigations and who had no prolonged apnea before, control narcoses were made to estimate the individual duration of apnea about two months later. The same amount of succinyldicholine was injected but without normal pseudocholinesterase; the apnea lasted about two hours.

FIGURE 4 shows the duration of apnea, and control measurements of pseudocholinesterase activity during narcosis, with the substrates benzoylcholine and ^{14}C-succinyldicholine. The first column group gives the control values before the first test narcosis; the second one those during the first test-narcosis, after application of the purified enzyme. In all cases the duration of apnea has been totally normalized, the time of relaxation being now eight minutes. The third group represents the values of the second test-narcosis, 20 hours later.

The significantly prolonged apnea during the second test narcosis (column group III) compared with the data of the first test narcosis, (column group II) cannot be understood only from the relatively small loss of serum activity. In one case, injections of half the amount of enzyme applied in these experiments, had no effect on the duration of apnea. This is explicable if one accepts that it is not only serum activity that is responsible for the short duration of apnea after succinyldicholine. High activity for succinyldicholine in the lung has been reported by Pilz.[9] Kalow[10] and Liddell[11] reported that pseudocholinesterase activity of various organs are controlled by the allele E_1^a. If these findings are also true for the lung – and if the data from Pilz are correct – one would expect that the enzyme activity of the lung participates in the degradation of the relaxant. Thus, a substitution of plasma activity only cannot reveal completely the

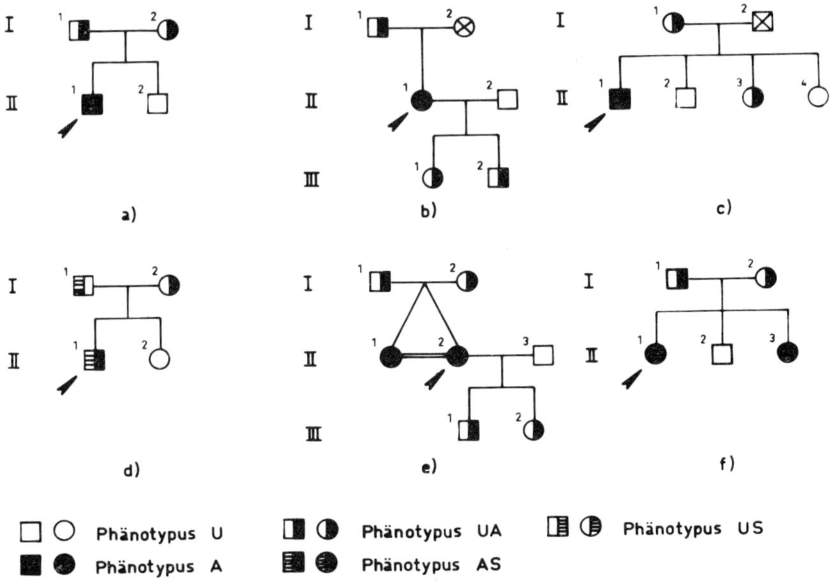

FIGURE 3. Segregation of phenotypes within the proband's families.

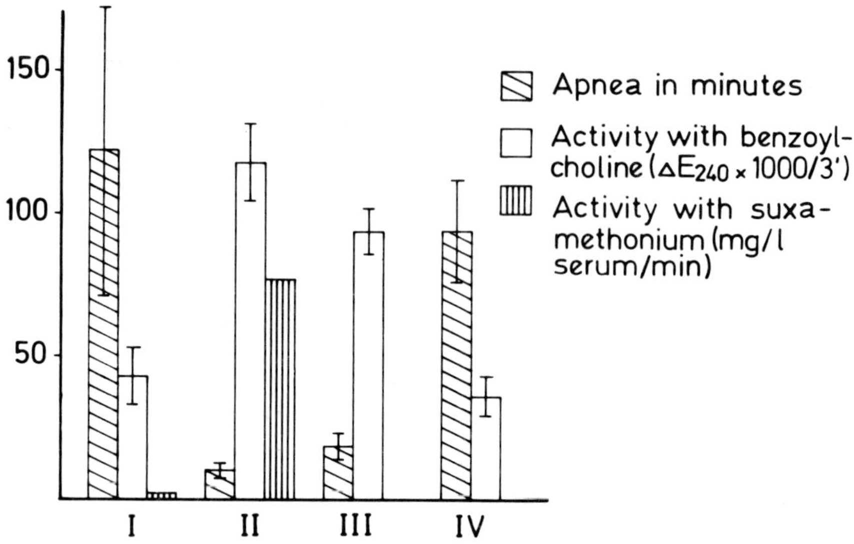

FIGURE 4. Data from narcoses: duration of apnea; activity with succinyldicholine and benzoylcholine.

physiological condition in persons of phenotype U. The control values for the three persons who had not been known as sensitive to suxamethonium before and who were found by screening tests are demonstrated by IV; as one would expect, they are sensitive to suxamethonium.

These data prove without doubt that normal human pseudocholinesterase in vitro and in vivo converts succinyldicholine and contributes to the short time of relaxation. The lyophilized pseudocholinesterase preparation, used in the described investigations, was prepared by the Behring Industry, and was found to be stable for more than six months at 4–8°C without loss of activity. Because of this property and the not too rare appearance of prolonged apnea after succinyldicholine (about 1:1500), and the possibility of estimating pseudocholinesterase variants within a short time, it can be recommended that anesthesiologists have these enzyme preparations among their antidotes.

Activation of Pseudocholinesterase by NH_4Cl: Differentiation of Phenotypes

At this point I wish to report some of our investigations with NH_4Cl. It has been shown by Svensmark[12] that ammoniumchloride activates the cholinesterases from serum as well as from liver by more than 200% in dilute phosphate buffer with benzoylcholine as substrate. Under special conditions one can get activation with serum of phenotype U and inhibition of the activity in serum of phenotype A. Using Kalow's assay[9] for DN-determination, but at 1 M ammoniumchloride, at a substrate concentration of 10^{-4} M benzoylcholine and or buffer concentration of 5 mM, one gets more than 200% activation for the serum activity of phenotype U, and an inhibition of the serum activity of phenotype A of 40–50%. Serum activity of phenotype UA is activated about 100%. There is no overlap. Large differences are also found using tris-buffer at low concentration, but are not as large as those found using phosphate-buffer.

Some Genetical Aspects of Acetylation of Isoniazid (Isonicotinic Acid Hydrazide; INH) in Rhesus Monkeys

We studied some biochemical properties of an INH-acetylating enzyme protein of liver homogenates from rhesus monkeys. Perhaps, the differing INH-conversion in this species and in the green cat is based on a polymorphism similar to that found in man. FIGURE 5 shows the distribution of the specific activity of the INH-acetylating liver enzyme in rhesus monkeys. The percentage of the slow-acetylating animals is about 44 percent.

The effects of the alleles Ac^R and Ac^S seem to be simply additive. The average value of specific activity of the heterozygotes was calculated from the mean values of both groups of homozygotes.

We studied, in 1962, the rapid or slow inactivation of INH in rhesus monkeys *in vivo* using alternatively C^{14}-labeled INH and C^{14}-acetyl coenzyme A with paper chromatography. The animal livers were checked for N-acetyltransferase activity using a spectrophotometric assay according to Jenne[13] but with N,S-diacetylcysteamine as the acetyl-group donor. The results showed good consistency in that a high plasma level of INH corresponded to low enzyme activity and vice versa.

The enzyme was purified from monkey livers about 460-fold by means of acetone precipitation and fractionation on DEAE-cellulose. The pH optimum

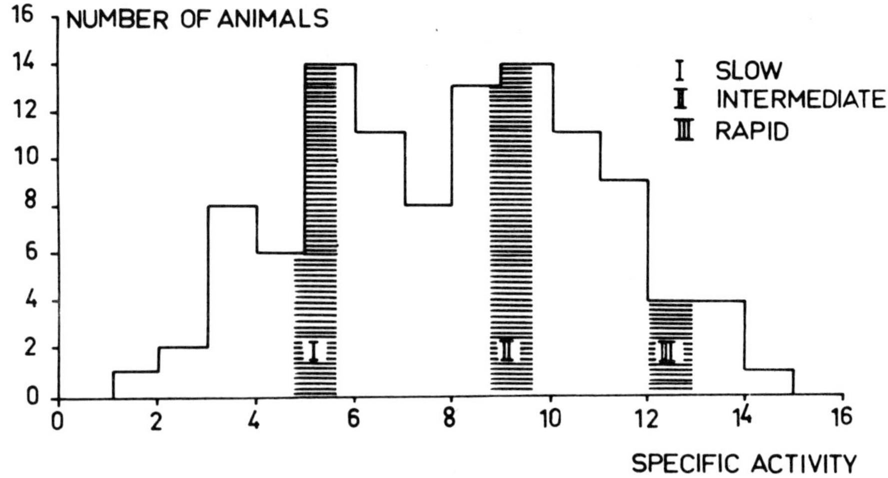

FIGURE 5. Frequency distribution of the specific activities of the N-acetyltransferase of rhesus monkeys.

Coreactant N,S-diacetyl-cysteamine	Km INH (Mole/l)	Coreactant INH	Km N,S-diacetyl-cysteamine (Mole/l)
9,3 × 10^{-5} M	45 × 10^{-5}	12 × 10^{-5} M	97 × 10^{-5}
27,9 × 10^{-5} M	100 × 10^{-5}	20 × 10^{-5} M	194 × 10^{-5}
186,0 × 10^{-5} M	250 × 10^{-5}	45 × 10^{-5} M	582 × 10^{-5}

FIGURE 6. Michaelis constants for INH and N,S-diacetylcysteamine with the N-acetyltransferase of rhesus monkeys.

was between 7, 5–9, 5, the RF-value in polyacrylamide-electrophoresis was about 0, 72. Measuring the K_M-values of acetyl coenzyme A and N,S-diacetylcysteamine, we ascertained that the affinity of the acetyl transferase is similar towards these acetyl group donors. In agreement with the results of Jenne[13] and Weber and Cohen,[14] the K_M-values are changing with the concentration of the coreactant (see FIGURE 6).

Substrate Specifity of N-Acetyltransferase from Rhesus Monkeys

To check qualitative differences between enzymes of high and low specific activity as well as the substrate specifity of the acetyltransferases, various compounds were examined. Concerning substrate specifity, we were able to show that aliphatic amines such as glucosamine, carnitine, choline, glutamic acid and others, which are usually acetylated in the organism, do not inhibit the INH-acetylating enzyme up to a concentration of 10^{-2} M. However, the aromatic compounds we examined, showed a different inhibition. The physiologically active compounds serotonine, tryptamine and probably thyroxine, and the drug Nepresol (dihydrazinophtalazine) show the highest affinity to the INH-acetylating system.

We were able to prove by radio-thin-layer chromatographic techniques in 1965 that serotonin is acetylated to acetyl-serotonine. At present we are investigating the possibility that these acetylases may be important in the metabolism of serotonin and tryptophan.

Structural and functional group correlations regarding affinity and mode of inhibition were considered (FIGURE 7). The different compounds are arranged in

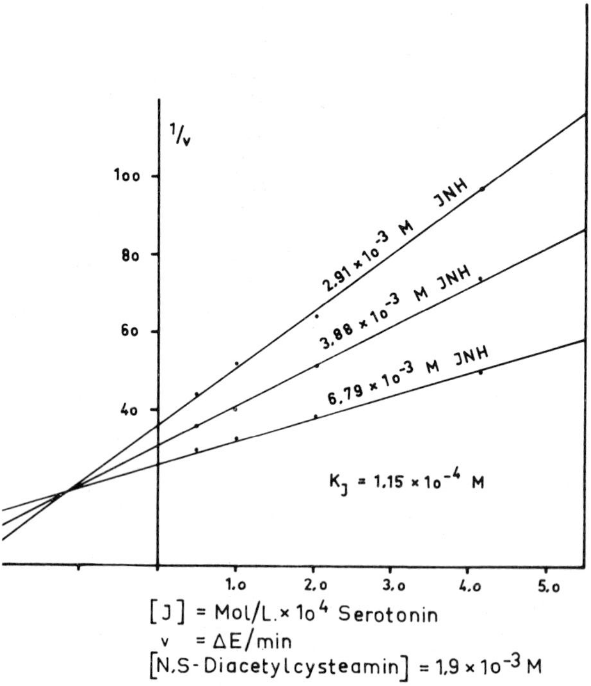

FIGURE 7. K_I-value and mode of inhibition of serotonin.

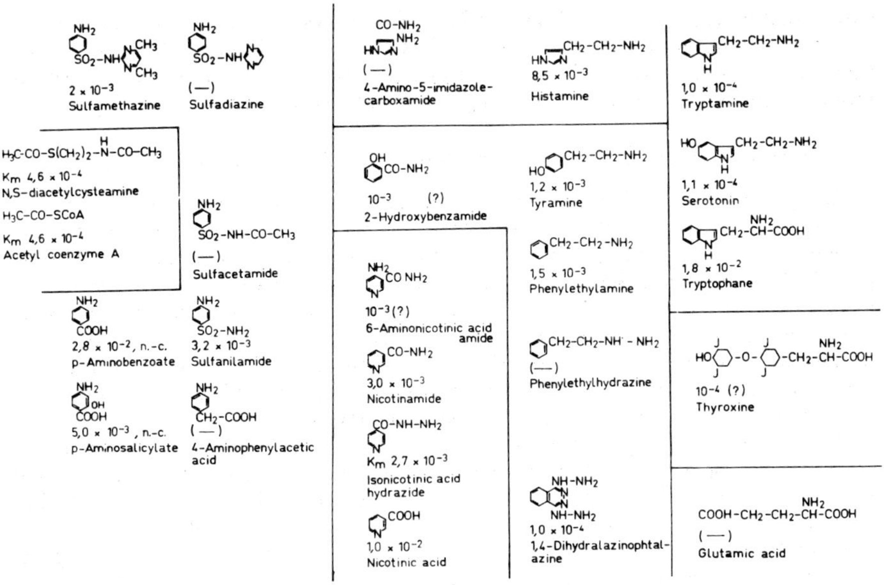

FIGURE 8. K_M- and K_I-values of various compounds regarding the enzymic conversion of INH.

FIGURE 8 in terms of various nuclei, side chains and specific groups. Comparing the competitive inhibitors serotonin, tyramine, phenylethylamine and histamine with tryptophan, we found the following: All compounds are characterized by an amino-group in the side chain, but they differ regarding the nucleus; tryptophan has an additional carboxylic group in the chain. Therefore, the basicity is diminished and the corresponding K_I-value is increased.

Another compound with an additional carboxylic group in the side chain, thyroxine, shows a lower K_I-value. However, we have to consider that the diphenylether of thyroxine may cause an induction influence – drawing the electrons toward the amino-group of the side chain. Compounds with similar chains, but without an aromatic nucleus, such as glutamic acid, show no influence in regard to enzymatic acetylation. Similar effects of a different structure were observed comparing the K_I-values of serotonin with that of tyramine, histamine and phenylethylamine – compounds which differ mainly in the nuclei.

It is of interest that other compounds with a carboxylic group, aside from tryptophan, such as p-aminobenzoic acid, phenyl acetic acid and nicotinic acid also show a very low affinity. However, hydroxylic groups in ortho position to the carboxylic group as in the case of p-aminosalicylic acid increase the affinity. Both the amide and hydrazide of nicotinic acid show an increase in affinity with a factor of ten. Two hydrazine groups, located next to the nucleus, cause an affinity of 10^{-4} M, as in the case of Nepresol (dihydrazinophtalazine). However, with a hydrazine group in the side chain, there is no affinity at all (e.g. phenylethylhydrazine). Analogous inhibitor values are to be found in the examined amides, with the exception of 4-amino-5-imidazol-carboxyamide.

As we have seen, enzyme preparations of different specific activities of rapid- and slow-acetylating animals, show similar qualitative properties, as in the purification factor, K_M-values of INH and N,S-diacetylcysteamine, inhibitor-constants of various compounds and pH-optima. These results are interpreted as an indication that the suggested qualitative differences of the acetylating system of rhesus monkeys are very small, corresponding to similar results in man.

Comparison of the N-Acetyltransferases of Monkey and Pigeon Liver

Comparing the well-studied arylamine acetylase of pigeon liver[15] and the N-acetyltransferase of rhesus liver (FIGURE 9), we found characteristic differences regarding the K_M-values of the model substance N,S-diacetylcysteamine, and INH as substrate; there are differences with a factor of about 100. However, we found the same K_M-values of both enzymes for acetyl-coenzyme A. While the arylamine acetylase of pigeon liver acetylates p-nitroaniline with high affinity to the substrate, there is no acetylating effect in the case of the liver enzyme from rhesus monkeys. Some other differences are found regarding the mode of inhibition with several compounds for these two enzymes.

After column chromatography in about 10% of the purified enzymes, we observed two peaks of activity. While the corresponding K_M-values are identical, the rate of inhibition by excessive substrate (INH) differs markedly. In eight cases out of 700 examined animals no acetylase activity at all was found with the usual test methods. This might be analogous to the so-called "silent gene" information in pseudocholinesterase polymorphism and other so-called defect-pathoproteinaemia. However, after purification by acetone fractionation, we calculated an original specific activity of about 5% of the average value of normal animals. Neither the K_M nor the rate of inhibition of excessive INH in these enzymes is different from that of the normal.

There are differences between the acetylating systems of lung and blood in

No.	Substrate	Structural formula	Conversion of substrates rhesus	Conversion of substrates pigeon	K_m-values (Mole/l) rhesus	K_m-values (Mole/l) pigeon
(9)	Acetyl coenzyme A	$H_3C{-}CO{-}SCoA$	+	+	$4{,}6 \times 10^{-4}$	$4{,}5 \times 10^{-4}$
(10)	N,S-diacetyl-cysteamine	$H_3C{-}CO{-}S(CH_2)_2{-}NH{-}CO{-}CH_3$	+	+	$4{,}6 \times 10^{-4}$	300×10^{-4}
(11)	Isonicotinic acid hydrazide	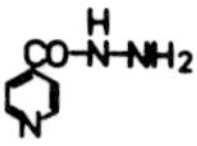	+	+	27×10^{-4}	$0{,}8 \times 10^{-4}$
(12)	p-Nitroaniline	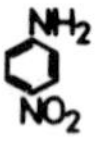	−	+	—	$0{,}6 \times 10^{-4}$
	Inhibitor				K_i-values (Mole/l) [Type of inhibition]	
(13)	p-Amino-benzoate	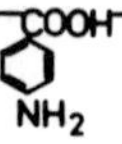	−	+	28×10^{-3} (non-competit.)	$0{,}83 \times 10^{-3}$ (competitive)
(14)	p-Amino-salicylate	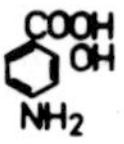	−	+	$5{,}0 \times 10^{-3}$ (non-competit.)	$0{,}93 \times 10^{-3}$ (competitive)
(15)	Sulfanil-amide	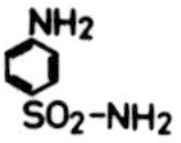	+	+	$3{,}2 \times 10^{-3}$ (competitive)	— (competitive)

FIGURE 9. K_M- and K_I-values of various substrates and inhibitors of the acetylating enzymes of rhesus monkeys and pigeons.

man and monkeys regarding the conversion of INH: in human beings small amounts are acetylated with acetyl coenzyme A, in monkeys this does not occur. The polymorphisms of acetyltransferases as well as those of pseudocholinesterases are illustrative of the fact that genes controlling the synthesis of enzyme proteins – the functions of which have not been explored – may cause unexpected variations in the metabolism of man.

References

1. Berry, W. K. 1960. Biochim. Biophys. (Amst.) **39:** 346.
2. Goedde, H. W. & K. Altland. 1968. Ann. N. Y. Acad. Sci. **149:** Art. 2.
3. Dietz, A. A., H. M. Rubinstein & T. Lubrano. 1966. Clin. Chem. **12:** 26.
4. Goedde, H. W., A. Doenicke & K. Altland. 1967. Pseudocholinesterasen: Pharmakogenetik, Biochemie, Klinik. Springer-Verlag, Berlin, Heidelberg, N. Y.
5. Kalow, W. 1966. Anaesthesist **15:** 13.
6. Thompson, J. C. & M. Whittaker. 1966. Acta Genet. (Basel) **16:** 209.
7. Borders, R. W., C. R. Steffen, W. K. Nowill & R. Martin. 1955. Anesthesiology **16:** 401.
8. Goedde, H. W., K. Altland & K. H. Scholler. 1966. Med. Klinik. In press.
9. Pilz, W. & H. Horlein. 1964. Hoppe Seylers Z. Physiol. Chem. **339:** 157.
10. Kalow, W. 1962. Pharmacogenetics. W. B. Saunders Co. Phila., London.
11. Liddell, J., G. E. Newman & D. F. Brown. 1963. Nature **198:** 1090.
12. Svensmark, O. 1963. Acta Physiol. Scand. **59:** 378.
13. Jenne, W. & P. D. Boyer. 1962. Biochim. Biophys. Acta (Amst.) **65:** 121.
14. Weber, W. W. & S. N. Cohen. 1967. Molecular Pharmacol. **3:** 266.
15. Tabor, H., H. H. Mehler & E. R. Stadtman. 1953. J. Biol. Chem. **204:** 127.

(NOTE: The figures in this paper may have been published elsewhere and it is through no fault of the publisher if permissions designating their reproduction have not been received. – Ed.)

DISCUSSIONS OF THE PAPER

Dr. Earl Usdin (*Atlantic Research Corp., Alexandria, Va.*): Was the Behring pseudocholinesterase you administered to patients who exhibited prolonged apnea prepared from human serum or plasma?

Dr. Goedde: Human plasma.

Dr. Usdin: Were there pronounced reactions resulting from the administration of this foreign protein?

Dr. Goedde: In some cases there was a relatively mild reaction.

Dr. Usdin: I should like to suggest that if there were reactions, it might be possible to eliminate them by administering the enzyme in microencapsulated form. Chang* has shown that such microencapsulated enzymes permit the substrate (which would be succinylcholine in this case) to reach the enzyme and the product to leave and still eliminate any antigenic reaction which administration of the enzyme normally contributes.

Dr. F. F. Foldes (*Montefiore Hospital, Bronx, N. Y.*): Dr. Clark and her associates pointed out several differences in the properties of the normal (NN) and atypical (DD) variants of plasma butyeylcholinesterase. One of the properties of the DD variant is that it hydrolyzes various substrates at relative rates which are different than that of the NN variant. All hitherto investigated substrates were hydrolyzed considerably more slowly by the DD than the NN variant and the relative hydrolysis rate of procaine was found to be the lowest.† Recently Dr. J. C. Smith of our laboratory found that in contrast to all other previously

* Chiang, T. M. *et al.* 1966. Canad. J. Physiol. Pharmacol. **44:** 115–128.

† Foldes, *et al.* 1963. Anesthesiology **24:** 208.

tested substrates tetracaine is hydrolyzed not slower, but somewhat faster by the DD than the NN variant. The divergence of the relative hydrolysis rate of procaine and tetracaine by the DD variant made possible the development of a method which allows the clearcut separation of not only the NN and DD but also that of the NN and ND variants.

The method consists of the ultraviolet spectrophotometric determination of the hydrolysis of procaine and tetracaine. Multiplying the ratio of the hydrolysis rates of procaine and tetracaine by 100 gives the P/T ratio. The P/T ratios as well as the dibucaine number (D.N.) determined in groups of subjects with NN, ND and DD variants (TABLE 1) indicated that the P/T ratio allows a more definite identification of the ND variant than the D.N. It is less influenced by inaccuracies in the determination of the enzymatic hydrolysis rates then the D.N. and is therefore more suitable for screening of a large population sample for ND variants than for the D.N.

TABLE 1

THE DIBUCAINE NUMBERS AND PROCAINE-TETRACAINE RATIOS OF VARIOUS GENOTYPES OF PLASMA CHOLINESTERASE

Genotype	Dibucaine No.		Procaine-Tetracaine Ratio	
	Mean ± SE	Range	Mean ± SE	Range
NN (23)	71.6 ± 0.6	66–77	366 ± 8	320–464
ND (24)	55.5 ± 1.0	46–62	196 ± 6	142–239
DD (18)	12.3 ± 1.1	6–25	40 ± 3	16–59

GLUCOSE-6-PHOSPHATE DEHYDROGENASE VARIANTS AND DRUG-INDUCED HEMOLYSIS*

Henry N. Kirkman

Department of Pediatrics
University of North Carolina School of Medicine
Chapel Hill, N. C.

INTRODUCTION

Deficiencies in activity of red cell glucose-6-phosphate dehydrogenase (G-6-PD) are among the most prevalent hereditary enzymic defects in man. In some populations, between 10 and 60 percent of the males are affected. Of significance for the present conference, however, is the susceptibility of such G-6-PD-deficient subjects to a hemolytic anemia that is induced by certain drugs and toxic substances. The possible mechanisms of this drug-induced hemolysis are discussed in greater detail elsewhere in this symposium.[1,2] This paper is a brief review of the abnormalities of human G-6-PD, with particular attention to any correlation between abnormal properties of the enzyme and clinical manifestations of the abnormality.

The antimalarial drug, pamaquine, has been known since 1926 to be capable of causing an acute hemolytic anemia in some people. Subsequent observations have revealed that such susceptible people are also sensitive to primaquine and to a number of other drugs (TABLE 1). Through the cross-transfusion experiments of Dern and coworkers, this susceptibility to primaquine-induced hemolysis was shown to be an intrinsic property of the red cells of susceptible subjects.[3] A clue to the nature of the defect appeared when Flanagan, Beutler, Dern and Alving found that the level of reduced glutathione (GSH) fell sharply in the red cells of sensitive subjects after several days of ingestion of the drug.[4] This fall occurred just before hemolysis in vivo. Beutler was able to reproduce this abnormal fall in GSH in vitro by incubating the blood of sensitive people with acetylphenylhydrazine.[5] This test made possible the identification of sensitive subjects even before they were exposed to drugs. It allowed Childs and coworkers to demonstrate that this abnormality is a sex-linked (or X-linked) trait with intermediate dominance,[6] a conclusion also obtained subsequently by studies of the G-6-PD defect, itself.[7,8] More recently, certain other chemicals have been found to diminish the level of GSH in sensitive cells during incubation in vitro.[9]

Many investigators now think that the drugs causing hemolysis, or the metabolic derivatives of these drugs, can exist in both an oxidized and reduced form and serve to increase the rate of oxidation of GSH within the red cells of normal and sensitive subjects. The metabolism of normal red cells is well suited to protect itself from such oxidative stresses. Glutathione reductase (FIGURE 1) regenerates GSH from oxidized glutathione (GSSG) by using NADPH, which, in turn, is generated by both G-6-PD and 6-phosphogluconate dehydrogenase (6-PGD). Carson and coworkers discovered that levels of G-6-PD are greatly reduced in sensitive cells, even when the affected subject is not exposed to drugs.[10] Subsequent studies have shown that the activity of glutathione reductase is not diminished in sensitive subjects. The impairment, then, seems to be an inability to meet the increased demand for NADPH that is imposed by the enhanced

* This study was supported by U. S. Public Health Service grant AM 11065 and Research Career Development Award 5 K03 AM 07992.

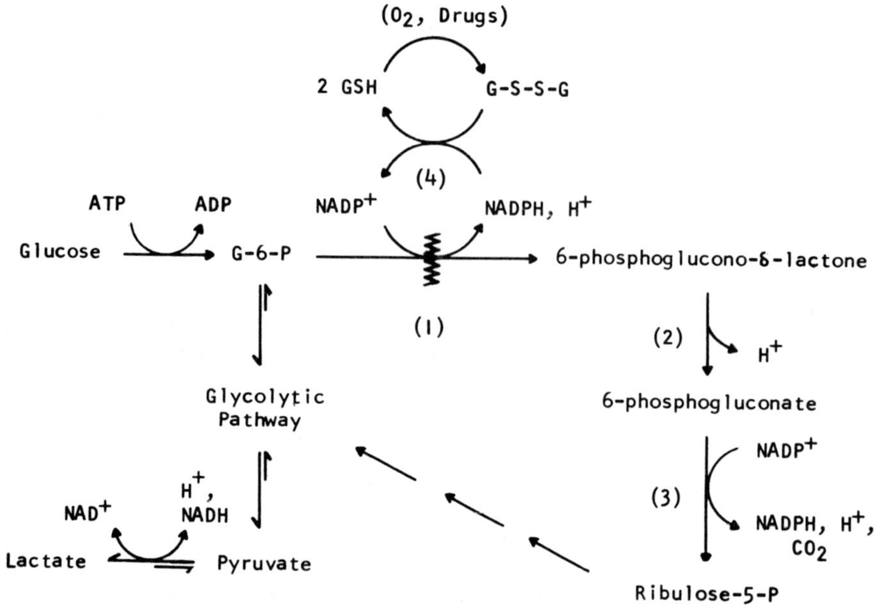

FIGURE 1. Metabolic pathways of G–6–P relevant to G–6–PD deficiency. (1) G–6–PD. (2) 6-phosphoglucono-δ-lactonase. (3) 6–PGD. (4) Glutathione reductase. Reaction (2) also occurs spontaneously.

oxidation of GSH. The mechanism of the hemolysis is not fully understood. During purification and assay, the presence of sulfhydryl-containing agents is often necessary for protection of the sulfhydryl groups of a large number of enzymes. That GSH may serve a similar important function in the red cell and may underlie the hemolytic mechanism is indicated by the observations that hemolytic anemias also result from primary deficiencies of glutathione[11] or glutathione reductase.[12]

In TABLE 1 appears a list of drugs and other agents known to be capable of causing acute hemolytic anemia in people whose red cells are deficient in activity

TABLE 1

DRUGS AND OTHER AGENTS THAT CAN CAUSE CLINICALLY SIGNIFICANT HEMOLYSIS IN G–6–PD–DEFICIENT PEOPLE

Acetanilid: 3.6 g	Nitrofurazone (Furacin): 1.5 g (C)
Phenylhydrazine: 30 mg	Nitrofurantoin (Furadantin): 400 mg
Sulfanilamide: 3.6 g	Furazolidone: 400 mg
Sulfacetamide	Furaltodone (Altofur): 1.0 g
Sulfapyridine: 4.0 g	Quinidine: 0.8 g (C)
Sulfamethoxypyridazine (Kynex): 2.0 g	Primaquine: 30 mg
Salicylazosulfapyridine (Azulfidine): 6.8 g	Pamaquine: 30 mg
Thiazolsulfone	Pentaquine
Diaminodiphenylsulfone: 200 mg	Quinocide: 30 mg
Trinitrotoluene (C)	Naphthalene
	Neosalvarsan: 600 mg
	Fava Beans

(C): Hemolysis observed principally in Caucasians.

of G-6-PD. The hemolytic potential of some drugs has been demonstrated by administration of these drugs to volunteers whose red cells are G-6-PD-deficient or who have received Cr^{51} labeled, G-6-PD-deficient cells. For some drugs in TABLE 1, however, the evidence stems only from hemolytic reactions observed in patients receiving the drugs.[13] In such instances, uncertainty sometimes exists whether the reaction entirely is attributable to the drug. For example, an acute hemolytic anemia has been observed occasionally when Caucasian G-6-PD-deficient subjects have received chloramphenicol. But this drug is used for the treatment of an infection, sometimes in combination with other drugs. For some drugs given to G-6-PD-deficient patients, the dosage may be important in determining whether or not severe hemolysis occurs. When G-6-PD deficiency may be present, attention to dosage seems particularly appropriate for sulfisoxazole (Gantrisin), for aspirin given to Caucasians, and for vitamin K given to newborn infants.[13]

Heterogeneity of G-6-PD Abnormalities

TABLE 1 designates several agents as probably causing hemolytic reaction more readily among G-6-PD-deficient Caucasians than among G-6-PD-deficient Negroes. Moreover, as determined by both clinical assessment and survival of labeled red cells, the severity and duration of hemolytic reaction seems greater among some G-6-PD-deficient Caucasians than among G-6-PD-deficient Negroes.[14,15] An even more obvious example of clinical heterogeneity of G-6-PD abnormalities is represented by the types of G-6-PD deficiency that are accompanied by congenital nonspherocytic hemolytic disease (CNHD). Such subjects, even without apparent exposure to drugs or toxic substances, have reticulocytosis and greatly shortened red cell survivals. They often have anemia. Additional evidence for heterogeneity of G-6-PD deficiency came from studies of Ramot, *et al.*[16] and of Marks and Gross,[17] who found the white cells of G-6-PD- deficient Mediterranean, Caucasian subjects to have a much greater deficiency of G-6-PD activity than white cells of G-6-PD-deficient Negroes.

Although some subjects have less than 1 percent of normal activity of G-6-PD, the enzyme is seldom so deficient as to prohibit isolation and characterization of the enzyme. The greatest amount of information on heterogeneity of G-6-PD abnormalities has come from such studies on the partially purified or highly purified enzyme (TABLE 2). Each 500 ml portion of normal human blood, however, contains only a few milligrams of G-6-PD. This limitation makes necessary large volumes of blood and over 20,000-fold purifications for the isolation of pure G-6-PD. Despite these handicaps, Yoshida has succeeded in obtaining peptide maps on normal G-6-PD (G-6-PD B) and G-6-PD A, a prevalent electrophoretic variant among American Negroes. He found a substitution of aspartic acid for asparagine, at a single amino acid residue of G-6-PD A.[18] Methods for obtaining the enzyme in comparable purity and amounts from G-6-PD-deficient subjects, however, have not been devised. Many of the characteristics shown in TABLE 2 have been obtained only with partially purified enzyme. Nevertheless, where family studies have been possible, the abnormal properties of the enzyme have followed the expected X-linked pattern of inheritance. The more prevalent variants of G-6-PD tend to be found among people whose ancestors lived in one of the tropical or semi-tropical areas of the Eastern Hemisphere (FIGURE 2).[13,19] G-6-PD deficiency occurs in much of Central and Western Africa and to a lesser extent in Southern Africa. Among Nigerian and North and South American Negroes, the enzyme of these deficient subjects has the phenotype G-6-PD A^-. Twelve

TABLE 2

VARIANTS OF HUMAN RED CELL G–6–PD

Variant[13]	Population	RBC activity, % of normal	Electrophoretic mobility % of normal	Km G-6-P μM	Km NADP μM	2dG-6-P utilization %	Thermo-stability	pH optima
			Common variants, in order of diminishing activity					
Normal B	All	(100)	(100)	50–78	2.9–4.4	< 4	(normal)	truncate
A	Negro	88	110	normal	normal	< 4	normal	truncate
Athens[30]	Greek	25	98	16–19	2.5–6.5	10–15	slightly increased	mildly biphasic
A⁻	Negro	8–20	110	normal	normal	< 4	normal	truncate
Canton	Cantonese	4–24	104–108	20–36	2.0–2.4	4–15	slightly reduced	mildly biphasic
Mediterranean	Greek, Sardinians, Sephardic Jews, Asiatic NW Indians	0–7	100	19–26	1.2–1.6	23–37	reduced	biphasic
			Uncommon variants, without apparent congenital nonspherocytic hemolytic disease					
"Madison"	Norwegian	100	70 (TEB) 90 (TRIS)	?	?	?	?	?
Baltimore-Austin	Negro	75	90 (TRIS)	68	3.1	< 4	normal	truncate
Ibaden-Austin	Negro	72	80	62–72	3.3	< 4	normal	truncate
Barbieri	Italian	40–50	135	increased	increased	?	normal	?

TABLE 2 (Continued)

Variant[13]	Population	RBC activity, % of normal	Electrophoretic mobility % of normal	Km G-6-P μM	Km NADP μM	2dG-6-P utilization %	Thermo-stability	pH optima
Uncommon variants, without apparent congenital nonspherocytic hemolytic disease								
Kerala	Asiatic SE Indian	50	75 (TEB) 90 (TRIS)	23	1.5	7.4	normal	mildly biphasic
Tel Hashomer	Tunisian Jew	25–40	60–70	30–40	?	normal	normal	mildly biphasic
Columbus	Negro	35	100	normal	normal	normal	?	?
Seattle	Welsh-Scottish ? Greek	8–21	90	15–25	2.4–2.8	7–11	normal	mildly biphasic
West Bengal	Asiatic Indian	9	90–94	31	6.6	4	normal	truncate
Markham[19]	New Guinea	1.5–10	105–108	4.4–6.3	?	162–222	?	very biphasic
Uncommon variants, with congenital nonspherocytic hemolytic disease								
Chicago	Western Europe	9–26	100	58–76	3.1–3.7	< 4	greatly reduced	truncate
Oklahoma	Western Europe	4–10	100	127–200	20	< 4	reduced	narrow peak
Ohio	Italian	2–16	110	slightly increased	slightly increased	normal	greatly reduced	?
Milwaukee[31]	Puerto Rico	0–4	90	224	?	< 4	?	narrow peak

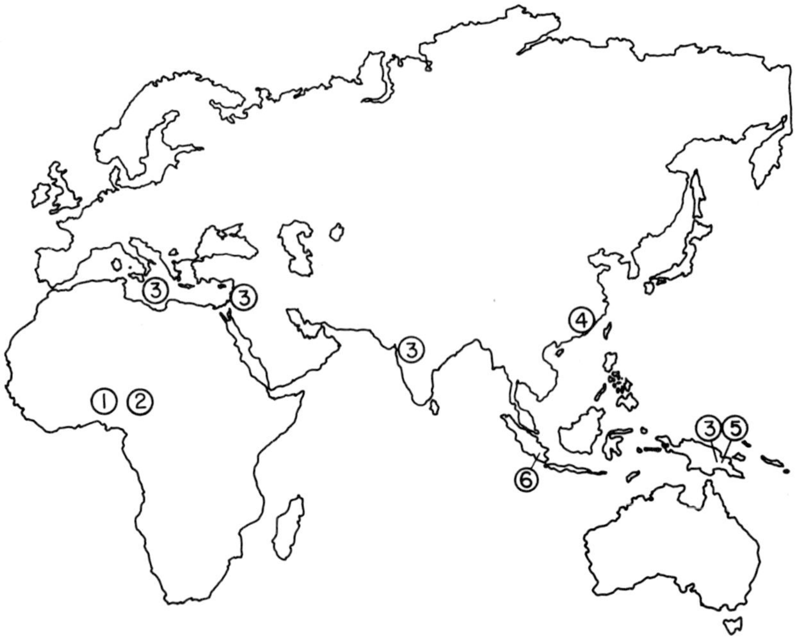

FIGURE 2. World distribution of relatively common variants of G–6–PD: (1) A, (2) A^-, (3) Mediterranean, (4) Canton, (5) Markham, (6) Indonesian. In Greece, other relatively common variants probably exist, as well as (3).

percent of North American Negro males have this type of G-6-PD. Another 22 percent of American Negro males have an electrophoretically similar but chromatographically distinguishable G-6-PD A.[13] This variant also may be present in Negroes from large areas of Africa. G-6-PD Mediterranean is distinguishable from the previously mentioned variants by many characteristics. Phenotypically identical forms of G-6-PD Mediterranean occur in Sardinia, Greece, Israel, Western India, and New Guinea. It may also be present in Turkey and Egypt. Other relatively common variants with distinctive properties are present among people from Canton and New Guinea.[19] In studies now in progress and in collaboration with Dr. L. I. Eng, the author finds another variant of G-6-PD, among G-6-PD-deficient males from Indonesia.

G-6-PD abnormalities may be classified into three very general clinical groups, those in which the abnormality results in : a) no symptoms, b) drug sensitivity without chronic reticulocytosis, and c) CNHD. Of the variants shown in TABLE 2, those in which the red cell activity is greater than 30 percent of normal generally are unaccompanied by hemolytic problems. Below this range of activity, however, only a poor correlation is found between the level of red cell G-6-PD and the severity or persistence of any accompanying hemolytic anemia.

G-6-PD Mediterranean subjects have red cell activities similar to those of two CNHD variants, yet have neither the persistent reticulocytosis nor recurrent anemia of the latter subjects (TABLE 3). Conversely, CNHD subjects with enzymic phenotype G-6-PD Chicago have red cell activities in the range of males with G-6-PD A^-, Canton, and Seattle, in whom chronic hemolytic disease

TABLE 3

SOME COMPARATIVE CHARACTERISTICS OF G–6–PD VARIANTS

G–6–PD Variant[13]	Relative Hemolysate Activity (%)	Relative V_{max} (%) / Km G–6–P (μM)	Thermostability In Vitro
	Not susceptible to drug-induced hemolytic anemia		
B	100	1.61	Normal
A	88	1.42	Normal
	Susceptible to drug-induced hemolytic anemia		
A^-	14	0.23	Normal
Canton	15	0.44	Slightly reduced
Mediterranean	3.0	0.12	Reduced
	Congenital non-spherocytic hemolytic disease		
Chicago	14	0.21	Greatly reduced
Oklahoma	4.4	0.031	Reduced
Ohio	2.7	0.029	Greatly reduced
Milwaukee[31]	0.5	0.003	?
	Others		
Seattle	13	0.53	Normal
Markham[19]	2.6	0.44	?

is not apparent. Little is known about the hemolytic propensity of subjects with G-6-PD Markham, but the hematocrit of their blood samples and the presence of this variant among clinically unselected subjects in New Guinea suggest that CNHD is unlikely. As with the G-6-PD Mediterranean subjects, however, these men have unusually low levels of activity of red cell G-6-PD. When consideration is given only to these activities, the discrepancies seem almost severe enough to raise doubt that G-6-PD could be the primary defect in these hemolytic problems. A realistic appraisal of enzyme function within human red cells, however, requires serious consideration of at least two other enzymic properties.

Michaelis-Menten Relationships

As with many enzymes, measurements of activity of G-6-PD are usually performed with concentrations of substrate far in excess of those occurring within the red blood cell. The use of high substrate concentrations in enzymic assays assures more nearly maximal and constant reaction rates, but the results may be misleading. This is especially a problem when intracellular concentrations of substrate fall close to, or below, the Michaelis constant (Km). Although in most instances the intracellular concentration of NADP exceeds the Km for NADP, the intracellular concentrations of G-6-P[20] can fall below the Km for that substrate. Genetically determined differences in Km among some variants of human red cell G-6-PD are as great as ten-fold. Failure to take these differences into consideration may result in an unrealistic estimate of relative activity. Thus, with a conventional assay, hemolysates of G-6-PD Oklahoma subjects have greater activity than those of G-6-PD Mediterranean subjects. Because of differences in Km, however, the opposite relationship would seem to exist at physiological concentrations of G-6-P (FIGURE 3). Although assays at

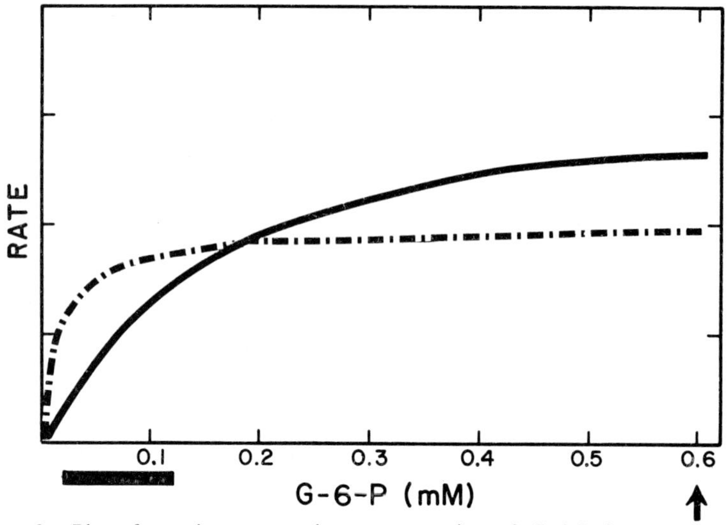

FIGURE 3. Plot of reaction rate against concentration of G–6–P for an enzyme with: (solid line) Km of 140 μM (G–6–PD Oklahoma), and (broken line) Km of 18 μM (G–6–PD Mediterranean). The curves have been constructed so that the relative rates at standard assay concentrations of G–6–P (arrow) are proportional to specific activities of hemolysates of the two variants. Solid bar: range of intracellular concentration of G–6–P.

G-6-P concentrations of 0.6 mM provide rates close to those of maximal velocity (V_{max}), rates at low substrate concentrations are more nearly proportional to the ratio V_{max}/Km. It may be significant that some of the previously mentioned discrepancies disappear when consideration is given to this ratio (TABLE 3).

Fincham and coworkers have reported that some mutants for glutamic dehydrogenase behave as though deficient in activity of this enzyme, despite nearly normal activity in assays carried out with high concentrations of substrate.[21] Similarly, Tedesco and Mellman measured argininosuccinate synthetase activity in lysates of cells cultured from normal subjects and from patients with citrullinemia At high concentrations of substrate the activities with citrullinemic and normal lysates were similar, but at lower concentrations of substrate a serious deficiency in the enzyme activity became apparent with citrullinemic lysates.[22]

Intracellular Stability of G-6-PD

Peculiar to the mammalian red cell is the cessation of protein synthesis very early in the life of the cell. Because of this condition, mere synthesis of an enzyme is not sufficient to insure its presence in the mature red cell: the enzyme must remain active during the several months of survival of each human red cell. In 1958, Marks and coworkers used a technique of differential osmotic shock to obtain hemolysates from red cells of different ages. Levels of G-6-PD of normal cells were found to fall moderately as the red cell aged.[23] More recently, other workers have found a moderate decay in activities of other enzymes of the aging, normal red blood cell. Marks has offered evidence that the decay in activity of G-6-PD from G-6-PD-deficient Negro males (G-6-PD A^-) is faster than normal.[17,24] Using another method of separating red cells by age, Powell, *et al.*, expanded these observations on red cells with normal G-6-PD and G-6-PD A$^-$.[25] Similar conclusions have been reached by Yoshida, Stamatoyannopoulos, and Motulsky[26] and, more recently, by Kirkman and Kennedy,[19] using mixtures of phthalate esters to fractionate red cells by the method of Danon and Marikovsky.[27] The abnormally rapid intracellular decay of G-6-PD A$^-$ has also been found recently by Piomelli and coworkers, who have used a gradient centrifugation method of separating red cells by age (Personal communication).

These findings illustrate how estimates of enzymic activity of unfractionated red cells fail to reflect how rapidly the activity of an enzyme may decay with age, or how low the activity of an enzyme may be in the very oldest red cells. This is especially true if survival of the red cell is limited by very low levels of activity of an enzyme. In FIGURE 4 are represented the decay curves for two hypothetical variants of a red cell enzyme. The activity of one enzyme has decayed so rapidly as to shorten red cell survival, yet the activity of this enzyme in an unfractionated sample of red cells would actually appear to be higher than that of the red cells having an enzyme variant with a more gradual rate of decay of activity. This is a consequence of the fact that the geometric mean of the first curve exceeds that of the second. For simplicity, the decay rates were assumed to be exponential and the proportion of red cells of each age was considered to be uniform up until the time of destruction at a critical age. Alternate models can be used, however, to illustrate the same conclusion, that a correlation may not exist between the activity of G-6-PD in unfractionated red cells and the severity of deficiency of G-6-PD in the very oldest cells.

Information is now available on the thermostability of a number of G-6-PD variants in vitro. With partially purified preparations, such assessment of ther-

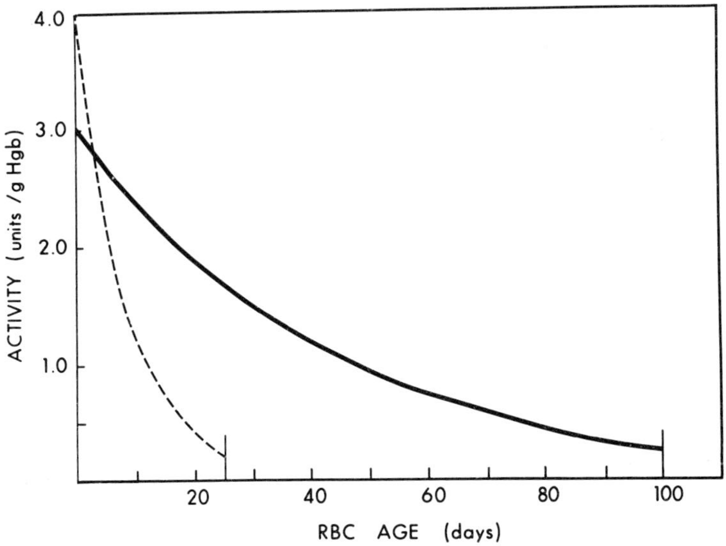

FIGURE 4. Curves depicting decay of red cell enzyme activity with red cell age, for two hypothetical variants.

mostability requires several precautions, including observations of mixed solutions of enzyme,[19] before the comparative thermostability or thermolability can be regarded as an intrinsic property of the enzyme. The thermostabilities listed in TABLE 3, for example, were determined in the author's laboratory by the same method. (A sample of Ohio-like G-6-PD, from the study of Grossman, *et al.*,[28] was kindly provided by Dr. F. E. Trobaugh.) Even with these precautions, however, large differences in thermostability can be demonstrated among G-6-PD variants. Further studies will be necessary for a determination of whether or not a consistent association exists between these thermostabilities and stability in vivo, but an association is already emerging between thermostability and manifestations, in that the variants with greatly reduced thermostability are among those giving rise to severe hemolytic disease.

Such observations on stability of G-6-PD variants, and particularly on stability in vivo, have helped to explain two puzzling features of G-6-PD A^- subjects. Their white cells have nearly normal activity for G-6-PD, yet the enzyme from their white cells has the same electrophoretic abnormality as the G-6-PD from their red cells. Presumably, the enzyme in the two types of cells is the same. Because the deficiency in red cells can be attributed to the lability of G-6-PD A^- in vivo, the white cells may be spared from this deficiency by the continuing synthesis of protein within white cells. A second puzzling feature of G-6-PD A^- subjects is the self-limited course of hemolysis which occurs even when the subject remains on primaquine for many weeks. This finding was shown earlier to be attributable to the fact that only the older red cells in a G-6-PD A^- subjects circulation were susceptible to hemolysis.[29] This phenomenon, in turn, can now be understood as being a possible consequence of the much lower levels of G-6-PD in older G-6-PD A^- red cells.

Summary

Various hemolytic disorders are associated with deficiencies in activity of human red cell glucose-6-phosphate dehydrogenase (G-6-PD). Among the many phenotypically distinct variants of G-6-PD, however, only a poor correlation is noted between the severity of the deficiency and the severity or duration of clinical manifestations. Better correlation may be seen when consideration is also given to Michaelis constants and to stability of the enzyme. In man, as in other species, Michaelis constants may be subject to such severe genetic alteration as to render obsolete the exclusive use of high concentrations of substrate in standard assays for enzymic activity. For the human red cell, consideration of thermostability and, especially, of stability in vivo of an enzyme is also necessary if the results of a standard assay for activity are not to be misleading. In the mature red cell, which has lost the ability to synthesize protein, the level of activity of a labile enzyme may be far lower in the older red cells than is reflected by the activity in an unselected population of red cells.

References

1. Carson, P. E. 1968. Hemolysis due to inherited erythrocyte enzyme deficiencies. This Annal.
2. Fraser, I. M. & E. S. Vesell. 1968. Effects of drugs and drug metabolites on erythrocytes from normal and glucose-6-phosphate dehydrogenase-deficient individuals. This Annal.

3. DERN, R. J., I. M. WEINSTEIN, G. V. LEROY, D. W. TALMAGE & A. S. ALVING. 1954. The hemolytic effect of primaquine. I. The localization of the drug-induced hemolytic defect in primaquine-sensitive individuals. J. Lab. Clin. Med. **43:** 303–309.

4. FLANAGAN, C. L., E. BEUTLER, R. J. DERN & A. S. ALVING. 1955. Biochemical changes in erythrocytes during hemolysis induced by aniline derivatives. J. Lab. Clin. Med. **46:** 814.

5. BEUTLER, E. 1957. The glutathione instability of drug-sensitive red cells. A new method for the in vitro detection of drug sensitivity. J. Lab. Clin. Med. **49:** 84–95.

6. CHILDS, B., W. ZINKHAM, E. A. BROWN, E. L. KIMBRO & J. V. TORBET. 1958. A genetic study of a defect in glutathione metabolism of the erythrocyte. Bull. Johns Hopkins Hosp. **102:** 21–37.

7. GROSS, R. T., R. E. HURWITZ & P. E. MARKS. 1958. An hereditary enzymatic defect in erythrocyte metabolism: glucose-6-phosphate dehydrogenase deficiency. J. Clin. Invest. **37:** 1176–1184.

8. SZEINBERG, A., C. SHEBA & A. ADAM. 1958. Enzymatic abnormality in erythrocytes of a population sensitive to *Vicia faba* or hemolytic anemia induced by drugs. Nature **181:** 1256.

9. KOSOWER, N. S., G. A. VANDERHOFF & I. M. LONDON. 1967. The regeneration of reduced glutathione in normal and glucose-6-phosphate dehydrogenase deficient human red blood cells. Blood **29:** 313–319.

10. CARSON, P. E., C. L. FLANAGAN, C. E. ICKES & A. S. ALVING. 1956. Enzymatic deficiency in primaquine sensitive erythrocytes. Science **124:** 484–485.

11. OORT, M., J. H. LOOS & H. K. PRINS. 1961. Hereditary absence of reduced glutathione in erythrocytes – a new clinical and biochemical entity? Vox Sanguinis **6:** 370–373.

12. LOEHR, G. W. & H. D. WALLER. 1962. Eine neue enzymopenische haemolytische Anaemie mit Glutathionreduktase- Mangel. Med. Klin. **57:** 1521–1525.

13. WORLD HEALTH ORGANIZATION SCIENTIFIC GROUP. 1967. Standardization of Procedures for the Study of Glucose-6-Phosphate Dehydrogenase. Wld. Hlth. Org. Techn. Report Ser. : 366.

14. GEORGE, J. N., D. A. SEARS, P. R. MCCURDY & M. E. CONRAD. 1967. Primaquine sensitivity in Caucasians: hemolytic reactions induced by primaquine in G–6–PD deficient subjects. J. Lab. Clin. Med. **70:** 80–93.

15. PANNACCIULLI, I., A. TIZIANELLO, F. AJMAR & E. SALVIDIO. 1965. The course of experimentally induced hemolytic anemia in a primaquine-sensitive Caucasian. A case study. Blood **25:** 92–95.

16. RAMOT, B., S. FISHER, A. SZEINBERG, A. ADAM, C. SHEBA & D. GAFNI. 1959. A study of subjects with erythrocytic glucose-6-phosphate dehydrogenase deficiency. II. Investigation of leukocytic enzymes. J. Clin. Invest. **38:** 2234–2237.

17. MARKS, P. A. & R. T. GROSS. 1959. Erythrocytic glucose-6-phosphate dehydrogenase deficiency: Evidence of differences between Negroes and Caucasians with respect to this genetically determined trait. J. Clin. Invest. **38:** 2253–2262.

18. YOSHIDA, A. 1967. A single amino acid substitution (asparagine to aspartic acid) between normal (B+) and the common Negro variant (A+) of human glucose-6-phosphate dehydrogenase. Proc. Natl. Acad. Sci. **57:** 835–840.

19. KIRKMAN, H. N., C. KIDSON & M. KENNEDY. 1968. Variants of human glucose-6-phosphate dehydrogenase. Studies of samples from New Guinea. *In* Hereditary Disorders of Erythrocyte Metabolism. E. Beutler, Ed. Grune & Stratton, Inc. N. Y. In press.

20. ROSE, I. A. & E. L. O'CONNELL. 1964. The role of glucose-6-phosphate in the regulation of glucose metabolism in human erythrocytes. J. Biol. Chem. **239:** 12–17.

21. FINCHAM, J. R. S. 1962. Genetically determined multiple forms of glutamic dehydrogenase in *Neurospora crassa*. J. Mol. Biol. **4:** 257–274.

22. TEDESCO, T. A. & W. J. MELLMAN. 1967. Argininosuccinate synthetase activity and citrulline metabolism in cells cultured from a citrullinemic subject. Proc. Natl. Acad. Sci. **57:** 829–834.

23. MARKS, P. A., A. B. JOHNSON, E. HIRSCHBERG & J. BANKS. 1958. Studies on the mechanism of aging of human red blood cells. Ann. N. Y. Acad. Sci. **75:** 85–105.

24. MARKS, P. A. 1961. (Discussion) Molecular Genetics and Human Disease. L. I. Gardner, Ed. 121–126. Charles C. Thomas, Springfield, Ill.

25. POWELL, R. D., G. J. BREWER, R. L. DEGOWIN & P. E. CARSON. 1966. Effects of glucose-6-phosphate dehydrogenase deficiency upon the host and upon host-drug-malaria parasite interactions. Military Med. **131:** 1039–1056.

26. YOSHIDA, A., G. STAMATOYANNOPOULOS & A. G. MOTULSKY. 1967. Negro variant of glucose-6-phosphate dehydrogenase deficiency (A^-) in man. Science **155:** 97–99.

27. DANON, D. & Y. MARIKOVSKY. 1964. Determination of density distribution of red cell population. J. Lab. Clin. Med. **64**: 668–674.
28. GROSSMAN, A., K. RAMANATHAN, P. JUSTICE, J. GORDON, N. T. SHAHIDI & D. Y. HSIA. 1966. Congenital nonspherocytic hemolytic anemia associated with erythrocyte glucose-6-phosphate dehydrogenase deficiency in a Negro family. Pediatrics **37**: 624–629.
29. DERN, R. J., E. BEUTLER & A. S. ALVING. 1954. The hemolytic effect of primaquine. II. The natural course of the hemolytic anemia and the mechanism of its self limited character. J. Lab. Clin. Med. **44**: 171–176.
30. STAMATOYANNOPOULOS, G., A. YOSHIDA, C. BACOPOULOS & A. G. MOTULSKY. 1967. Athens variant of glucose-6-phosphate dehydrogenase. Science **157**: 831–833.
31. WESTRING, D. W. & A. V. PISCIOTTA. 1966. Anemia, cataracts, and seizures in a patient with glucose-6-phosphate dehydrogenase deficiency. Arch. Int. Med. **118**: 385–390.

HEMOLYSIS DUE TO INHERITED ERYTHROCYTE ENZYME DEFICIENCIES

Paul E. Carson

Department of Medicine and the Section on Genetics and International Health
University of Chicago, Chicago, Ill.

The term, pharmacogenetics, is especially apt when applied to the development of our knowledge of the inherited erythrocyte enzyme deficiencies which result in increased hemolytic susceptibility. We discovered glucose-6-phosphate dehydrogenase (G6PD) deficiency in this context as part of the study of primaquine-induced hemolysis.[1,2] Subsequently, several genetically determined erythrocytic deficiencies have been reported in association with increased hemolytic susceptibility and representative examples are given in TABLE 1.[3–12] The discovery of additional deficiencies is readily predictable. The division into two groups shown in TABLE 1 is a clinical rather than a biochemical distinction, although as indicated both in the Table and in FIGURE 1, showing the biochemical relationships, the groups naturally fall into disorders of the pentose phosphate pathway as opposed to those of the glycolytic pathway. Normally, the pentose phosphate pathway is relatively inactive and hexokinase deficiency would be expected, therefore, to present like other deficiencies of the glycolytic pathway. Although glutathione (GSH) is not an enzyme, its deficiency is considered to be an enzymatic defect of synthesis.

The clinical distinction between the two groups arises from the following considerations. All of the deficiencies so far reported for enzymes of the glycolytic pathway have, to the best of my knowledge, been sought for and found in patients with chronic nonspherocytic hemolytic anemia. Furthermore, there is apparently no evidence that deficiencies of the glycolytic pathway result in increased susceptibility to drug-induced hemolysis, and, whether these deficiencies can occur without spontaneous hemolytic anemia is questionable. Certainly if a genetic defect in the glycolytic pathway were to be found in an individual without clinical evidence of hematological abnormality, testing the blood from this subject for increased hemolytic susceptibility to pharmacological agents would be very important.

On the other hand, with the possible exception of glutathione deficiency, the elements of the oxidative reactions of the pentose phosphate pathway can be deficient in individuals who do not have clinically evident hematological abnormality. In G6PD deficiency this is the rule rather than the exception. In these individuals the increased hemolytic susceptibility is revealed even during health by ingestion of agents such as primaquine, various other drugs, or fava beans.[2] From the pharmacological point of view we can say, therefore, that most of the results of the last few years which might appropriately be discussed in this monograph have been found in the conditions associated with defects of the pentose phosphate pathway rather than those of the glycolytic pathway and the remainder of this paper will be devoted primarily to the pentose phosphate pathway.

Until recently the inclusion of 6-phosphogluconic dehydrogenase (6PGD) deficiency in the list of those susceptible to primaquine-induced hemolysis was tentative. In the case reported by Dern, *et al.*[13] only partial deficiency was found and the patient was also heterozygous for G6PD deficiency. We have now had an opportunity, however, to test the hemolytic susceptibility of blood from the

TABLE 1

GENETIC DEFICIENCIES OF GLUCOSE CATABOLISM ASSOCIATED WITH HEMOLYSIS

Pentose Phosphate Pathway	Glycolytic Pathway
Glucose-6-phosphate Dehydrogenase[1]	Hexokinase[8]
Glutathione reductase [3,4]	Triose isomerase[9]
Glutathione[5]	Glyceraldehyde-3-phosphate Dehydrogenase[10]
6-Phosphogluconic Dehydrogenase[6,7]	2-3 Diphosphoglyceromutase[11]
	Pyruvate kinase[12]

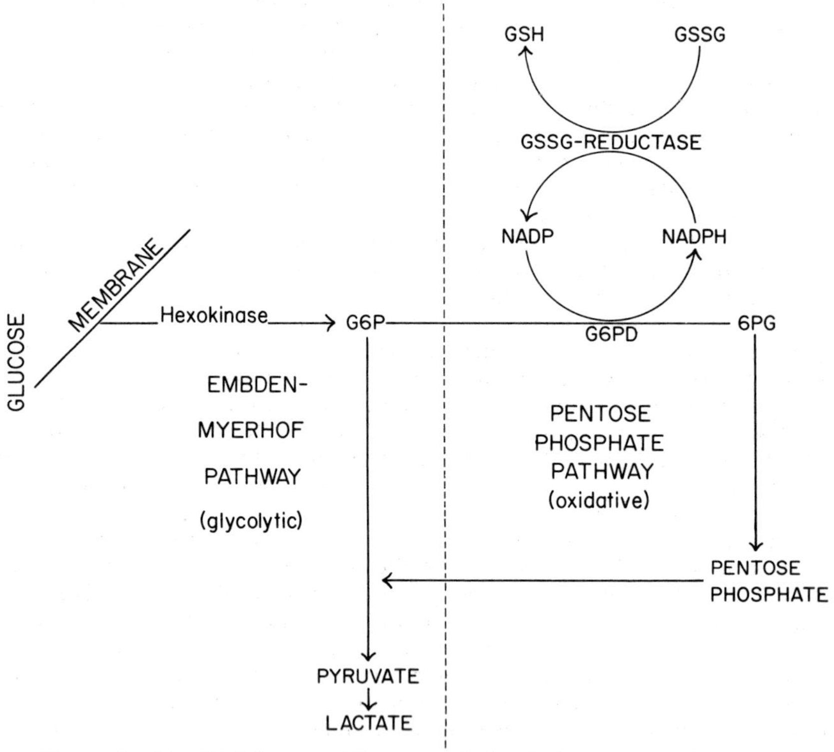

FIGURE 1. Simplified diagram of glucose catabolism in the human erythrocyte.

individual with virtually complete 6PGD deficiency discovered by Parr in London.[2,6] With his and Turnbull's cooperation blood obtained from this patient, who has no clinically evident hematological abnormality, was sent to us, labeled with Cr^{51} and given to two compatible recipients, one of whom received 30 mg of primaquine base daily, and the other who received no drug. In the recipient who received primaquine, the half-life of the erythrocytes of this blood was reduced to 14 days, from a normal of well over 20 days. The control recipient unfortunately had a typical minor incompatibility reaction after 14 days. However, the extrapolation of his previously normal curve indicated an expected half-life of well over 20 days. These results indicate that 6PGD deficiency also can exist without evident clinical hematological abnormality but with increased hemolytic susceptibility to primaquine. The hemolysis induced, incidentally, was comparable to the hemolysis observed in individuals with intermediate erythrocytic G6PD levels, i.e., it was not as severe as in individuals with fully expressed G6PD deficiency.[14]

This discussion would be incomplete without a brief review of the typical picture of primaquine-induced hemolysis. For this purpose I have chosen to describe some of the results we have obtained recently with the use of diaminodiphenylsulfone (DDS), a substance which has a primaquine-like hemolytic effect in G6PD deficient individuals, but unlike primaquine causes hemolysis in nondeficient normal individuals. The testing of DDS was conducted to evaluate its potential usefulness as an antimalarial agent in the treatment of chloroquine resistant falciparum malaria. This substance has, of course, been used for many years in treatment of leprosy, is currently also being used extensively in certain dermatological disorders and is considered to have potential value for treatment of other conditions.

The data are presented in FIGURE 2 showing the hemolysis induced during the administration of 200 mg per day of DDS to a healthy Negro male G6PD deficient volunteer.[15] This hemolysis appears to be entirely analogous to the

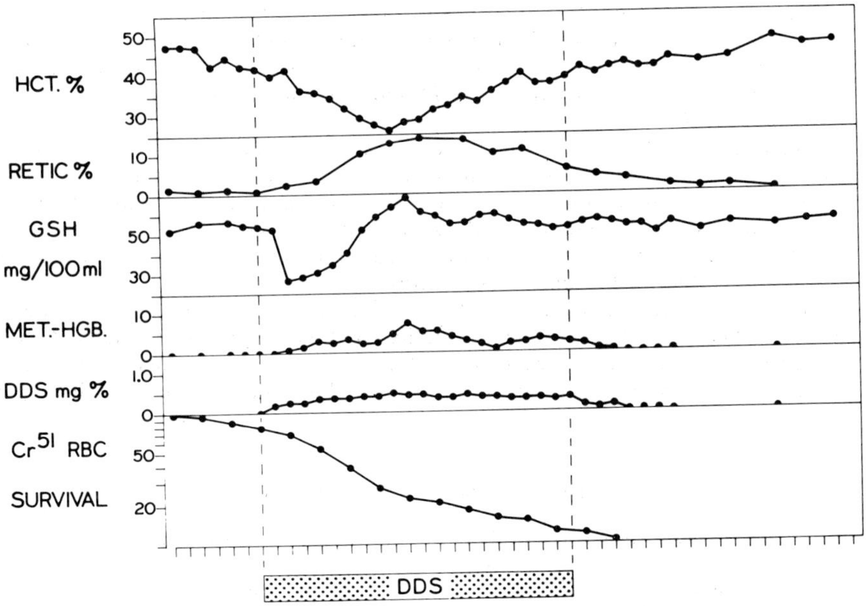

FIGURE 2. Hemolysis induced in a male Negro G-6-PD deficient volunteer during the daily administration of 200 mgm of DDS. (Reprinted by permission from Military Medicine, Supplement, Vol. 131, September 1966, Number 9.)

standard hemolysis induced by the administration of 30 mg daily of primaquine base.[2] Similar quantitative clinical investigations in Caucasian and Oriental G6PD deficient subjects are almost unavailable. There is evidence, however, that they are more susceptible to drug-induced hemolysis, as expected from lower erythrocytic and tissue assays for G6PD than in Negro subjects.[2]

The typical changes which occur in the blood glutathione are also shown in FIGURE 2.[15] A low blood glutathione was the first biochemical abnormality found in individuals then known as primaquine sensitive.[16] Subsequently, it was reported by Flanagan, *et al.*[17] that glutathione was unstable during hemolysis induced by primaquine and this is also observed during the administration of DDS. After the initial precipitous drop in the blood glutathione, a rise occurs even though drug is continued and there is an overshoot before return to baseline values. This fall, discovered during clinical testing, was taken up by Beutler into a test, in vitro, for G6PD deficiency using acetylphenylhydrazine and designated the glutathione stability test.[18]

Unlike primaquine, DDS induces hemolysis in normal as well as in G6PD deficient individuals.[15,19,20] The course of the hemolysis is, however, quite different and initially instead of a fall in GSH there is a rise beginning before the onset of measurable reticulocytosis. The hemolysis appears to be two-phased; during the second phase it becomes accelerated, the glutathione then falls below the baseline and takes several weeks to return to normal.

Although the course of the hemolysis induced by DDS differs in normal and in G6PD deficient individuals the hemolytic effect of DDS can be differentiated from its antimalarial effect. The administration of paraaminobenzoic acid blocks the antimalarial effect of DDS but does not prevent or alter the course of hemolysis induced by DDS in either normal or G6PD deficient subjects.[15] The mechanism for the hemolysis induced by DDS is not yet known and measurements of other parameters such as glutathione reductase activity have not shown any change in either normal or G6PD deficient individuals during the administration of DDS.

Data such as these have led to extensive investigations on blood in vitro in attempts to establish the relationship of glutathione to G6PD, glutathione reductase, glutathione peroxidase, methemoglobin reduction, etc. It is not my purpose to review this subject, but I would like to bring up one additional phenomenon of glutathione stability which we observed some years ago but have never reported and which still requires explanation.

Some of the consequences of G6PD deficiency for the red cell are shown in TABLE 2. When a substance such as methylene blue or phenazine methosulfate is added to buffered intact normal red cell systems containing glucose, the glucose metabolism is shunted through the normally dormant pentose phosphate path-

TABLE 2

PROPERTIES OF G6PD DEFICIENT CELLS

Intact Erythrocytes		Hemolysate	
O_2 uptake	↓	O_2 uptake	↓
CO_2 production	↓	CO_2 production	↓
Glucose utilization	↓	G-6-P utilization	↓
Methemoglobin reduction	↓	Methemoglobin reduction	↓
GSH stability	↓	GSH stability	?

way. In G6PD deficient red cells the response of this pathway is only minimally available, and compared to normal red cells oxygen uptake, CO_2 production, glucose utilization, and methemoglobin reduction via the NADPH pathway are decreased. So also is the glutathione stability. In hemolysates of red cells entirely similar results can be obtained if glucose-6-phosphate and NADP instead of glucose, are added to the system, with, however, one exception. In such systems, even though deficient in G6PD, glutathione stability remains quite steady. We do not know the explanation for this anomalous phenomenon first found by Dr. Murray Kuhr, working in our laboratory while he was still a medical student, but I believe further work on this phenomenon is warranted.[21,22]

Another set of investigations that we have pursued through several years has involved the study of stromal effects on hemolysate enzymes. Curiously, the effects found as indicated in TABLE 3 have been for G6PD,[23–25] 6PGD,[25,26] and glutathione reductase,[2,27,25,28] whereas similar experiments with some of the enzymes of the glycolytic pathway have shown no effects.[29] These stromal effects were originally found during incubation of whole hemolysates compared to the incubation of stroma-free hemolysates. The mechanisms for each of these effects are different and have considerable basic interest at the molecular level. In addition some of them, at least, appear to be significant physiologically and clinically.

The first of these effects to be found was the differential inactivation of G6PD. The mechanism for this inactivation was eventually determined to be the destruction of NADP by stromal NADPase. As already explained by Dr. Kirkman, NADP is necessary for the stability of G6PD, and its removal from this molecule by any one of several means results in its inactivation.[30]

The second effect, on 6PGD, was found originally in control systems being used in the investigation of the G6PD inactivation.[25] When both stromata and NADP were present in hemolysate incubation systems, 6PGD invariably was partially inactivated even though G6PD was simultaneously protected by the added NADP. Then it was found that the change in activity of 6PGD was accompanied by an alteration in its electrophoretic pattern, suggesting structural change in the enzyme itself.[26] Finally, in work recently completed in our laboratory by Dr. Franco Ajmar, details of which will be presented elsewhere, we have found that the effect on 6PGD also is associated with stromal NADPase, but indirectly through the action of one of the products of the reaction of stromal NADPase with NADP, phosphoadenosine-diphosphateribose (P-ADPR).[31] The steps can be symbolized as follows:

$$\text{NADP} \xrightarrow{\text{stromal NAD(P)ase}} \text{P-ADPR} \quad (1)$$

$$\text{P-ADPR} + \text{6-PGD} \longrightarrow \textit{6-PGD mod.} \quad (2)$$

where *6-PGD mod.* represents the altered enzyme.

We do not yet know the significance of this molecular phenomenon although it should be useful in the elucidation of the structure of the enzyme molecule. That this system participates in the intracellular regulation of the pentose phosphate pathway is a possibility, although we have not as yet succeeded in reversing the second reaction. Another area which should be looked into is whether release of NADPase at times of tissue injury by production of P-ADPR might be of pathological significance, especially since it has recently been described as having inhibitory effects on NADP dependent systems.[32]

The third stromal effect is an apparent activation of glutathione reductase. This effect can now be considered in a larger context of several features of gluta-

TABLE 3

STROMAL EFFECTS IN HEMOLYSATES

Present	Absent
Glucose-6-phosphate Dehydrogenase	Pyruvate kinase
6-Phosphogluconic Dehydrogenase	Glyceraldehyde-3-phosphase Dehydrogenase
Glutathione reductase	Lactic dehydrogenase

thione reductase, which when integrated, begin to clarify the role of this enzyme in human physiology. Some of these features are listed in TABLE 4, and are as follows:

1. The function of the enzyme is to reduce oxidized glutathione. In addition Scott, *et al.* have reported after partial purification of the glutathione reductase of human erythrocytes that the enzyme is also a dihydrolipoic dehydrogenase.[33] For practical purposes the reaction is stoichiometric,[34] and has even been used to determine oxidized glutathione.

2. Erythrocytic glutathione reductase does not decrease with increasing age of circulating human erythrocytes.[35,36] This is in contrast to many red cell enzymes such as G6PD[37] and pyruvate kinase[38,39] which have increased activities in reticulocytes and young cells compared to older cells. As will appear from subsequent considerations there could be a physiological release of activity of the enzyme with increasing cell age although until further evidence is obtained, a reasonable explanation is that this is a relatively more stable enzyme molecule. Alterations of erythrocytic glutathione reductase activity, therefore, like those found in several situations to be described below, are "real" rather than due to a cell age phenomenon.

3. Glutathione reductase deficiency has been reported to be associated with primaquine-induced hemolysis[2,3,25] and with chronic nonspherocytic hemolytic anemia.[4] Furthermore, in whole body studies after the injection of glucose-1-C^{14} or glucose-6-C^{14} there is a depression of the expired $C^{14}O_2$ similar to that found in G6PD deficient individuals.[25,40]

4. The erythrocytic glutathione reductase activity in G6PD deficient subjects is increased consistently compared to the values for normal subjects with remarkably little overlap.[2,25,41,42] Highly significant increases have also been found in the erythrocytic glutathione reductase activity from patients with maturity

TABLE 4

SOME FEATURES OF GLUTATHIONE REDUCTASE

(1) Function—to reduce GSSG, "irreversibly"
(2) Activity in red cells not correlated with red cell age
(3) Deficiency associated with primaquine-induced hemolysis, hemolytic anemia, and altered glucose metabolism
(4) Increased in G-6-PD deficiency, diabetes, and gout
(5) "Activated" by stromata in hemolysates of normal but not of G-6-PD deficient red cells
(6) Decreased sensitivity to inhibition by CrO_4 in G-6-PD deficient red cells
(7) "Activated," in vivo, during administration of nicotinic acid
(8) Decreased in S. E. Asian populations

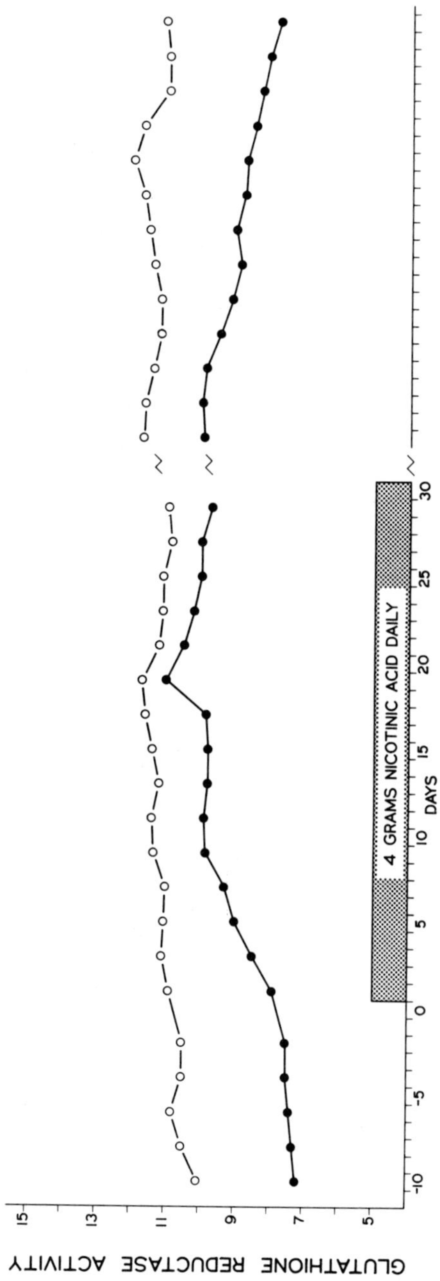

FIGURE 3. Effects of the administration of nicotinic acid on erythrocytic glutathione reductase activity.

○-○-○ G-6-PD deficient subjects.
●-●-● Non-G-6-PD deficient subjects.

onset diabetes[43] and gout,[44,45] although there is more overlap with normal values.

5. The apparent activation of glutathione reductase found during incubation of hemolysates with stromata occurs only in hemolysates from blood of non-G6PD deficient individuals. In hemolysates of blood from G6PD deficient individuals with already elevated glutathione reductase activity no increase is apparent in this experiment. Using carefully prepared hemoglobin-free stromata we can show that the stromata both of G6PD deficient and of normal red cells have the capacity to cause this apparent activation in hemolysates from normal blood, but not in hemolysates from G6PD deficient erythrocytes. This seems to indicate that the difference is intrinsic in the hemolysate and not in the stromata. Release of inhibition has not been ruled out as the mechanism for the "activation."

6. Reports from two laboratories indicate that the inhibition of erythrocytic glutathione reductase by chromate is less in G6PD deficient blood than in normal blood.[46,47] This has been suggested to be associated with the relative availability of reduced NADP.[46]

7. In studies conducted on the effect of the administration of 4 grams of nicotinic acid per day to healthy normal volunteers we have recently found, as shown in FIGURE 3, that a marked increase occurs in the erythrocytic glutathione reductase of the normal subjects but not of the G6PD deficient subjects.[48] This increase occurs without reticulocytosis or other evidence for alteration in mean cell age of the circulating erythrocytes. Furthermore, in studies for which the data will be reported elsewhere we have found that after the plateau of the increased glutathione reductase activity is reached, the hemolysates of blood from these individuals are no longer activated by incubation with stromata.[49] Of additional interest are the marked changes of carbohydrate metabolism in these individuals during the administration of nicotinic acid which include increased fasting blood glucoses and impaired glucose tolerance curves,[48,50] thus once again correlating increased erythrocytic glutathione reductase activity with altered carbohydrate metabolism.

8. Finally, as part of population studies recently undertaken in cooperation with Llewellyn J. Legters and the U.S. Army Medical Research Team (WRAIR)[51] we have measured the erythrocytic glutathione reductase activity in 255 Southeast Asians and a control group of 88 Caucasion and Negro American personnel.[52] The preliminary results are shown in TABLE 5. Several significant comparisons are apparent.

a) The non-G6PD deficient members of this population with hemoglobin AA have a significantly decreased ($p < 0.001$) erythrocytic glutathione reductase activity compared to the control subjects.

b) There is an even more pronounced depression of this enzyme activity in the subjects with hemoglobin AE or EE.

c) The hemoglobin E effect is significant within the overall Southeast Asian population, i.e., the erythrocytic glutathione reductase activity of the group with hemoglobin AE is significantly lower ($p < 0.001$) than this activity in the group with hemoglobin AA. Analyses of eight subgroups, however, revealed that in one of them this effect was not present and larger numbers will be required to definitely establish a hemoglobin E effect. (Without exception, *all* subgroups with hemoglobin AA had significantly low erythrocytic glutathione reductase activity.)

d) In marked contrast to these differences the presence of G6PD deficiency again results in elevated glutathione reductase activity regardless of hemoglobin type.

TABLE 5

POPULATION STUDY OF GLUTATHIONE REDUCTASE ACTIVITY*

Hemoglobin Type	Control	S. E. Asian Population
AA	0.87 ± 0.15 (n = 88)	0.71 ± 0.19† (n = 255)
AE		0.57 ± 0.17‡ (n = 72)
EE		0.48 ± 0.08 (n = 9)
AA (G-6-PD deficient)	1.30 ± 0.06 (n = 3)	1.18 ± 0.14 (n = 12)
AE (G-6-PD deficient)		1.18 ± 0.13 (n = 7)
EE (G-6-PD deficient)		1.12 (n = 1)

* Determined by the method of Long & Carson[43] with a final pH of 6.8–7.2. Values are referred to a final hemoglobin concentration in the cuvette of 0.105 Gms/100 ml. For conversion to I.U. multiply by approximately 10. The same batches of reagents were used for all analyses reported in this table.

† These values by Student's "t" test are highly significant compared to the control group ($p < 0.001$). The significance is unchanged if the activities are referred to numbers of cells instead of to hemoglobin.

‡ The significance of these values compared to the values for the S. E. Asian group with hemoglobin AA is also $p < 0.001$. See text for comment on subgroups, however.

Preliminary analysis of the subgroups of this population indicates that a subgroup of apparently better nutritional status than the others had the highest glutathione reductase. The values in a great many of these subjects correspond to those which are thought in this country and in Europe to result in increased hemolytic susceptibility. Whether these individuals are susceptible to primaquine-induced hemolysis, however, has not been determined. Determination of hemoglobin A_2 levels in this group was not done and the incidence of thalassemia is not yet known for these groups. If a recent report[53] suggesting that hemoglobin A_2 is increased in patients with malaria should be confirmed, the incidence of thalassemia in these areas would be difficult to ascertain and, of course, previous population studies of the incidence of thalassemia performed in malarious areas might have to be reinterpreted.

Five bloods from the Southeast Asian groups (one hemoglobin AA, three hemoglobin AE, and one hemoglobin EE, averaging 53% of the mean of the control group) were checked for stromal "activation" of glutathione reductase. All but one reached levels within the control range, two above and two below the mean (a degree of activation considerably greater than that which we have found in our normal local subjects). This suggests that the depressed erythrocytic glutathione reductase activity in these subjects is not intrinsic but may be due to an extrinsic inhibitory factor. In the G6PD deficient subjects such a factor would be absent, greatly diminished, or unavailable.

In addition to the changes in erythrocytic glutathione reductase activity which can be proven and which I have summarized, I should comment that in various bloods of hospital patients we have not infrequently found apparently significant increases of this enzyme activity. Some of these are isolated cases, none are in sufficient number or well enough controlled to establish significance but among those conditions which I believe deserve investigation are uremia, burns, and pregnancy.

Further studies of these and other population groups in various parts of the world will contribute to our understanding of the role of glutathione reductase. The full story of the role of glutathione reductase in human physiology is far from complete but the various features discussed indicate that this enzyme could play a regulatory role in carbohydrate metabolism as well as in defense against hemolysis, and also suggest that a factor or factors as yet unknown may exist which are capable in their turn of regulating this enzyme activity.

In conclusion, I have tried to present some of the pharmacogenetic aspects of enzyme deficiencies, particularly those of the pentose phosphate pathway, and to present a preliminary exploration of some of the possible relationships among them with respect not only to hemolytic susceptibility but also to carbohydrate metabolism and general physiology. Once again the value and necessity for working at molecular, cellular, clinical, and population levels in the elucidation of the meaning of these phenomena are reinforced.

Acknowledgments

This work was supported by U. S. Public Health Service Grant No. HE 06078, and by U. S. Army Contracts No. DA-49–193-MD-2413 and DA-49–007–968.

P. E. Carson is a Research and Career Development Awardee of U. S. Public Health Service.

This paper is contribution number 350 from the Army Research Program on Malaria.

References

1. Carson, P. E., C. L. Flanagan, C. E. Ickes & A. S. Alving. 1956. Enzymatic deficiency in primaquine sensitive erythrocytes. Science **124**: 484.
2. Carson, P. E. & H. Frischer. 1966. Glucose-6-phosphate dehydrogenase deficiency and related disorders of the pentose phosphate pathway. Am. J. Med. **41**: 744.
3. Carson, P. E., G. J. Brewer & C. E. Ickes. 1961. Decreased glutathione reductase with susceptibility to hemolysis. J. Lab. & Clin. Med. **58**: 840.
4. Lohr, G. W. & H. D. Waller. 1962. Eine neue enzymopenische hämolytische Anämie mit Glutathionreduktase-Mangel. Med. Klin. **36**: 1521.
5. Oort, M., J. A. Loos & H. K. Prins. 1961. Hereditary absence of reduced glutathione in the erythrocytes — a new clinical and biochemical entity. Vox Sang. **6**: 370.
6. Parr, C. W. 1966. Erythrocyte phosphogluconate dehydrogenase polymorphism. Nature **210**: 487.
7. Brewer, G. J. & R. J. Dern. 1964. A new inherited enzymatic deficiency of human erythrocytes: 6-phosphogluconate dehydrogenase deficiency. Am. J. Human Genet. **16**: 472.
8. Valentine, W. N., F. A. Oski, D. E. Paglia, M. A. Baughan, A. S. Schneider & J. L. Naiman. 1967. Hereditary hemolytic anemia with hexokinase deficiency. Role of hexokinase in erythrocyte aging. New Eng. J. Med. **276**: 1.
9. Valentine, W. N., A. S. Schneider, M. A. Baughan, D. E. Paglia & H. L. Heins, Jr. 1966. Hereditary hemolytic anemia with triosephosphate isomerase deficiency. Studies in kindreds with coexistent sickle cell trait and erythrocyte glucose-6-phosphate dehydrogenase deficiency. Am. J. Med. **41**: 27.
10. Harkness, D. R. 1966. A new erythrocytic enzyme defect with hemolytic anemia: Glyceraldehyde-3-phosphate dehydrogenase deficiency. J. Lab. & Clin. Med. **68**: 879.
11. Schröter, W. 1965. Kongenitale nichtspärocytare hämolytische Anämie bie 2,3-Diphosphoglyceratmutase-Mangel der Erythrocyten im frühen Säuglingsalter. Klin. Wchnschr. **43**: 1147.
12. Valentine, W. N., K. R. Tanaka & S. Miwa. 1961. A specific erythrocyte glycolytic enzyme defect (pyruvate kinase) in three subjects with congenital non-spherocytic hemolytic anemia. Trans. Assoc. Am. Physicians. **74**: 100.

13. Dern, R. J., G. F. Brewer, R. E. Tashian & T. B. Shows. 1966. Hereditary variation of erythrocytic 6-phosphogluconate dehydrogenase. J. Lab. & Clin. Med. **67**: 255.
14. Carson, P. E., C. Parr, A. L. Turnbull, H. Frischer & J. E. Bowman. 1967. Unpublished observations.
15. McNamara, J. V., R. B. Eppes, R. D. Powell & P. E. Carson. 1966. The effects of para-aminobenzoic acid on the hemolytic effects of 4,4′-diaminodiphenylsulfone. Military Med. **131**: 1057.
16. Beutler, E., R. J. Dern, C. L. Flanagan & A. S. Alving. 1955. The hemolytic effect of primaquine. VII. Biochemical studies of drug-sensitive erythrocytes. J. Lab. & Clin. Med. **45**: 286.
17. Flanagan, C. L., E. Beutler, R. J. Dern & A. S. Alving. 1955. Biochemical changes in erythrocytes during hemolysis induced by aniline derivatives. J. Lab. & Clin. Med. **46**: 814.
18. Beutler, E., M. Robson & E. Buttenwieser. 1957. The mechanism of glutathione destruction and protection in drug-sensitive and non-sensitive erythrocytes. *In vitro* studies. J. Clin. Invest. **36**: 617.
19. DeGowin, R. L., R. B. Eppes, R. D. Powell & P. E. Carson. 1965. Studies of sulfone-induced hemolysis. Clin. Res. **13**: 270.
20. DeGowin, R. L., R. B. Eppes, R. D. Powell & P. E. Carson. 1966. The haemolytic effects of diaphenylsulfone (DDS) in normal subjects and in those with glucose-6-phosphate-dehydrogenase deficiency. Bull. World Health Organ. **34**: 671.
21. Kuhr, M. & P. E. Carson. Unpublished data.
22. Kuhr, M. 1965. The relation of glutathione stability to G6PD deficiency. Univ. Chicago Medical Alumni Bull. **21**: 18.
23. Carson, P. E., S. L. Schrier & A. S. Alving. 1956. Inactivation of glucose-6-phosphate dehydrogenase in human erythrocytes. J. Lab. Clin. Med. **48**: 794.
24. Carson, P. E., S. L. Schrier & R. W. Kellermeyer. 1959. Glucose-6-phosphate dehydrogenase and human erythrocytes: Characteristics of glucose-6-phosphate dehydrogenase from normal and primaquine-sensitive erythrocytes. Nature **184**: 1291.
25. Carson, P. E., G. T. Okita, H. Frischer, J. Hirasa, W. K. Long & G. J. Brewer. 1963. Patterns of hemolytic susceptibility and metabolism. Proc. 9th Congr. Europ. Soc. Haemat., Lisbon : 655.
26. Carson, P. E., F. Ajmar, F. Hashimoto & J. E. Bowman. 1966. Electrophoretic demonstration of stromal effects on haemolysate glucose-6-phosphate dehydrogenase and 6-phosphogluconic dehydrogenase. Nature **210**: 813.
27. Carson, P. E., W. K. Long & C. E. Ickes. 1961. Activation of glutathione reductase (GCCGR) in hemolysates by stromata. Fed. Proc. **20**: 64.
28. Carson, P. E., B. Scharrer, B. Morgan & F. Ajmar. 1967. *In vitro* activation of glutathione reductase. J. Clin. Invest. **46**: 1044.
29. Carson, P. E. & N. Blau. Unpublished data.
30. Kirkman, H. N. 1959. Glucose-6-phosphate dehydrogenase and human erythrocytes. Nature **184**: 1291.
31. Ajmar, F., B. Scharrer, F. Hashimoto & P. Carson. 1968. Interrelation of stromal NAD(P)ase and human erythrocytic 6-phosphogluconic dehydrogenase. Proc. Natl. Acad. Sci. **59** No. 2 : 538–545.
32. Ben-Hayyim, G., A. Hochman & M. Avron. 1967. Phosphoadenosine diphosphate ribose, a specific inhibitor of nicotinamide adenine dinucleotide phosphate enzymes. J. Biol. Chem. **242**: 2837.
33. Scott, E. M., I. W. Duncan & V. Ekstrand. 1963. Purification and properties of glutathione reductase of human erythrocytes. J. Biol. Chem. **238**: 3928.
34. Carson, P. E. 1960. Glucose-6-phosphate dehydrogenase deficiency in hemolytic anemia. Fed. Proc. **19**: 995.
35. Bonsignore, A., G. Fornaini, A. Fantoni, G. Leoncini & P. Segni. 1964. Relationship between age and enzymatic activities in human erythrocytes from normal and fava bean sensitive subjects. J. Clin. Invest. **43**: 834.
36. Powell, R. D., G. J. Brewer, R. L. DeGowin & P. E. Carson. 1966. Effects of glucose-6-phosphate dehydrogenase deficiency upon the host and upon host-drug-malaria parasite interactions. Military Med. **131**: 1039.
37. Marks, P. A. & A. B. Johnson. 1958. Relationship between the age of human erythrocytes and their osmotic resistance: a basis for separating young and old erythrocytes. J. Clin. Invest. **37**: 1542.
38. Powell, R. D. & R. L. DeGowin. 1965. Relationship between activity of pyruvate kinase and age of the normal human erythrocyte. Nature **205**: 507.

39. POWELL, R. D. & R. L. DEGOWIN. 1965. Studies on the activity of pyruvate kinase in hemolysates of normal and glucose-6-phosphate dehydrogenase-deficient erythrocytes. Ann. Intern. Med. **62:** 1086.
40. CARSON, P. E. & G. T. OKITA. 1963. Metabolic patterns of hemolytic susceptibility. J. Clin. Invest. **42:** 922.
41. SCHRIER, S. L., R. W. KELLERMEYER, P. E. CARSON, C. E. ICKES & A. S. ALVING. 1958. The hemolytic effect of primaquine. IX. Enzymatic abnormalities in primaquine-sensitive erythrocytes. J. Lab. Clin. Med. **52:** 109.
42. EPPES, R. B., G. J. BREWER, R. L. DEGOWIN, J. V. MCNAMARA, C. L. FLANAGAN, S. L. SCHRIER, A. R. TARLOV, R. D. POWELL & P. E. CARSON. 1966. Oral glucose tolerance in Negro men deficient in glucose-6-phosphate dehydrogenase. New Eng. J. Med. **275:** 855.
43. LONG, W. K. & P. E. CARSON. 1961. Erythrocyte glutathione reductase activity in diabetes. Biochem. Biophys. Res. Comm. **5:** 934.
44. LONG, W. K. 1962. Red blood cell glutathione reductase in gout. Science **138:** 991.
45. LONG, W. K. 1967. Glutathione reductase in red blood cells: Variant associated with gout. Science **155:** 712.
46. KOUTRAS, G. A., A. S. SCHNEIDER, M. HATTORI & W. N. VALENTINE. 1965. Studies on chromated erythrocytes. Mechanisms of chromate inhibition of glutathione reductase. Brit. J. Haemat. **11:** 360.
47. ZURCHER, C. Doctoral Thesis. 1967. Enige Onderzoekingen Betreffende de reactie van normale en abnormale erythrocyten met chromaat. (with a summary in English) University of Amsterdam.
48. MCNAMARA, J. V., H. FRISCHER, K. H. RIECKMANN, T. A. STOCKERT, R. D. POWELL & P. E. CARSON. 1967. Increased activity of erythrocyte glutathione reductase during administration of nicotinic acid. J. Lab. Clin. Med. **70:** 989.
49. CARSON, P. E., B. MORGAN & D. DEJOHNETTE. Unpublished data.
50. STOCKERT, T., A. M. LAWRENCE, H. FRISCHER, J. V. MCNAMARA, K. H. RIECKMANN, R. D. POWELL & P. E. CARSON. Unpublished data.
51. BOWMAN, J. E., L. J. LEGTERS, P. E. CARSON, A. J. COTTINGHAM, S. C. BOONE & E. J. COLWELL. In preparation.
52. CARSON, P. E., J. E. BOWMAN, L. J. LEGTERS, A. J. COTTINGHAM, S. C. BOONE & E. J. COLWELL. In preparation.
53. ARENDS, T. 1967. High concentrations of haemoglobin A_2 in malaria patients. Nature **215:** 1517.

EFFECTS OF DRUGS AND DRUG METABOLITES ON ERYTHROCYTES FROM NORMAL AND GLUCOSE-6-PHOSPHATE DEHYDROGENASE-DEFICIENT INDIVIDUALS

Ian M. Fraser* and Elliot S. Vesell

Section on Pharmacogenetics
Laboratory of Chemical Pharmacology
National Heart Institute
Bethesda, Md.

Introduction

The preceding papers by Kirkman (1967) and Carson (1967) describe genetic, biochemical and clinical aspects of glucose-6-phosphate dehydrogenase (G-6-PD) deficiency. Attention is focused in this presentation on some pharmacological facets of the drug-induced hemolytic anemia occurring in individuals with G-6-PD deficient erythrocytes. Emphasis is placed on the role of certain drug metabolites in the hemolytic process.

The precise mechanism responsible for hemolysis in G-6-PD deficient erythrocytes remains obscure. It occurs with apparent spontaneity or following ingestion of various drugs. Oxidant effects of these compounds have been postulated (Kalow, 1962; Marks, 1964; Cohen & Hochstein, 1964, 1965; Harley, 1966; Carson & Frischer, 1966; Beutler, 1967; Aebi, 1967). Drugs causing hemolysis in vivo exhibit much lower activity in vitro. Certain metabolites of these drugs have been implicated in producing either hemolysis, increased fragility or isolated metabolic derangements in erythrocytes from man or other species. Some significant aspects of these investigations will be reviewed below.

The present study is an analysis in vitro relating a series of metabolic events to the hemolytic process. It presents the first demonstration that certain drug metabolites cause increased mechanical fragility in erythrocytes known to be G-6-PD deficient. This investigation therefore makes available a testing system in vitro for screening compounds which may exert hemolytic effects in vivo.

An early contribution by Earle *et al.* (1948) described an interesting effect of the 8-aminoquinoline, pamaquine, on human erythrocytes. A dose-related methemoglobinemia in patients receiving this drug was observed. However, pamaquine, in concentrations existing in vivo, failed to produce methemoglobinemia in vitro. Severe hemolytic reactions occurred in about 6% of Negro, but not in Caucasian, patients. A significant increase in the mechanical fragility of the erythrocytes was reported in three of ten patients of unspecified nationality who were receiving pamaquine. The greatest change occurred in a patient identified as a Negro male who developed a severe hemolytic anemia. These observations of Earle *et al.* (1948) were made before G-6-PD deficiency was discovered as the genetic defect in the majority of drug-induced hemolytic reactions. In subsequent studies on primaquine-sensitive Negro males, Beutler *et al.* (1954) reported that no significant alteration of the osmotic or mechanical fragility of the erythrocytes could be detected during a hemolytic episode produced by primaquine administration.

Brodie and Udenfriend (1950), associates of Earle, Bigelow, Zubrod and Kane in the investigation of antimalarials at Goldwater Memorial Hospital, sug-

* Present address: Dept. of Pharmacology, School of Medicine, Loma Linda University, Loma Linda, Calif.

gested that a metabolite of pamaquine was responsible for the methemoglobinemia and hemolytic effects. Brodie and Udenfriend observed that a few drops of urine or plasma from humans or dogs receiving pamaquine produced methemoglobin when added to hemolyzed cells and hemolysis when added to intact erythrocytes. Two metabolites were demonstrated. One was an unstable compound, probably a 5-hydroxy derivative, which acted by reversible conversion to quinonimine. It possessed the property of inducing methemoglobinemia and hemolysis.

Josephson *et al.* (1951a, b) isolated the 5,6-quinoline-quinone metabolite of pamaquine from tissues and droppings of treated chickens. Antimalarial and methemoglobin-producing properties of this metabolite in vitro were approximately 16-fold greater than those of pamaquine. No hemolytic activity was reported.

The metabolism of pentaquine, another 8-aminoquinoline antimalarial, has been studied in the rhesus monkey (Elderfield & Smith, 1953; Smith, 1956). The 6 methoxy group was rapidly dealkylated; 5-hydroxylation and N-dealkylation also occurred. On the basis of these studies Alving *et al.* (1962) suggested a pathway for pentaquine degradation, a modified version of which is shown in FIGURE 1, including possible N-dealkylation. Alving *et al.* (1962) suggested that the quinoline-quinone derivative was the metabolite accounting for most of the antimalarial activity and also in G-6-PD deficient individuals for the methemoglobinemia and hemolysis produced by such 8-aminoquinoline antimalarials as pamaquine, pentaquine and primaquine. However, direct experimental evidence implicating this or other metabolites in the differential effect on G-6-PD deficient and normal erythrocytes was lacking.

The metabolism of acetanilide, which also produces hemolytic reactions much more readily in G-6-PD deficient than in normal individuals (Dern *et al.*, 1955; Carson & Frischer, 1966; Beutler, 1959, 1966), has been extensively studied and several metabolites have been identified as shown in FIGURE 2 (Brodie & Axelrod, 1949; Williams, 1959; Welch *et al.*, 1966; Kiese, 1966). New aspects of the metabolism of acetanilide are described in a subsequent paper of this conference (Shahidi, 1967).

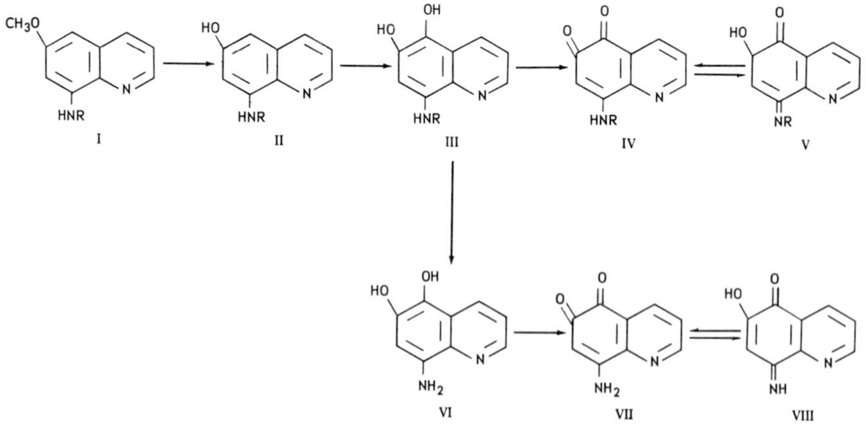

FIGURE 1. Pathways for metabolism of primaquine and related 8-aminoquinoline antimalarials (based on Elderfield & Smith, 1953; Smith, 1956; Alving *et al.*, 1962).

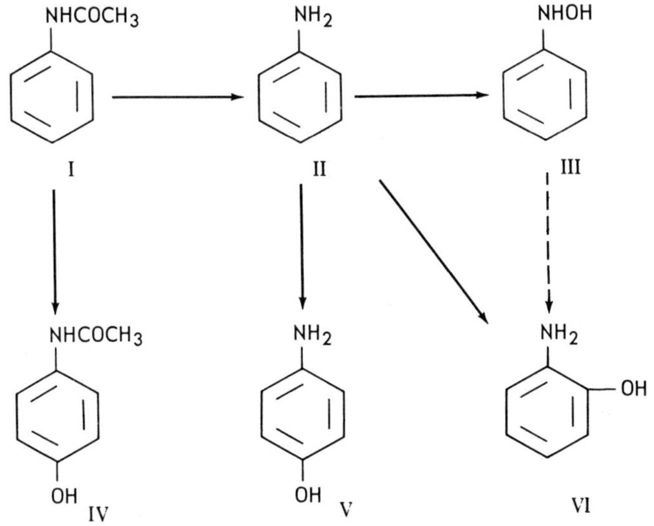

FIGURE 2. Pathways of acetanilide metabolism (based on Brodie & Axelrod, 1949; Williams, 1959; Welch *et al.*, 1966; Kiese, 1966). Solid arrows indicate better established reactions than these shown by broken arrows.

Hemolysis of G-6-PD deficient erythrocytes was not observed in vivo when small doses of p-aminophenol or larger doses of p-hydroxyacetanilide were administered (Dern *et al.*, 1955; Beutler, 1959). Shahidi and Treichel (1967) have recently reported that 2-hydroxyphenetidine, a metabolite of acetophenetidine, exhibited in vitro a selective hemolytic effect on G-6-PD deficient human erythrocytes.

In an extensive review Kiese (1966) has emphasized the importance of N-hydroxylation in producing methemoglobin-forming substances from aniline derivatives. Metabolites such as p-aminophenol formed by C-hydroxylation are also active in methemoglobin formation but in most cases are probably less potent and of less significance. Kiese (1966) formulated a scheme for an enzymatically catalyzed cyclic formation of methemoglobin in erythrocytes exposed to phenylhydroxylamine and oxygen. FIGURE 3 is a modified diagram of this mechanism. Reduction of nitrosobenzene to phenylhydroxylamine requires a supply of NADPH generated by G-6-PD. In accord with the hypothesis of Kiese (1966), red cells severely deficient in G-6-PD exhibit very little methemoglogin formation when treated with nitrosobenzene (Löhr and Waller (1961)).

Wagner *et al.* (1964) demonstrated additional effects of phenylhydroxylamine on rabbit erythrocytes. A marked decrease in the glutathione content occurred rapidly following treatment of rabbit erythrocytes with 5×10^{-4} or 5×10^{-3} M phenylhydroxylamine. Higher concentrations of phenylhydroxylamine produced hemolysis two hours after treatment under aerobic but not semi-anaerobic, conditions.

Degowin *et al.* (1966) reported that diaphenylsulfone (DDS) caused more hemolysis in G-6-PD deficient than in normal individuals. Hjelm and de Verdier (1965) showed that a metabolite of DDS in plasma rather than DDS itself was responsible for methemoglobin formation. They also observed that incubation of

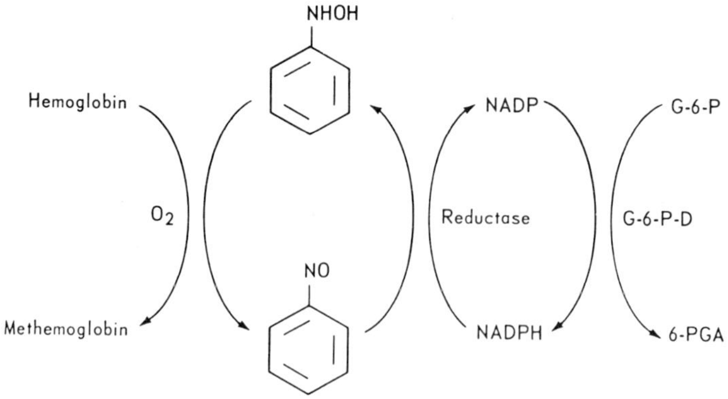

FIGURE 3. Mechanism for cyclic interconversion of nitrobenzene and phenylhydroxylamine with accompanying methemoglobin formation in erythrocytes (based on Kiese, 1966).

DDS with a rat liver microsome preparation converted DDS to a substrate capable of producing methemoglobin in cattle erythrocytes. Hjelm and de Verdier suggested that a nitroso or hydroxylamino metabolite was formed by the action of microsomal enzymes in rat liver. This hypothesis is in accord with the work of Kiese and others (Kiese, 1966; Uehleke, 1964; Debackere & Uehleke, 1964) who have shown that by both N- and C-hydroxylation, microsomal enzymes catalyze the production of methemoglobin-forming metabolites from various aniline derivatives.

Thus several types of drugs cause hemolytic reactions in G-6-PD deficient individuals by being metabolized to hydroxylated intermediates. These intermediates possess considerably greater oxidant properties than the parent compounds. The work reviewed above shows that under certain conditions these metabolites are capable of producing methemoglobin, glutathione-depletion and hemolysis in vitro and therefore parallel the effect in vivo of the parent drugs in G-6-PD deficient individuals (Beutler, 1966).

In a further endeavor to assess the mechanism of action of drug metabolites in causing hemolysis, we have studied in vitro the effect of several possible or "model" drug metabolites on a variety of parameters of red cell function. Among the parameters chosen were mechanical fragility, osmotic fragility, glutathione levels, methemoglobin formation and the NADP/NADPH ratio. The principal metabolites employed were 8-amino-5,6-quinolinediol (AQD), 5,6-dihydroxypentaquine (8-(5-isopropylaminopentylamino)-5,6-quinolinediol) (DHPQ), p-aminophenol (AP) and nitrosobenzene (NB).

We have also extended the previous work of Brodie and Udenfriend (1950) with pamaquine in a similar study with primaquine in the dog.

MATERIALS AND METHODS

Healthy adult mongrel female dogs, anesthetized with pentobarbital, were used in attempts to detect methemoglobin formation and hemolytic metabolites of primaquine in the urine. Urine was collected at hourly intervals from an indwelling catheter and tested immediately or deep-frozen for subsequent use. After several control urine specimens had been collected, primaquine phosphate dissolved in isotonic sodium chloride solution was administered i.v. over a 30 to 60 minute period. Washed canine erythrocytes were used to test for hemolytic and methemoglobin-forming metabolites in canine urine because Brodie and Udenfriend (1950) reported canine erythrocytes were more sensitive than human erythrocytes to metabolites of pamaquine. Urine collected 2 to 4 hours after the i.v. administration of primaquine phosphate (10 mg/kg) was mixed with an equal volume of a 50% suspension of washed canine erythrocytes in isotonic sodium chloride solution buffered with 0.01 M phosphate at pH 7.4 (Frankel & Reitman, 1963). The suspensions were then incubated at 37°C in a Dubnoff metabolic shaking bath. Determinations of the extent of hemolysis were made at hourly intervals.

Human blood specimens from patients at D. C. General Hospital and the N. I. H. Clinical Center were screened for G-6-PD deficiency by a modification of the method of Sass *et al.* (1966), and assayed for G-6-PD activity by a modification of the method of Bishop (1966). All G-6-PD deficient subjects were Negro. Before use in experiments in vitro the erythrocytes from fresh blood were separated by centrifugation and washed twice in isotonic sodium chloride solution buffered with 0.01 M phosphate at pH 7.4 (Frankel & Reitman, 1963). The erythrocytes were incubated for two hours at 37°C in a Dubnoff metabolic shaking bath as a 35% suspension in isotonic sodium chloride solution buffered at pH 7.4 with the addition of 10 mM glucose and various drugs or drug metabolites where indicated.

Mechanical fragility was determined by modifications of the method described in Page and Culver (1960). Alterations consisted of extension of the test period to two hours and increase of the speed to 60 rpm with a radius of rotation of 11 cm. The procedure for osmotic fragility was that described in Frankel and Reitman (1963). Glutathione was measured by the fluorometric method of Cohn and Lyle (1966) and methemoglobin by the procedure of Robin and Harley (1964). The NADP and NADPH were determined by the sensitive enzymatic recycling procedure with fluorometric assay developed by Lowry *et al.* (1961) and previously employed successfully with human erythrocytes by Gross *et al.* (1966).

Results

Hemolytic and Methemoglobin-Forming Metabolite(s) of Primaquine in the Dog

Extensive hemolysis (up to 100%) occurred when canine erythrocytes were incubated with canine urine collected between 2 and 4 hours after i.v. administration of primaquine phosphate. Figure 4 shows the results of a representative experiment. Erythrocytes incubated in urine collected prior to primaquine administration were hemolyzed much more slowly and to a lesser extent (up to 51%) than during incubation with urine collected between 2 to 4 hours after primaquine administration (Figure 4). An aliquot of the same suspension of canine erythrocytes incubated in saline instead of urine showed negligible hemolysis. Considerable methemoglobin formation was observed during the incubation of the erythrocytes with urine collected following primaquine administration. Much less methemoglobin formation was observed during the incubation with control urine. In preliminary attempts to extract and purify an active metabolite, we encountered problems of instability, reported previously by Brodie and Udenfriend (1950) in their search for metabolites of pamaquine.

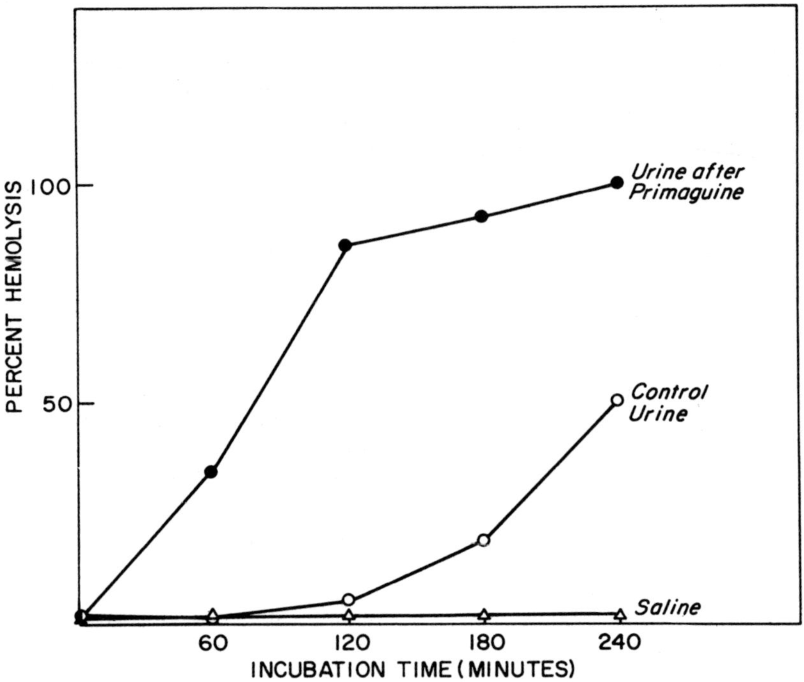

FIGURE 4. Hemolysis of canine erythrocytes incubated at 37°C in urine collected over a one hour period before (control urine) or a two to four hour period after i.v. administration of primaquine (10 mg/kg) to a dog. The incubation mixture consisted of urine and an equal volume of a 50% suspension of canine erythrocytes in 0.85% sodium chloride solution buffered with phosphate pH 7.4, 0.01 M.

Effects of Metabolites of Primaquine and Pentaquine on Normal and G-6-PD Deficient Human Erythrocytes

The effect of 8-amino-5,6-quinolinediol (AQD) on the mechanical fragility of normal and G-6-PD deficient human erythrocytes was examined initially within a range of concentrations from 10^{-4} M to 5×10^{-4} M. A small increase in fragility was detected at 10^{-4} M; the maximum increase occurred at 2.5×10^{-4} M. Accordingly, a concentration of 2.5×10^{-4} M was used in further studies with this agent and in comparing its effects to those of primaquine (PQ) and 5,6-dihydroxypentaquine (DHPQ).

TABLE 1 summarizes the alterations of mechanical fragility produced by these agents. Primaquine (PQ) did not increase the mechanical fragility either of normal or of G-6-PD deficient erythrocytes, but AQD and DHPQ did increase the mechanical fragility of both types of erythrocytes. The increase produced by AQD and DHPQ was significantly greater with G-6-PD deficient than with normal erythrocytes ($p < 0.05$). G-6-PD deficient control cells hemolyzed significantly less than normal control cells ($p < 0.01$). Therefore, a ratio of percent hemolysis in treated erythrocytes to percent hemolysis in control erythrocytes as shown in FIGURE 5 was employed in the belief that it provided a more meaningful comparison. The difference between this ratio was normal erythrocytes and for G-6-PD deficient erythrocytes was not significant for PQ ($p > 0.05$), significant

TABLE 1

EFFECTS OF PRIMAQUINE (PQ), 8-AMINO-5,6-QUINOLINEDIOL (AQD) AND 5,6-DIHYDROXYPENTAQUINE (DHPQ), EACH AT A CONCENTRATION OF 2.5×10^{-4} M, ON THE MECHANICAL FRAGILITY OF NORMAL AND G-6-PD DEFICIENT ERYTHROCYTES

Drug	Erythrocyte Type	No. of Specimens	Percent Hemolysis Control	Percent Hemolysis Treated	t-Test p-Value
PQ	Normal	11	14.7 ± 0.8	15.7 ± 1.0	< 0.025
	Deficient	12	9.6 ± 0.7	12.2 ± 0.8	< 0.001
AQD	Normal	6	13.1 ± 0.8	12.3 ± 0.8	> 0.05
	Deficient	6	9.3 ± 0.8	8.4 ± 0.7	> 0.05
DHPQ	Normal	5	13.7 ± 1.9	14.7 ± 2.2	< 0.05
	Deficient	5	9.5 ± 0.1	12.0 ± 0.5	< 0.01

for DHPQ ($p < 0.025$), and highly significant for AQD ($p < 0.001$) (FIGURE 5).

Reduced glutathione (GSH) of erythrocytes (FIGURE 6) was measured in the same experiments as those in which mechanical fragility was determined (FIGURE 5). PQ produced only a slight decrease of GSH either in normal or in G-6-PD deficient erythrocytes. AQD and DHPQ markedly decreased the GSH content of G-6-PD deficient erythrocytes but only slightly decreased that of normal erythrocytes. This difference between normal and G-6-PD deficient erythrocytes treated either with AQD or with DHPQ was highly significant ($p < 0.001$).

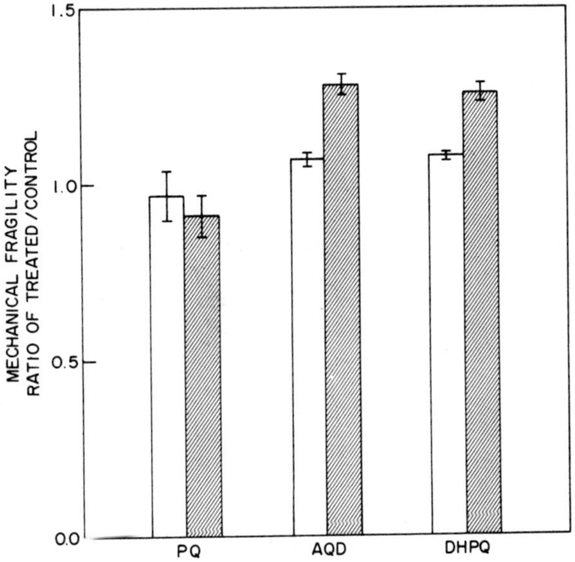

FIGURE 5. The effect of primaquine (PQ), 8 amino-5,6-quinolinediol (AQD) and 5,6-dihydroxypentaquine (DHPQ), each at a concentration of 2.5×10^{-4} M, on the mechanical fragility of normal (open bars) and G-6-PD deficient (cross-hatched bars) erythrocytes. The results are expressed as the ratio of the percent hemolysis of cells exposed to drug to the percent hemolysis of control cells. A ratio of 1.0 indicates no effect. The values shown are means from the same specimens given in TABLE 1; small vertical lines indicate the standard error of the mean. The difference between normal and deficient erythrocytes is not significant for PQ ($p > 0.05$), significant for DHPQ ($p = 0.025$) and highly significant for AQD ($p = 0.001$).

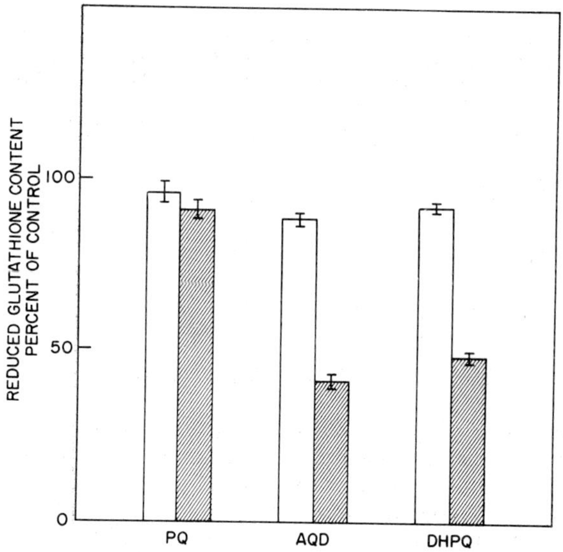

FIGURE 6. The effect of primaquine (PQ), 8-amino-5,6-quinolinediol (ADQ) and 5,6-dihydroxypentaquine (DHPQ), each at a concentration of 2.5×10^{-4} M, on the reduced glutathione content of normal (open bars) and G-6-DP deficient (cross-hatched bars) erythrocytes. Results are expressed as the percent of the reduced glutathione content of control cells. Small vertical lines indicate the standard error of the mean. These results were obtained with the same specimens that were used to obtain data given in FIGURE 5. The difference between normal and deficient erythrocytes is not significant for PQ ($p > 0.05$), but highly significant for AQD and DHPQ ($p < 0.001$).

Methemoglobin formation was measured in the same experiments as those in which mechanical fragility (FIGURE 5) and GSH (FIGURE 6) were determined. Methemoglobin formation occurred with both AQD and DHPQ. The percentage formed was approximately twice as great in G-6-PD deficient as in normal erythrocytes (FIGURE 7), a highly significant difference ($p < 0.001$). Negligible amounts of methemoglobin were generated in cells treated with PQ.

The effect of 2.5×10^{-4} M AQD on the concentrations of NADPH and NADP was measured in erythrocytes from five normal and six G-6-PD deficient individuals. The results are summarized in TABLE 2. The concentration of NADPH in both normal and G-6-PD deficient erythrocytes was significantly decreased by treatment with AQD ($p < 0.05$). No equivalent increase in NADP was detected, probably because concentration changes of 4–5 μM are at the borderline of sensitivity of the method at total concentrations of NADP of 40–60 μM. FIGURE 8 shows the ratio of NADPH and NADP. The ratio in normal untreated calls was significantly higher than that in G-6-PD deficient untreated erythrocytes ($p < 0.002$). Treatment with AQD decreased this ratio significantly in normal erythrocyte ($p < 0.05$) and even more significantly in G-6-PD deficient erythrocytes ($p < 0.001$). Proportionately the decrease was greater in G-6-PD deficient than in normal erythrocytes, although the absolute decrease in the ratio was similar in both types of cell.

For comparison with mechanical fragility, osmotic fragility was examined at the same concentration of PQ and AQD (2.5×10^{-4} M). As shown in FIGURE 9,

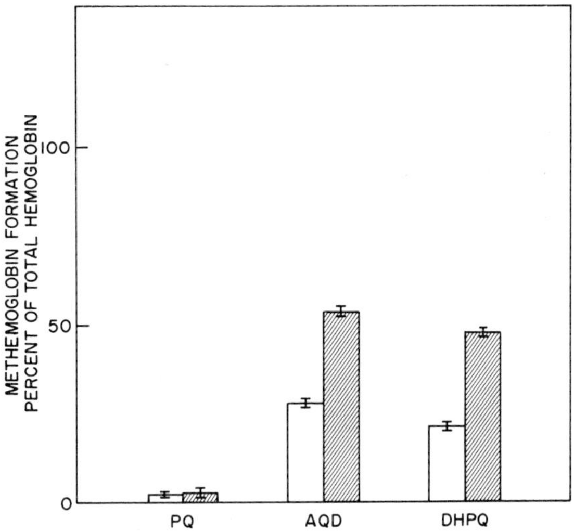

FIGURE 7. The effect of primaquine (PQ), 8-amino-5,6-quinolinediol (AQD) and 5,6-dihydroxypentaquine (DHPQ), each at a concentration of 2.5×10^{-4} M, on methemoglobin formation in normal (open bars) and G-6-DP deficient (cross hatched bars) erythrocytes. Small vertical lines indicate the standard error of the mean. These results were obtained with the same specimens that were used to obtain data given in FIGURES 5 and 6. The difference between normal and deficient erythrocytes is not significant for PQ ($p > 0.05$), but highly significant for AQD and DHPQ ($p < 0.001$).

TABLE 2

EFFECT OF 8-AMINO-5,6-QUINOLINEDIOL (AQD) (2.5×10^{-4} M) ON CONCENTRATIONS OF NADPH AND NADP IN NORMAL AND G-6-PD DEFICIENT ERYTHROCYTES

Erythrocyte Type	Nucleotide Form	No. of Specimens	Concentration (μM) in Control	+ AQD	t-Test p-Value
Normal	NADPH	5	21.7 ± 1.9	16.1 ± 0.8	< 0.05
	NADP	5	45.3 ± 1.7	43.4 ± 0.6	> 0.05
Deficient	NADPH	6	11.6 ± 1.1	7.2 ± 1.0	< 0.025
	NADP	6	62.6 ± 2.4	63.8 ± 3.9	> 0.05

exposure to these agents produced little, if any, change in osmotic fragility in normal or G-6-PD deficient erythrocytes. At a higher concentration of AQD (5×10^{-3} M), a small percentage (7%) of the cells hemolyzed and a significant increase in osmotic fragility occurred both in normal and in G-6-PD deficient erythrocytes.

Effects of Aniline Derivatives on Normal and G-6-PD Deficient Erythrocytes

A comparison of the effect of acetanilide (AA), p-aminophenol (AP) and nitrosobenzene (NB) on mechanical fragility, GSH content and methemoglobin formation in normal and G-6-PD deficient erythrocytes was made. Each of these

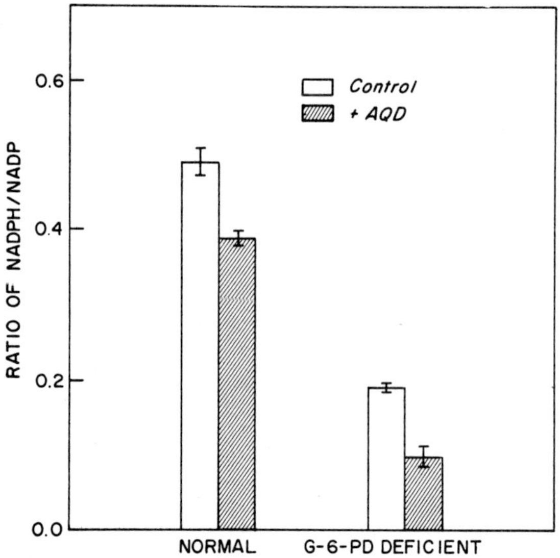

FIGURE 8. The effect of 8-amino-5,6-quinolinediol (2.5×10^{-4} M) on the NADPH/NADP ratio of normal and G-6-PD deficient erythrocytes. The values shown are from the same specimens given in TABLE 2. Small vertical lines indicate the standard error of the mean. The ratio in normal control erythrocytes is significantly different from that in deficient control erythrocytes ($p < 0.002$). AQD produced a significant decrease in the ratio in normal erythrocytes ($p < 0.05$) and a highly significant decrease in the ratio in deficient erythrocytes ($p < 0.001$).

compounds was investigated at a concentration of 10^{-3} M. The results of the mechanical fragility tests are summarized in TABLE 3. Whereas acetanilide (AA) had no significant effect ($p > 0.05$), both AP and NB significantly increased mechanical fragility in both normal and G-6-PD deficient erythrocytes ($p < 0.025$). As in the studies with PQ, AQD and DHPQ, the mechanical fragility of normal control erythrocytes was significantly greater than that of G-6-PD deficient control erythrocytes ($p < 0.05$). Consequently, the ratio of percent hemolysis in treated erythrocytes to percent hemolysis in control erythrocytes shown in FIGURE 10 provided the most valid basis for comparing normal and G-6-PD deficient erythrocytes. The difference between this ratio for normal erythrocytes and G-6-PD deficient erythrocytes was not significant for AA ($p > 0.05$), but quite significant for AP ($p < 0.02$) and NB ($p < 0.05$) (FIGURE 10).

GSH content and methemoglobin formation were measured in the same experiments as those in which mechanical fragility was determined (FIGURES 11 and 12). AP and NB, but not AA, markedly decreased the GSH content of both normal and G-6-PD deficient erythrocytes. The decrease in GSH produced by AP or NB in normal erythrocytes was not significantly different from that produced in G-6-PD deficient erythrocytes ($p > 0.05$). Extensive methemoglobin formation occurred with AP and even more with NB. AA was essentially inactive (FIGURE 12). With AP, methemoglobin formation was slightly, but significantly greater in G-6-PD deficient than in normal erythrocytes ($p < 0.002$). With NB, methemoglobin formation was slightly less in G-6-PD deficient than in normal erythrocytes, but the difference was not statistically significant ($p > 0.05$).

For comparison with mechanical fragility, osmotic fragility was measured at the same concentration of AP and NB (10^{-3} M). As shown in FIGURE 13, AP produced a small change in osmotic fragility but there was no significant difference between normal and G-6-PD deficient erythrocytes. NB caused no change in the osmotic fragility of normal or G-6-PD deficient erythrocytes.

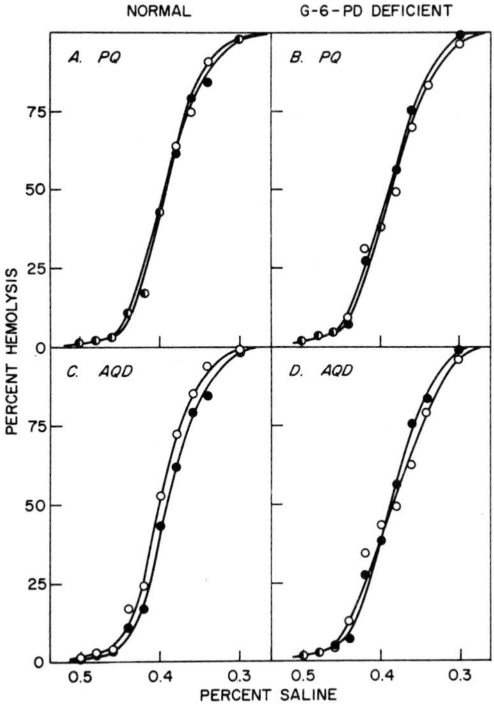

FIGURE 9. The effect of primaquine (PQ) and 8-amino-5,6-quinolinediol (AQD), each at a concentration of 2.5×10^{-4} M, on the osmotic fragility of normal and G-6-PD deficient erythrocytes. Curves for control cells are shown by solid circles and for drug treated cells by open circles.

TABLE 3

EFFECT OF ACETANILIDE (AA), P-AMINOPHENOL (AP) AND NITROSOBENZENE (NB), EACH AT A CONCENTRATION OF 10^{-3} M, ON THE MECHANICAL FRAGILITY OF NORMAL AND G-6-PD DEFICIENT ERYTHROCYTES

Drug	Erythrocyte Type	No. of Specimens	Percent Hemolysis Control	Percent Hemolysis Treated	t-Test p-Value
AA	Normal	5	12.5 ± 0.8	11.8 ± 0.8	> 0.05
	Deficient	5	9.8 ± 0.3	10.3 ± 0.6	> 0.05
AP	Normal	7	14.5 ± 1.1	16.5 ± 1.7	< 0.025
	Deficient	7	9.3 ± 0.8	13.3 ± 1.0	< 0.005
NB	Normal	5	13.3 ± 1.3	17.7 ± 1.8	< 0.01
	Deficient	4	10.2 ± 0.2	15.9 ± 0.5	< 0.005

Discussion

The most significant and novel aspect of these results is the increased mechanical fragility of G-6-PD deficient human erythrocytes produced by each of the four drug metabolites tested. In all cases erythrocytes deficient in G-6-PD exhibited greater hemolysis than normal erythrocytes. Metabolites were active in concentrations at which the parent drugs were ineffective. These results suggest that mechanical fragility is a more useful model than any proposed previously for the study of hemolysis produced in vivo by drugs and drug metabolites. Indeed, prior to the present experiments, no system employed in vitro had established differences between normal and G-6-PD deficient erythrocytes that could be clearly related to hemolysis following exposure to relatively low and more nearly physiologic concentrations of drugs or their metabolites. The increased mechanical fragility of G-6-PD deficient erythrocytes on exposure to various drug metabolites in vitro may well indicate, therefore, the hemolytic properties that these metabolites possess in vivo. Thus a test system for screening drugs and drug metabolites in vitro according to their effect on mechanical fragility appears feasible.

After the early studies of Meltzer and Welch (1884) and Rous and Turner (1916) tests of mechanical fragility have been favorably evaluated and discussed by several investigators (Shen *et al.*, 1944; Stewart *et al.*, 1950; Goldbloom *et al.*, 1953; Schubothe & Fok, 1960; Fok & Schubothe, 1960) as a model in vitro for

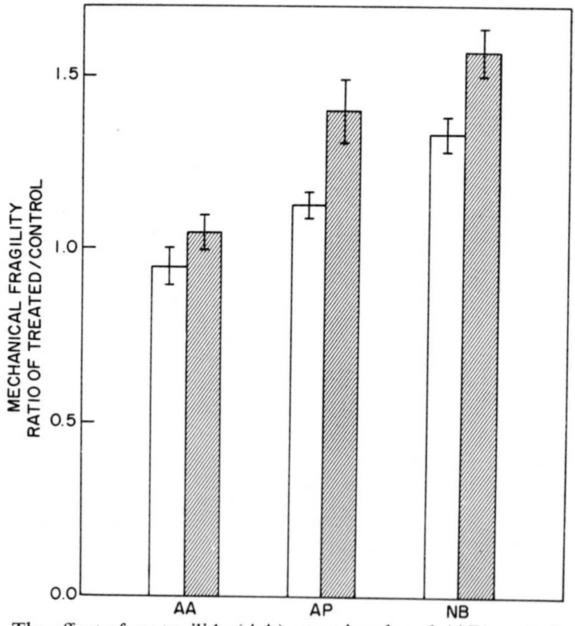

FIGURE 10. The effect of acetanilide (AA), p-aminophenol (AP) and nitrosobenzene (NB), each at a concentration of 10^{-3} M, on the mechanical fragility of normal (open bars) and G-6-PD deficient (cross hatched bars) erythrocytes. The results are expressed as in FIGURE 5 (see caption). Values shown are means from the same specimens given in TABLE 3; small vertical lines indicate the standard error of the mean. The difference between normal and G-6-PD deficient erythrocytes is not significant for AA ($P > 0.05$), but significant for AP and NB ($p < 0.05$).

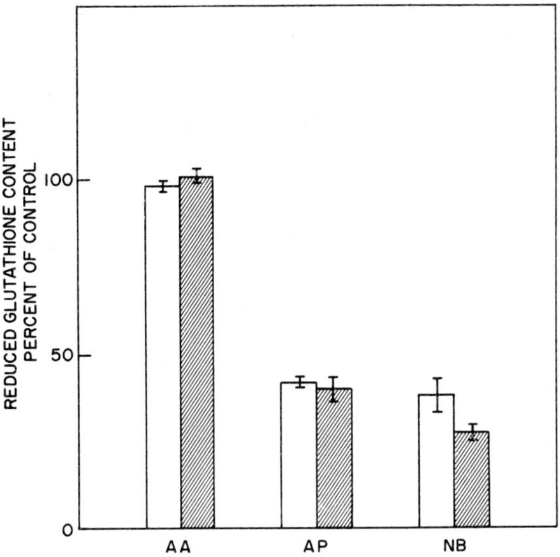

FIGURE 11. The effect of acetanilide (AA), p-aminophenol (AP), and nitrosobenzene (NB), each at a concentration of 10^{-3} M, on the reduced glutathione (GSH) content of normal (open bars) and G-6-PD deficient (cross hatched bars) erythrocytes. Results are expressed as the percent of reduced glutathione content of control cells. Small vertical lines indicate the standard error of the mean. These results were obtained with the same specimens that were used to obtain data given in FIGURE 10. The decrease in GSH produced by AP and NB in normal erythrocytes was not significantly different from that produced in deficient erythrocytes ($p > 0.05$).

conditions existing in vivo. In particular, the mechanical fragility test appears to simulate the destruction of erythrocytes in vivo better than does the osmotic fragility test. Stewart *et al.* (1950) showed that the mechanical fragility of dog erythrocytes increased with the aging of the cell. The suggestion of Rous and Robertson in 1917 (Rous & Robertson, 1917; Robertson & Rous, 1917; Rous, 1923) that the chief means of erythrocyte destruction is by fragmentation still enjoys general acceptance (Wintrobe, 1961). Weed and Reed (1966) have reviewed recent work on erythrocyte fragmentation in the circulation and emphasized its importance in several clinical disorders. They suggest that fragmentation plays a significant role in the drug-induced hemolysis of G-6-PD deficiency. Greenberg and Wong (1961) and Salvidio *et al.* (1967) have shown that intravascular hemolysis represents the major mechanism for destruction of G-6-PD deficient erythrocytes in individuals receiving primaquine, although sequestration of slightly damaged cells by the spleen is also involved, particularly in cases of severe G-6-PD deficiency.

Mechanical fragility has certain limitations as an in vitro model of the destructive process occurring in vivo. Fok and Schubothe (1960) have suggested that in the test red cells are traumatized indirectly by currents generated from rolling movements of the beads and from physical surface forces of the beads and flask. These phenomena may only approximate circulatory conditions in vivo. Furthermore, in the test as we have performed it, 10–20% of normal or G-6-PD deficient cells are fragmented in a two-hour-period in contrast to the much slower fragmentation rate of the oldest cells in the circulation. Finally numerous variables involved in the test limit its reproducibility in successive determinations. Despite these limitations, the results of its use in the present study afford a new example of its potential value.

The drug metabolites were more active than the parent compounds in increasing mechanical fragility and methemoglobin content and decreasing glutathione content of erythrocytes. Erythrocytes from G-6-PD deficient individuals showed greater alterations than normal erythrocytes. The metabolites or probable metabolites used in our experiments were chosen as models because their structures suggested that they might possess greater redox properties than the parent drugs. As shown earlier (FIGURE 1) the 5,6-dihydroxy-8-aminoquinolines can be converted to quinones or quinonimines, possibly in a reaction involving hemoglobin and oxygen. Kiese (1966) has reviewed evidence for formation of a quinonimine from p-aminophenol and its role in the production of methemoglobin. As discussed previously (FIGURE 3), nitrosobenzene can be converted by the erythrocyte to phenylhydroxylamine. This in turn reacts with hemoglobin and oxygen to yield an oxidant intermediate with production of methemoglobin and reformation of nitrosobenzene. By contrast, the parent drug, such as primaquine and acetanilide, are not readily converted by the erythrocyte to forms with such high redox potential. Some authors (Kalow, 1962; Marks, 1964; Cohen & Hochstein, 1964, 1965; Carson & Frischer, 1966; Beutler, 1967; Aebi, 1967) have attributed oxidant characteristics to the parent drugs, including the ability to generate hydrogen peroxide. However, the model metabolites we have studied are probably converted to oxidant intermediates. Shahidi and Treichel (1967) have recently reached the same conclusion; they attribute the hemolytic action of

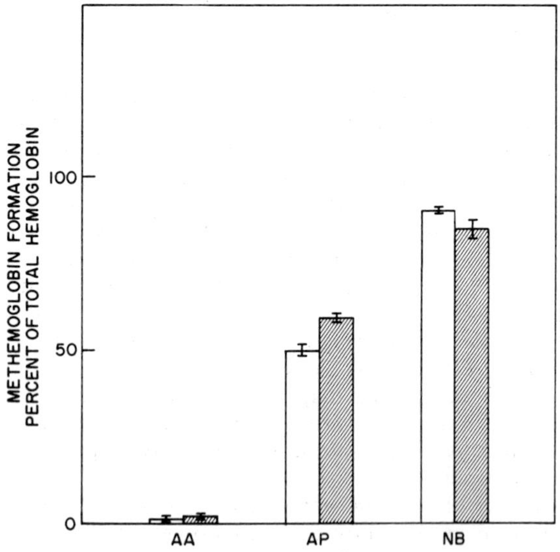

FIGURE 12. The effect of acetanilide (AA), p-aminophenol (AP), and nitrosobenzene (NB), each at a concentration of 10^{-3} M, on methemoglobin formation in normal (open bars) and G-6-PD deficient (cross hatched bars) erythrocytes. Small vertical lines indicate the standard error of the mean. These results were obtained with the same specimens that were used to obtain data shown in FIGURE 10. The difference between methemoglobin formation in deficient erythrocytes is significant with AP ($p < 0.002$), but not significant with NB ($p > 0.05$).

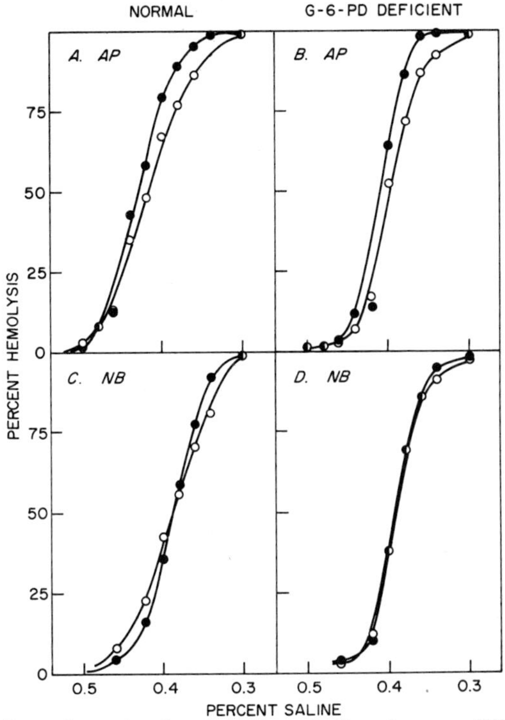

FIGURE 13. The effect of p-aminophenol (AP) and nitrosobenzene (NB), each at a concentration of 10^{-3} M, on the osmotic fragility of normal and G-6-PD deficient erythrocytes. Curves for control cells are shown by solid circles and for drug treated cells by open circles.

acetophenetidin to the o-hydroxy metabolite. Kosower *et al.* (1965) and Kosower and Kosower (1967) suggest participation of oxidant intermediates or free radicals in decreasing the reduced glutathione content of G-6-PD deficient erythrocytes following exposure to phenylhydrazine and 3,4-dihydroxyphenylalanine.

The primary mechanism whereby drug metabolites increase mechanical fragility may involve direct oxidant effects on the membrane or intracellular metabolic events including alterations of the reduced glutathione content, NADPH/NADP ratio and methemoglobin content.

Ever since the discovery by Beutler (1957) of the glutathione instability of drug-sensitive red cells, considerable emphasis has been placed on the role of depletion of reduced glutathione in the hemolytic process (Beutler, 1966; Dausset & Contu, 1966; Aebi, 1967). With 8-amino-5,6-quinolinediol (AQD) and 5,6 dihydroxypentaquine (DHPQ), our data show a good correlation between decreased levels of reduced glutathione and increased mechanical fragility of the erythrocytes. However, there was no such close correlation in the case of p-aminophenol (AP) and nitrosobenzene (NB). Also, a lower concentration of p-aminophenol (5×10^{-4}) was found to decrease the reduced glutathione content of G-6-PD deficient erythrocytes almost as markedly as did 10^{-3} M p-aminophenol without an accompanying significant increase in mechanical fragility. The decrease in the NADPH/NADP ratio produced by 8-amino-5,6-quinolinediol (AQD) was proportionately more significant in G-6-PD deficient than in normal cells and thus correlates with the difference in effects on the mechanical fragility. However, since the reduced glutathione content is closely dependent on this ratio, studies with p-aminophenol and nitrosobenzene might be anticipated to reveal the same lack of correlation with this ratio as was found for reduced glutathione. Methemoglobin formation also was closely correlated with changes in mechanical fragility produced by 8-amino-5,6-quinolinediol (AQD) and 5,6-dihydroxy-pentaquine (DHPQ) but was not so well correlated with those produced by p-aminophenol (AP) and nitrosobenzene (NB).

Such parameters of red cell function as reduced glutathione content, NADPH/NAPD ratio and methemoglobin formation are generally more affected by drug metabolites than by the parent drugs and are more altered in G-6-PD deficient than in normal erythrocytes. However, in our experiments alterations in these intracellular metabolites appeared not to be directly related to changes in mechanical fragility. The consistently increased mechanical fragility of G-6-PD deficient erythrocytes on exposure to each of four drug metabolites may thus represent a direct oxidant effect of these agents or their intermediates on the erythrocyte membrane. Changes in mechanical fragility may therefore be employed as a test in vitro for drugs and drug metabolites suspected of possessing hemolytic activity in vivo.

These experiments also suggest a modified view of the sequence of events leading to drug induced hemolysis in vivo:

1. Metabolism of the drug to a product with greater redox properties.
2. Conversion of this metabolite to an oxidant intermediate by the erythrocyte.
3. Oxidant damage to the erythrocyte membrane, possibly by oxidation of reduced sulfhydryl groups.
4. Increased fragmentation of older erythrocytes in the circulation resulting from this membrane damage.

In this view increased sensitivity of G-6-PD deficient erythrocytes to hemolysis by drug metabolites may result from decreased capacity to regenerate or protect reduced sulfhydryl groups in the membrane. The fall in reduced glutathione is secondary to a lower level of NADPH which, in turn, is attributable to G-6-PD deficiency. Methemoglobin production and possibly further hemoglobin denaturation may be side actions of oxidant intermediates formed from drug metabolites.

Summary and Conclusions

Hydroxylated metabolites of primaquine and acetanilide increased the mechanical fragility of G-6-PD deficient erythrocytes much more than that of normal erythrocytes. In some cases, they decreased glutathione content and increased methemoglobin content more markedly in G-6-PD deficient than in normal erythrocytes. Parent drugs were inactive at the same concentrations. These results suggest that drug metabolites are converted in the erythrocyte to oxidant intermediates capable of damaging the membrane of G-6-PD deficient cells. Mechanical fragility is suggested as a valuable technique in studying metabolic differences between normal and G-6-PD deficient erythrocytes and for testing drug metabolites in vitro for hemolytic actions that they might exert in vivo.

Acknowledgments

We gratefully acknowledge the advice of Drs. Bernard B. Brodie, James R. Gillette and N. Raphael Shulman. Dr. Paul R. McCurdy of the D. C. General Hospital made available routine hematology specimens.

Dr. R. O. Clinton of the Sterling-Winthrop Research Institute, Rensselaer, New York supplied primaquine phosphate; Dr. S. Archer of the same Institute had 8-amino-5,6-quinolinediol synthesized for us. Dr. Bing T. Poon of the Walter Reed Army Institute of Research, Washington, D. C. supplied the 5,6-dihydroxy-pentaquine. Dr. Arthur K. Cho kindly recrystallized nitrosobenzene.

This investigation was supported in part by a Public Health Service Fellowship No. 1–F3-GM-32,366–01 from the National Institute of General Medical Sciences. Computational aid was rendered by the Scientific Computation Facility of Loma Linda University supported in part by Grant FR-00276–03 from the Special Research Resources Division, National Institutes of Health, United States Public Health Service.

References

Aebi, H. E. 1967. Ann. Rev. Biochem. **36:** 271.

Alving, A. S., R. D. Powell, G. J. Brewer & J. D. Arnold. 1962. *In* Drugs, Parasites and Hosts. Eds. L. G. Goodwin & R. H. Nimmo-Smith. J. A. Churchill Ltd., Lond.

Beutler, E. 1957. J. Lab. Clin. Med. **49:** 84.

Beutler, E. 1959. Blood **14:** 103.

Beutler, E. 1966. *In* The Metabolic Basis of Inherited Disease. 2nd Ed., Eds. J. B. Stanbury, J. B. Wyngaarden & D. S. Fredrickson. McGraw-Hill, N. Y.

Beutler, E. 1967. Amer. J. Clin. Pathol. **47:** 303.

Beutler, E., R. J. Dern & A. S. Alving. 1954. J. Lab. Clin. Med. **44:** 177.

Bishop, C. 1966. J. Lab. Clin. Med. **68:** 149.

Brodie, B. B. & J. Axelrod. 1949. J. Pharmacol. **97:** 58.

Brodie, B. B. & S. Udenfriend. 1950. Proc. Soc. Exp. Biol. Med. **74:** 845.

Carson, P. E. 1967. Ann. N. Y. Acad. Sci. This Annal.

Carson, P. E. & H. Frischer. 1966. Amer. J. Med. **41:** 744.

Cohen, G. & P. Hochstein. 1964. Biochemistry **3:** 895.

Cohen, G. & P. Hochstein. 1965. J. Pharmacol. **147:** 139.

Cohn, V. H. & J. Lyle. 1966. Anal. Biochem. **14:** 434.

Dausset, J. & L. Contu. 1967. Ann. Rev. Med. **18:** 55

Debackere, M. & H. Uehleke. 1964. Proc. European Soc. for the Study of Drug Toxicity **4:** 40.

Degowin, R. L., R. B. Eppes, R. D. Powell & P. E. Carson. 1966. Bull. Wld. Hlth. Org. **35:** 165.

Dern, R. J., E. Beutler & A. S. Alving. 1955. J. Lab. Clin. Med. **45:** 30.

Earle, D. P. Jr., F. S. Bigelow, C. G. Zubrod & C. A. Kane. 1948. J. Clin. Invest. **27** (No. 3, pt. 2): 121.

Elderfield, R. C. & L. L. Smith. 1953. J. Amer. Chem. Soc. **75:** 1022.

Fok, F. P.-T. & H. Schubothe. 1960. Brit. J. Haemat. **6:** 355.

Frankel, S. & S. Reitman, Eds. 1963. Gradwohl's Clinical Laboratory Methods and Diagnosis, Vol. **2:** 1134. C. P. Mosby Co. St. Louis.

Goldbloom, R. B., E. Fischer, J. Reinhold & D. Y.-Y. Hsia. 1953. Blood **8:** 165.

Greenberg, M. S. & H. Wong. 1961. J. Lab. Clin. Med. **57:** 733.

Gross, R. T., E. A. Schroeder & B. W. Gabrio. 1966. J. Clin. Invest. **45:** 249.

Harley, J. D. 1966. Nature **210:** 1164.

Hjelm, M. & C.-H. de Verdier. 1965. Biochem. Pharmacol. **14:** 1119.

Josephson, E. S., D. J. Taylor, J. Greenberg & A. P. Ray. 1951a. Proc. Soc. Exp. Biol. Med. **76:** 700.

Josephson, E. S., J. Greenberg, D. J. Taylor & J. L. Bami. 1951b. J. Pharmacol. **103:** 7.

Kalow, W. 1962. Pharmacogenetics. W. B. Saunders Co. Phil.

Kiese, M. 1966. Pharmacol. Rev. **18:** 1091.

Kirkman, H. N. 1967. Ann. N. Y. Acad. Sci. This Annal.

Kosower, N. S. & E. M. Kosower. 1967. Nature **215:** 285.

KOSOWER, N. S., G. VANDERHOFF, E. M. KOSOWER & P. C. HUANG. 1965. Biochem. Biophys. Res. Comm. **20:** 469.
LÖHR, G. W. & H. D. WALLER. 1961. Dtsch. med. Wschr. **86:** 27.
LOWRY, O. H., J. PASSONNEAU, D. W. SCHULZ & M. K. ROCK. 1961. J. Biol. Chem. **236:** 2746.
MARKS, P. A. 1964. *In* The Red Blood Cell. Eds. C. Bishop & D. M. Surgenor. Academic Press, N. Y.
MELTZER, S. J. & W. H. WELCH. 1884. J. Physiol. **5:** 255.
PAGE, L. B. & P. J. CULVER. 1960. A Syllabus of Laboratory Examinations in Clinical Diagnosis. Harvard Univ. Press, Cambridge. p. 123.
ROBERTSON, O. H. & P. ROUS. 1917. J. Exper. Med. **25:** 665.
ROBIN, H. & J. D. HARLEY. 1964. Austral. Ann. Med. **13:** 313.
ROUS, P. 1923. Physiol. Rev. **3:** 75.
ROUS, P. & O. H. ROBERTSON. 1917. J. Exper. Med. **25:** 651.
ROUS, P. & J. R. TURNER. 1916. J. Exper. Med. **23:** 219.
SALVIDIO, E., I. PANNACCIULLI, A. TIZIANELLO & F. AJMAR. 1967. New England J. Med. **276:** 1339.
SASS, M. D., C. J. CARUSO & D. R. AXELROD. 1966. J. Lab. Clin. Med. **68:** 156.
SHAHIDI, N. T. 1967. Ann. N. Y. Acad. Sci. This Annal.
SHAHIDI, N. T. & I. TREICHEL. 1967. J. Clin. Invest. **46:** 1116.
SCHUBOTHE, H. & F. P.-T. FOK. 1960. Brit. J. Haemat. **6:** 350.
SHEN, S. C., W. B. CASTLE & E. M. FLEMING. 1944. Science **100:** 387.
SMITH, C. C. 1956. J. Pharmacol. **116:** 67.
STEWART, W. B., J. M. STEWART, M. J. IZZO & L. E. YOUNG. 1950. J. Exper. Med. **91:** 147.
UEHLEKE, H. 1964. Proc. European Soc. for the Study of Drug Toxicity **4:** 140.
WAGNER, J., P. HYKEŠ, V. JANATA & K. KÁCL. 1964. Acta Biol. Med. Germ. Suppl. **3:** 312.
WEED, R. I. & C. F. REED. 1966. Amer. J. Med. **41:** 681.
WELCH, R. M., A. H. CONNEY & J. J. BURNS. 1966. Biochem. Pharmacol. **15:** 521.
WILLIAMS, R. T. 1959. Detoxication Mechanisms. 2nd Ed. John Wiley & Sons, Inc., N. Y.
WINTROBE, M. M. 1961. Clinical Hematology. 5th Ed. Lea & Febiger, Phila. p. 167.

HEREDITARY METHEMOGLOBINEMIA, TOXIC METHEMOGLOBINEMIA AND THE REDUCTION OF METHEMOGLOBIN*

Ernst R. Jaffé† and Gertrude Neumann

Department of Medicine, Albert Einstein College of Medicine, Bronx Municipal Hospital Center, N. Y.

INTRODUCTION

Methemoglobin or ferrihemoglobin in which the iron of the heme moiety is in the ferric form is incapable of binding molecular oxygen reversibly. Normally, less than one percent of the total hemoglobin in human erythrocytes is methemoglobin.[1] This concentration is maintained as the result of an equilibrium between the rate at which hemoglobin is oxidized and the rate at which methemoglobin is reduced (FIGURE 1). In this scheme, 'a' represents the oxidation of hemoglobin, a reaction which may be increased by many drugs and chemicals,[2,3] either directly or after conversion to "active" metabolites. The symbol, 'b', represents processes within the erythrocytes, such as glutathione (GSH) peroxidase[4,5] or catalase,[6] which protect hemoglobin against oxidation. An increase in the concentration of methemoglobin can result from exposure to agents which increase the rate of oxidation, 'a', and which may overwhelm the protective mechanisms, 'b'. Once methemoglobin is formed within erythrocytes, it can be reduced to hemoglobin by enzymatic or other processes represented by arrow 'c'.[7] The degree of methemoglobinemia will be determined by the extent to which 'a-b' exceeds 'c'. The duration and severity of the methemoglobinemia will be influenced by the metabolism of the methemoglobin-forming drugs, by the mechanisms which protect hemoglobin, and by the ability of the erythrocytes to reduce methemoglobin. All of these processes probably are affected by genetically determined factors. This paper will be concerned only with the reduction of methemoglobin composed of normal polypeptide chains and not with hemoglobin M.[8]

The reduction of methemoglobin in human erythrocytes appears to depend, primarily, on the activity of a DPNH-dependent methemoglobin reductase system.[7–9] Three other pathways capable of reducing methemoglobin are present in human erythrocytes, but appear to be less important. The relative contribution made by each of the pathways can be calculated from data reported by Scott and his associates.[10] The system of greatest importance, the DPNH-methemoglobin reductases (DPNH dehydrogenase I and II), can account for 67 percent of the rate, while ascorbic acid can account for 16 percent, GSH for 12 percent and TPNH-methemoglobin reductase for perhaps 5 percent. Sass and his associates[11] have recently described a patient without methemoglobinemia whose erythrocytes, although deficient in TPNH-methemoglobin reductase activity, are able to reduce nitrite-induced methemoglobin to hemoglobin at a normal rate in vitro. This TPNH-methemoglobin reductase system, therefore, may be an auxiliary pathway which requires an artificial electron carrier, such as methylene blue, to become effective in reducing methemoglobin to hemoglobin.

* The studies reported in this paper were supported by grant HE–10041 from the National Heart Institute, U.S.P.H.S.

† Career Scientist of the Health Research Council of the City of New York (I–169).

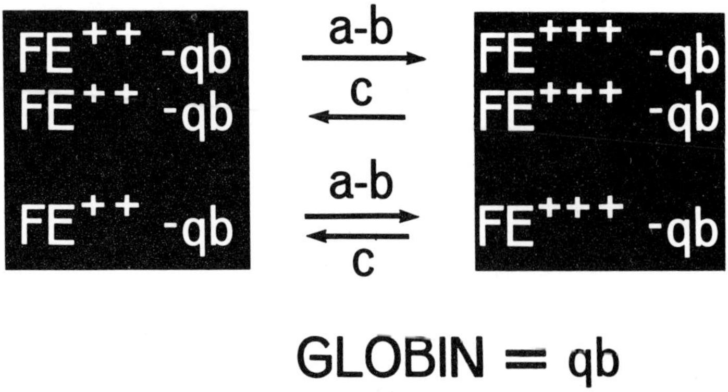

FIGURE 1. Schematic representation of the intracellular equilibrium between hemoglobin (Fe^{++}-gb) and methemoglobin (Fe^{+++}-gb).

Reduction of Methemoglobin in Intact Human Erythrocytes

The ability of human erythrocytes to reduce methemoglobin can be demonstrated readily in vitro. After most of the hemoglobin is converted to methemoglobin by treatment with sodium nitrite, the erythrocytes are washed repeatedly and are incubated with glucose or inosine or twice the molar concentration of L (+) sodium lactate in a suitable buffer solution.[12] Incubation of normal erythrocytes results in the *net* reduction of methemoglobin at a rate of about 5 to 6 percent per hour for the first 5 to 6 hours. After 22 to 24 hours of incubation, almost all of the methemoglobin has been reduced. Incubation without added substrate results in minimal reduction. When the erythrocytes of a patient with hereditary methemoglobinemia associated with a deficiency in DPNH-methemoglobin reductase activity are used, only limited reduction of methemoglobin is observed. The extent of reduction in these cells with added substrates is comparable to the rate of reduction in normal erythrocytes without substrate. Intermediate rates of reduction can be demonstrated with erythrocytes with intermediate levels of activity of DPNH-methemoglobin reductase.[12,13] Determinations of the activities of other enzymes, glucose utilization and concentrations of cofactors in erythrocytes deficient in DPNH-methemoglobin reductase activity have failed to reveal other consistent abnormalities.[9] Erythrocytes of severely deficient subjects, however, produce less pyruvate[14] and more lactate[15] than do normal cells when nitrite-treated erythrocytes are incubated with glucose, because more DPNH is available in these cells to reduce pyruvate to lactate when not used for the reduction of methemoglobin. The degree of impairment in the ability of intact erythrocytes to reduce methemoglobin tends to parallel the degree of DPNH-methemoglobin reductase deficiency, although a precise correlation cannot be shown.[13] It should be noted that the determination of DPNH-methemoglobin reductase activity is based on an *indirect* method. The rate of reduction of an artificial receptor, the dye, 2,6-dichlorobenzenone indophenol, is determined in the presence of excess added DPNH in hemolysates prepared from nitrited erythrocytes.[16]

Activation of the TPNH-methemoglobin reductase system can be demonstrated by including small amounts of methylene blue in the incubation medium.[12,14] Rapid reduction of methemoglobin then occurs in normal erythrocytes and in erythrocytes with various degrees of DPNH-methemoglobin reductase deficiency with glucose as substrate.[12,13] This finding strengthens the thesis that the TPNH-methemoglobin reductase system does not play a major role in human erythrocytes in the absence of an artificial electron carrier.

These observations support the concept that the hereditary methemoglobinemia associated with a severe deficiency in DPNH-methemoglobin reductase activity is the consequence of the loss of about two-thirds of the normal capacity to reduce methemoglobin. The disorder appears to be transmitted as an autosomal characteristic. Individuals with clinically apparent methemoglobinemia are presumed to be homozygotes and their erythrocytes are severely deficient in DPNH-methemoglobin reductase activity. Subjects without significant methemoglobinemia but with erythrocytes containing intermediate levels of activity of DPNH-methemoglobin reductase are thought to be heterozygotes.

A decreased ability to reduce nitrite-induced methemoglobin is also seen with intact erythrocytes obtained from cord blood.[17,18] The decrease is comparable to that observed with erythrocytes from subjects heterozygous for DPNH-methemoglobin reductase deficiency. Decreased levels of DPNH-methemoglobin reductase activity have been described in studies of erythrocytes from cord blood.[19,20] Significant methemoglobinemia does not normally occur in either newborn infants or adults heterozygous for DPNH-methemoglobin reductase deficiency, but slightly elevated concentrations of methemoglobin have been reported as being present in the blood of both types of subjects.[21–23] Newborn infants, however, are unusually susceptible to the development of toxic methemoglobinemia. This increased susceptibility may be contributed to by the decreased DPNH-methemoglobin reductase activity. Although clinical examples have not yet been encountered, children and adults heterozygous for DPNH-methemoglobin reductase deficiency also may be more susceptible to the effects of agents which produce toxic methemoglobinemia. Further investigations along these lines are warranted.

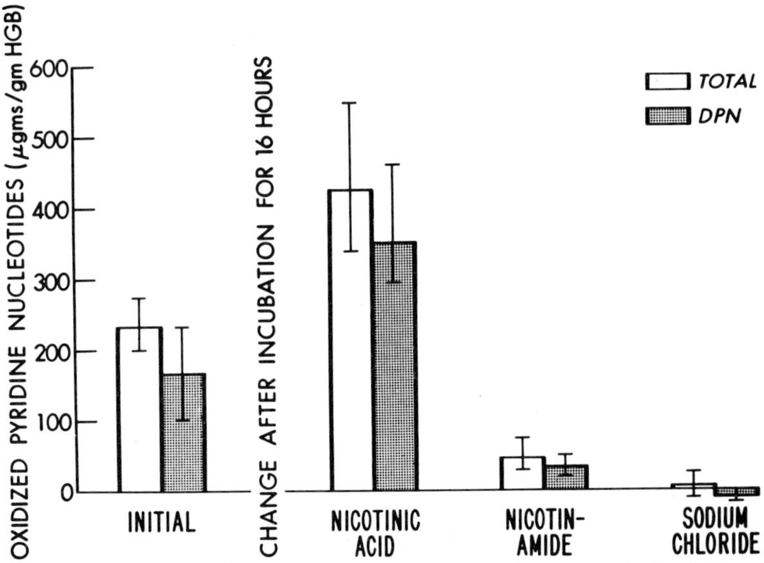

FIGURE 2. Concentrations of total oxidized pyridine nucleotides and of DPN in washed human erythrocytes before incubation and the changes in the concentrations after incubation for 16 hours with the media described in the text. The average values obtained for 11 separate experiments are shown and the ranges are indicated by the narrow lines.

Effect of Increased DPN Content on the Reduction of Methemoglobin

The availability of oxidized pyridine nucleotides may influence the metabolic activity of various tissues. The addition of DPN to whole homogenates of rat and mouse liver, kidney, heart and brain has been shown to enhance the oxidation of glucose via the Embden-Meyerhof pathway.[24] The effect of altered intracellular concentrations of DPN on the reduction of methemoglobin in human erythrocytes, therefore, has been investigated.[25]

Washed erythrocytes, obtained from normal individuals and from subjects homozygous and heterozygous for DPNH-methemoglobin reductase deficiency, were incubated at 37° C for 16 hours with nicotinic acid, glucose, glutamine and inorganic phosphate as described previously.[26] Incubation with this medium resulted in an increase in the concentration of total oxidized pyridine nucleotides in all three types of cells to levels almost three times those present prior to incubation (FIGURE 2). The initial concentration of about 230 μg of oxidized pyridine nucleotides per g of hemoglobin was increased by an average of 420 μg per gram. Approximately 83 percent of this increase could be accounted for by

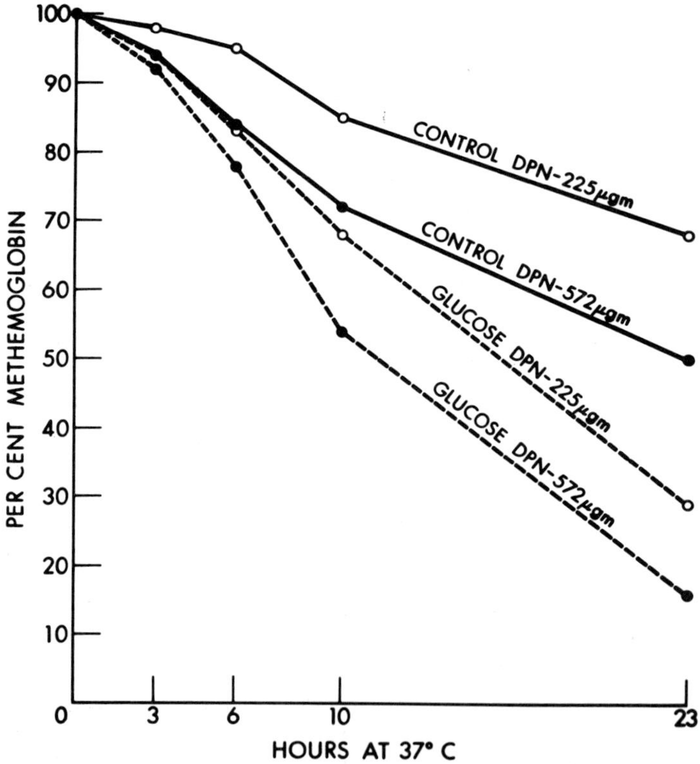

FIGURE 3. Reduction of methemoglobin in normal human erythrocytes during incubation without added substrate (Control) or with 0.012 M Glucose. Erythrocytes in suspensions labeled DPN-225 μgm were preincubated for 16 hours with the nicotinamide-containing medium, while those labeled DPN-572 μgm were preincubated with the nicotinic acid-containing medium.

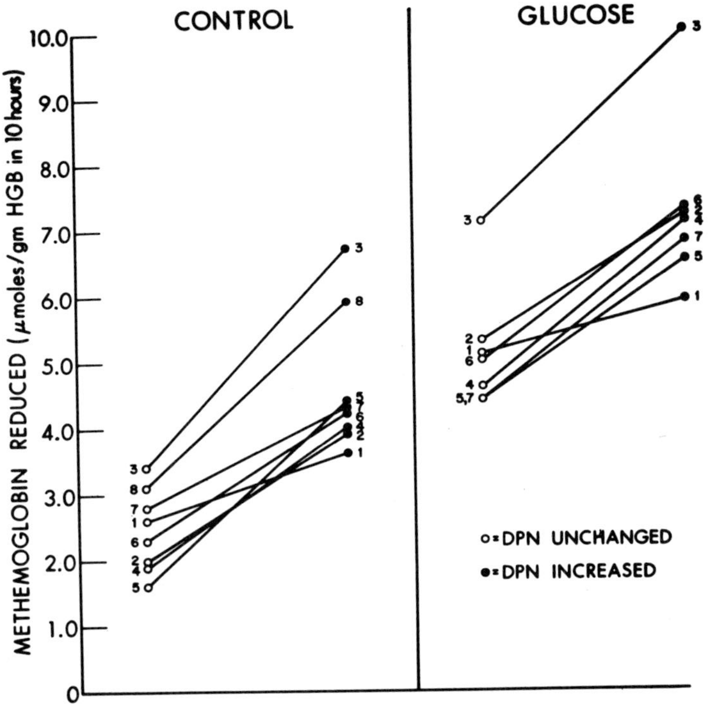

FIGURE 4. Reduction of methemoglobin by normal human erythrocytes during 10 hours of incubation without added substrate (Control) or with 0.012 M Glucose with concentrations of DPN as indicated. Results obtained in paired samples of the same experiment are numbered and are connected by lines.

an increase in the concentration of DPN. When the nicotinic acid in the medium was replaced by an equimolar amount of nicotinamide, the increase in DPN was only about 10 percent of that observed with nicotinic acid. No increase or even a slight decrease in DPN content occurred when neither nicotinic acid nor nicotinamide was present. These preincubated erythrocytes were treated with equal volumes of 0.072 M sodium nitrite in an isotonic solution to convert most of the hemoglobin to methemoglobin. The cells were then washed six times and were incubated without added substrate or with 0.012 M glucose in an isotonic sodium chloride-sodium phosphate buffer solution with shaking at 37° C. The packed cell volume was about 16 percent.

The results of a typical experiment with normal erythrocytes are shown in FIGURE 3. Reduction of methemoglobin was progressive and nearly linear during the initial 10 hours of incubation. Since the differences in the rates of reduction were less striking during the subsequent 13 hours, the values obtained after 10 hours were used for all calculations. Reduction of methemoglobin occurred in the control suspension without added substrate, presumably from utilization of lactate and other substrates which had accumulated during the period of preincubation and which were not removed by the subsequent washings. The rate of reduction in the suspension with the increased DPN concentration was about 1.9 times greater than that in the suspension with the unaltered DPN content. Reduction was twice as rapid in the suspension with added glucose as in the suspension without added substrate. The rate was about 1.5 times greater in the suspension with glucose and an increased concentration of DPN than in the comparable suspension with a normal content of DPN. The increased rate of reduction of methemoglobin was not due to the breakdown and metabolism of the newly synthesized DPN, for the concentrations of DPN were not altered significantly after the 10 hour period of reincubation.

The results of eight experiments without added substrate and seven with added glucose performed with normal erythrocytes are summarized in FIGURE 4. The rate of reduction of methemoglobin, expressed as micromoles reduced per gram of total hemoglobin during 10 hours, was consistently higher in erythrocyte suspensions with increased concentrations of DPN. As expected, the rates were always higher when glucose was present. Differences in the rates of reduction between erythrocytes preincubated with nicotinamide or sodium chloride alone were not observed.

When erythrocytes with extremely low or intermediate levels of DPNH-methemoglobin reductase activity were preincubated with the nicotinic acid-containing medium, the increases in total oxidized pyridine nucleotides and in DPN were identical to those observed with normal erythrocytes. The very low rate of reduction of methemoglobin in erythrocytes severely deficient in DPNH-methe-

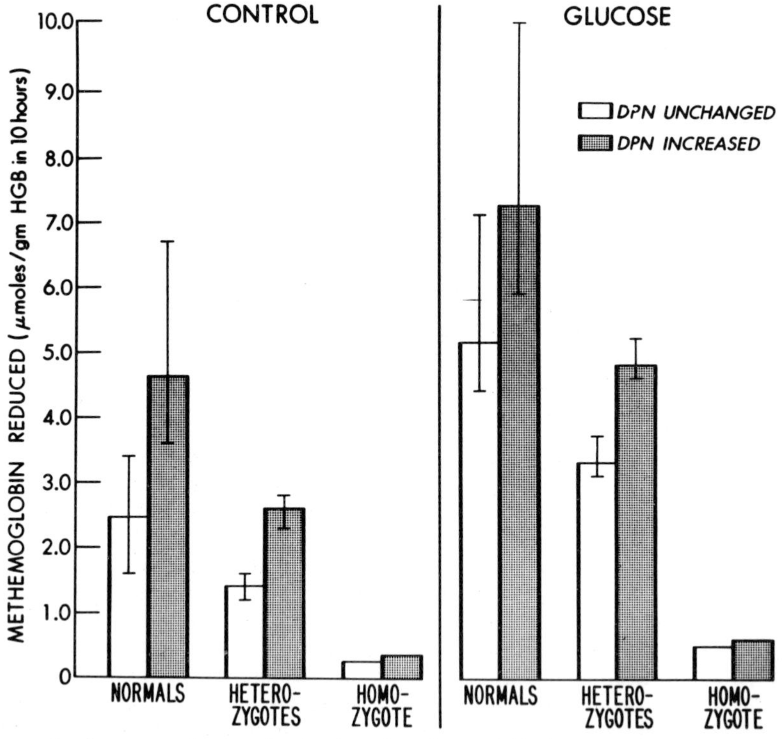

FIGURE 5. Summary of rates of reduction of methemoglobin in normal human erythrocytes (8 Control without added substrate, 7 with 0.012 M Glucose), erythrocytes with intermediate levels of activity of DPNH-methemoglobin reductase (3 subjects, Heterozygotes) and erythrocytes severely deficient in DPNH-methemoglobin reductase activity (1 subject, 2 experiments, Homozygote) with concentrations of DPN as indicated. Ranges are indicated by narrow lines.

moglobin reductase activity was not influenced significantly by the increased content of DPN, without or with glucose (FIGURE 5). The erythrocytes of three subjects who had been shown to be heterozygous for DPNH-methemoglobin reductase deficiency did demonstrate increased rates of reduction of methemoglobin when the DPN content was increased. The rates, however, failed to reach the levels observed with erythrocytes from normal subjects.

The increased DPN content in the erythrocytes preincubated with the nicotinic acid-containing medium may have permitted the generation of more DPNH, mediated through the activity of lactic dehydrogenase or glyceraldehyde-3-phosphate dehydrogenase. Substrates for these enzymes would be provided by the metabolism of added glucose and of lactate or other organic phosphate esters which had accumulated in the cells during the initial period of incubation. The increased supply of DPNH could then have been utilized by the DPNH-methemoglobin reductase system to reduce methemoglobin more rapidly. Participation of the TPNH-methemoglobin reductase system in these experiments could not be excluded, but the acceleration of reduction observed when methylene blue was added to the suspensions was not affected by increased concentrations of oxidized pyridine nucleotides. Although the rate of reduction of methemoglobin was influenced by the concentration of DPN, the level of activity of the DPNH-methemoglobin reductase system appeared to be more important in determining the rate at which methemoglobin would actually be reduced in intact human erythrocytes.

The Role of Reduced Glutathione in the Reduction of Methemoglobin

Differences of opinion about the role of the pentose phosphate shunt pathway in the reduction of methemoglobin in human erythrocytes have been expressed.[7] Strömme and Eldjarn[27] have interpreted the results of their studies as indicating that whatever reduction of methemoglobin results from the activity of this pathway can be explained by the direct, nonenzymatic reduction of methemoglobin by GSH. Although GSH can reduce methemoglobin to hemoglobin in vitro, the rate and efficiency of this reaction is limited.[7] Jacob and Jandl[28] have concluded that methemoglobin has little, if any, effect on the activity of the pentose phosphate shunt pathway which is influenced by the ratio of oxidized glutathione to GSH.

This question was reinvestigated by treating normal human erythrocytes with sufficient N-ethyl maleimide (NEM) to bind all of the GSH in the cells, presumably by forming an irreversible complex.[29] Erythrocytes, washed once with phosphate-buffered sodium chloride solution, were incubated at 37° C for 10 minutes with either an equal volume of sodium chloride-sodium phosphate buffer alone or with this buffer containing 3 to 5 μmoles per ml of NEM and were then washed once more. After incubation at room temperature for 20 minutes with equal volumes of 0.145 M sodium nitrite solution and washing six times, 16 percent suspensions without and with substrates were prepared in an isotonic glycylglycine-sodium phosphate buffer, pH 7.4.[12] The suspensions were incubated at 37° C with shaking. Concentrations of GSH were determined by the nitroprusside method[30] and concentrations of methemoglobin were measured by the method of Evelyn and Malloy.[31] Clear filtrates obtained after adding one volume of each erythrocyte suspension to 6 volumes of cold 2 percent perchloric acid were used for the determination of glucose (Boehringer glucose UV-test), ribose of inosine,[32] lactate[33] and pyruvate[34] before and after various periods of incubation.

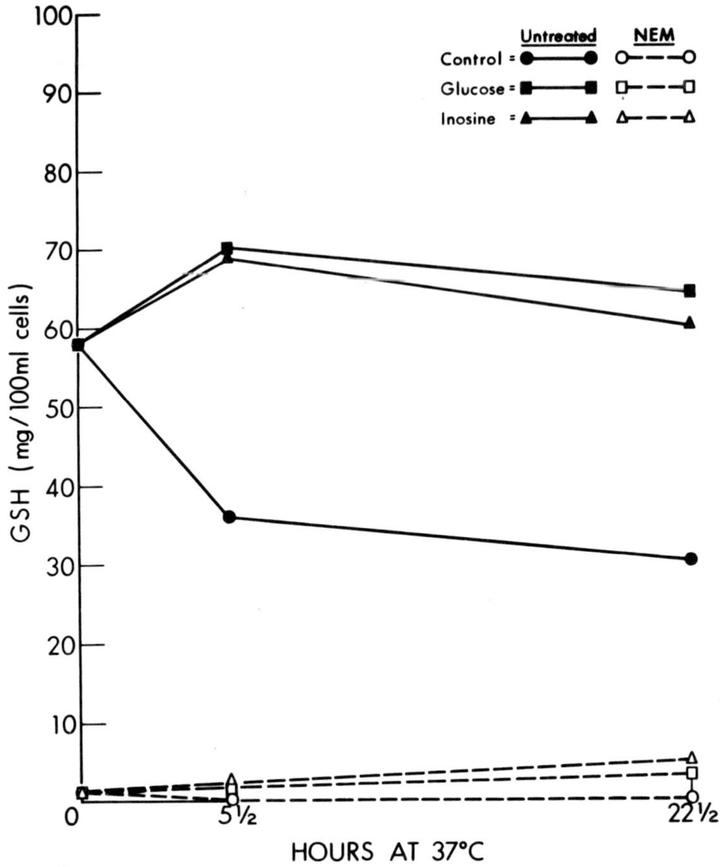

FIGURE 6. Concentrations of GSH in nitrite-treated, normal human erythrocytes before and after incubation without added substrate (Control) and with 0.012 M Glucose or Inosine after preincubation with 3 μmoles of N-ethyl maleimide (NEM) per ml of erythrocytes or with phosphate-buffered sodium chloride solution (Untreated).

The data obtained in a representative experiment are shown in FIGURES 6 and 7 and TABLE 1. The concentration of GSH was reduced to near zero by preincubation with NEM and remained negligible during the subsequent 22½ hours of incubation (FIGURE 6). The concentration of GSH was reduced from 77 mg per 100 ml of erythrocytes in the whole blood to 58 mg per 100 ml by treatment with nitrite alone. During incubation without substrate, a further decline in the concentration of GSH occurred in erythrocytes not preincubated with NEM. Regeneration of GSH, however, did occur upon incubation with 0.012 M glucose or inosine. The rate of reduction of methemoglobin with glucose as substrate was decreased by about 33 percent in the NEM-treated erythrocytes during the initial 5½ hours of incubation (FIGURE 7). Reduction with inosine was not inhibited significantly by NEM. Utilization of glucose during this period was inhibited by 21 percent by NEM, and the formation of lactate plus pyruvate was decreased by 40 percent (TABLE 1). Utilization of the ribose moiety of

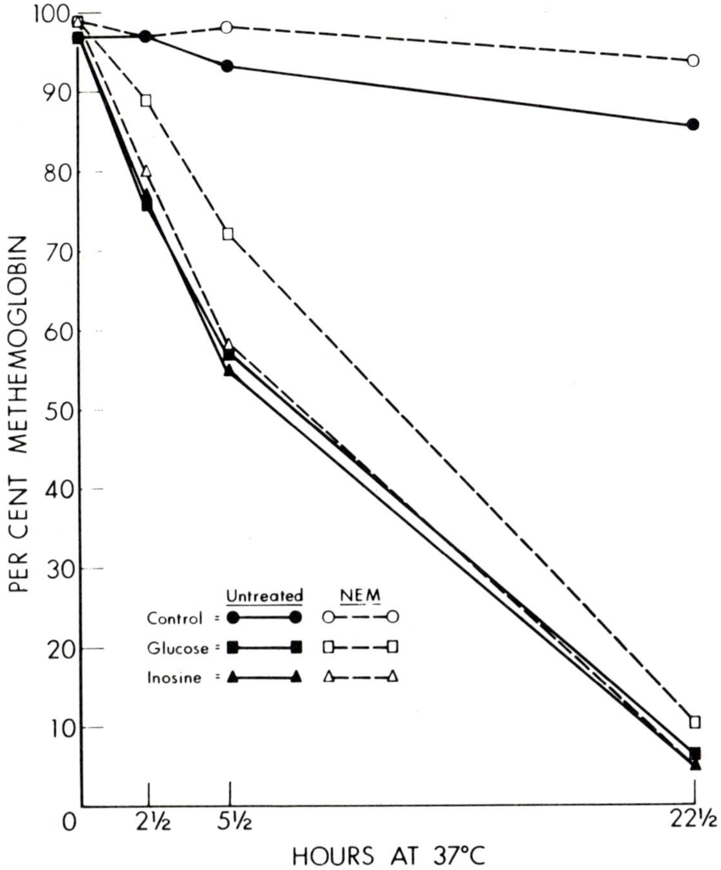

FIGURE 7. Reduction of methemoglobin in the nitrite-treated, normal human erythrocytes under the conditions described in the legend for FIGURE 6.

TABLE 1

UTILIZATION OF GLUCOSE AND RIBOSE OF INOSINE AND PRODUCTION OF LACTATE AND PYRUVATE DURING INCUBATION OF NITRITE-TREATED ERYTHROCYTES AFTER PREINCUBATON WITHOUT AND WITH N-ETHYL MALEIMIDE

	Incubation at 37° C for:					
	5½ hrs μmoles/ml cells		% inhibi-tion	22½ hrs μmoles/ml cells		% inhibi-tion
	Control	NEM*		Control	NEM*	
Glucose utilization	19.9	15.8	21	42.0	35.7	15
Ribose of inosine utilization	35.1	35.8	0	—	—	—
Lactate with glucose	26.6	14.5	45	74.7	58.2	22
Lactate with inosine	48.4	47.0	3	—	—	—
Pyruvate with glucose	1.7	2.6	0	4.2	3.1	26
Pyruvate with inosine	0.1	0.1	0	—	—	—
Lactate + pyruvate with glucose	28.3	17.1	40	78.9	61.3	22
Lactate + pyruvate with inosine	48.5	47.1	3	—	—	—

* Erythrocytes preincubated for 10 minutes with 3 μmoles N-ethyl maleimide per ml of cells.

inosine and the formation of lactate from inosine were not inhibited significantly by treatment of the erythrocytes with NEM. After 22½ hours of incubation, the effects of NEM on glucose utilization, lactate plus pyruvate formation and the reduction of methemoglobin were less striking.

Inhibition of the reduction of methemoglobin by NEM when glucose is the substrate can be explained by inhibition of glycolysis with decreased generation of DPNH, probably secondary to a direct or indirect effect of NEM on the activity of such essential enzymes as hexokinase, aldolase and glyceraldehyde-3-phosphate dehydrogenase.[35] Utilization of the ribose moiety of inosine does not require hexokinase activity and is not impaired by NEM. Essentially normal reduction of methemoglobin, therefore, can occur with inosine. Under the conditions of these experiments, GSH does not appear to be required for the reduction of methemoglobin. These findings also are consistent with the observation that the reduction of methemoglobin in human erythrocytes deficient in glucose-6-phosphate dehydrogenase activity is not impaired.[36]

Conclusions

The ability of human erythrocytes to reduce methemoglobin is determined, primarily, by the level of activity of a DPNH-methemoglobin reductase system, provided that the generation of DPNH is not impaired. The studies reviewed here do not explain the relationship between the formation of methemoglobin and the destruction of human erythrocytes upon exposure to certain drugs. Toxic methemoglobinemia may actually result more from the combined effects of enhanced oxidation of hemoglobin and excessive demands on protective mechanisms, the 'a-b' of FIGURE 1, than from inhibition of the pathways for the reduction of methemoglobin. Impairment of the glycolytic activity of erythrocytes by drugs or their metabolites, however, may inhibit both the protective mechanisms and the means for reduction of methemoglobin. In toxic methemoglobinemia associated with hemolysis, the formation of methemoglobin may take place coincidentally with irreversible alterations in essential structural components of the erythrocyte membrane that actually lead to hemolysis. Except for the decreased oxygen-carrying capacity of the blood and, under certain conditions, an alteration in the oxygen dissociation curve of hemoglobin,[9] the presence of methemoglobin by itself does not appear to have an adverse effect on the function and survival of human erythrocytes.

References

1. FINCH, C. A. 1948. Methemoglobinemia and sulfhemoglobinemia. New Engl. J. Med. **239:** 470.
2. BODANSKY, O. 1951. Methemoglobinemia and methemoglobin-producing compounds. Pharmacol. Rev. **3:** 144.
3. KIESE, M. 1966. The biochemical production of ferrihemoglobin-forming derivatives from aromatic amines, and mechanisms of ferrihemoglobin formation. Pharmacol. Rev. **18:** 1091.
4. MILLS, G. C. 1959. The purification and properties of glutathione peroxidase of erythrocytes. J. Biol. Chem. **234:** 502.
5. COHEN, G. & P. HOCHSTEIN. 1963. Glutathione peroxidase: The primary agent for the elimination of hydrogen peroxide in erythrocytes. Biochemistry (Wash.) **2:** 1420.
6. AEBI, H., J. P. HEININGER & E. LAUBER. 1964. Methämoglobinbildung in Erythrocyten durch Peroxideinwirkung. Versuche zur Beurteilung der Schutzfunktion von Katalase und Glutathionperoxidase. Helv. Chim. Acta **47:** 1428.
7. JAFFÉ, E. R. 1964. Metabolic processes involved in the formation and reduction of methemoglobin in human erythrocytes. *In* The Red Blood Cell. C. Bishop & D. M. Surgenor, Eds. : 397–422. Academic Press. N. Y. & Lond.

8. JAFFÉ, E. R. & P. HELLER. 1964. Methemoglobinemia in man. *In* Progress in Hematology. C. V. Moore & E. B. Brown, Eds. **4**: 48–71. Grune & Stratton, N. Y.
9. JAFFÉ, E. R. 1966. Hereditary methemoglobinemias associated with abnormalities in the metabolism of erythrocytes. Am. J. Med. **41**: 786.
10. SCOTT, E. M., I. W. DUNCAN & V. EKSTRAND. 1965. The reduced pyridine nucleotide dehydrogenases of human erythrocytes. J. Biol. Chem. **240**: 481.
11. SASS, M. D., C. J. CARUSO & M. FARHANGI. 1966. First case of TPNH-methemoglobin reductase deficiency. Blood **28**: 989.
12. JAFFÉ, E. R. 1968. DPNH-methemoglobin reductase (diaphorase). *In* Biochemical Methods in Red Cell Genetics. J. J. Yunis, Ed. : In press. Academic Press, N. Y. & Lond.
13. JAFFÉ, E. R., G. NEUMANN, H. ROTHBERG, F. T. WILSON, R. M. WEBSTER & J. A. WOLFF. 1966. Hereditary methemoglobinemia with and without mental retardation. A study of three families. Am. J. Med. **41**: 42.
14. GIBSON, Q. H. 1948. The reduction of methaemoglobin in red blood cells and studies on the cause of idiopathic methaemoglobinaemia. Biochem. J. **42**: 13.
15. JAFFÉ, E. R. 1959. The reduction of methemoglobin in human erythrocytes incubated with purine nucleosides. J. Clin. Invest. **38**: 1555.
16. SCOTT, E. M. & I. V. GRIFFITH. 1959. The enzymic defect of hereditary methemoglobinemia: diaphorase. Biochim. Biophys. Acta **34**: 584.
17. KÜNZER, W. & D. SCHNEIDER. 1953. Zur Aktivität der reduzierenden Fermentsysteme in den Erythrozyten junger Säuglinge. Acta Haematol. (Basel) **9**: 346.
18. LEE, W. M., F. E. BRAGG, II & E. R. JAFFÉ. 1967. Reduction of methemoglobin in human adult and cord blood erythrocytes incubated with glucose or inosine. Proc. Soc. Exptl. Biol. Med. **124**: 214.
19. ROSS, J. D. 1963. Deficient activity of DPNH-dependent methemoglobin diaphorase in cord blood erythrocytes. Blood **21**: 51.
20. MCDONALD, C. D., JR. & T. H. J. HUISMAN. 1962. A comparative study of enzymic activities in normal adult and cord blood erythrocytes as related to the reduction of methemoglobin. Clin. Chim. Acta **7**: 555.
21. KRAVITZ, H., L. D. ELEGANT, E. KAISER & B. M. KAGAN. 1956. Methemoglobin values in premature and mature infants and children. Am. J. Diseases Children **91**: 1.
22. CAWEIN, M., C. H. BEHLEN, II, E. J. LAPPAT & J. E. COHN. 1964. Hereditary diaphorase deficiency and methemoglobinemia. Arch. Internal Med. **113**: 578.
23. FIALKOW, P. J., J. A. BROWDER, R. S. SPARKES & A. G. MOTULSKY. 1965. Mental retardation in methemoglobinemia due to diaphorase deficiency. New Engl. J. Med. **273**: 840.
24. WENNER, C. E., D. F. DUNN & S. WEINHOUSE. 1953. A study of glucose oxidation in whole tissue homogenates. J. Biol. Chem. **205**: 409.
25. JAFFÉ, E. R. & G. NEUMANN. 1966. Effect of increased DPN content on the reduction of methemoglobin in human erythrocytes. Federation Proc. **25**: 704b.
26. JAFFÉ, E. R. & G. NEUMANN. 1965. The synthesis of pyridine nucleotides in fresh and stored human erythrocytes. Transfusion **5**: 412.
27. STRÖMME, J. H. & L. ELDJARN. 1962. The role of the pentose phosphate pathway in the reduction of methaemoglobin in human erythrocytes. Biochem. J. **84**: 406.
28. JACOB, H. S. & J. H. JANDL. 1966. Effects of sulfhydryl inhibition on red blood cells. III. Glutathione in the regulation of the hexose monophosphate pathway. J. Biol. Chem. **241**: 4243.
29. MORELL, S. A., V. E. AYERS, T. J. GREENWALT & P. HOFFMAN. 1964. Thiols of the erythrocyte. I. Reaction of N-ethylmaleimide with intact erythrocytes. J. Biol. Chem. **239**: 2696.
30. BEUTLER, E. 1957. The glutathione instability of drug-sensitive red cells. A new method for the *in vitro* detection of drug sensitivity. J. Lab. Clin. Med. **49**: 84.
31. EVELYN, K. A. & H. T. MALLOY. 1938. Microdetermination of oxyhemoglobin, methemoglobin, and sulfhemoglobin in a single sample of blood. J. Biol. Chem. **126**: 655.
32. MEJBAUM, W. 1939. Über die Bestimmung kleiner Pentosemengen, insbesondere in Derivaten der Adenylsäure. Z. Physiol. Chem. **258**: 117.
33. BARKER, S. B. & W. H. SUMMERSON. 1941. The colorimetric determination of lactic acid in biological material. J. Biol. Chem. **138**: 535.
34. FRIEDEMANN, T. E. & G. E. HAUGEN. 1943. Pyruvic acid. II. The determination of keto acids in blood and urine. J. Biol. Chem. **147**: 415.
35. JACOB, H. S. & J. H. JANDL. 1962. Effects of sulfhydryl inhibition on red blood cells. I. Mechanism of hemolysis. J. Clin. Invest. **41**: 779.
36. JAFFÉ, E. R. 1963. The reduction of methemoglobin in erythrocytes of a patient with congenital methemoglobinemia, subjects with erythrocyte glucose-6-phosphate dehydrogenase deficiency, and normal individuals. Blood **21**: 561.

DISCUSSION OF THE PAPER

DR. MOTULSKY (*University of Washington*): I would like to mention a case that was studied recently by Drs. Finch and Rittrisen in Seattle which may be of interest in view of what has been said. This was a soldier of white extraction with a glucose-6-phosphate dehydrogenase deficiency who was given a test dose of primaquine. He developed a severe methemoglobenemia (35–40% methemoglobin) and mild hemolysis as shown by a reticulocytosis and a shortened red cell life according to chromium 51 studies.

Further analyses showed that he had about 20% of the mean activity of glutathione reductase. So here there is a peculiar coincidence of possibly two defects, a not too severe one of methemoglobin reductase and one of glutathione reductase, the combination producing a severe methemoglobenemia.

Later, he was rechallenged with a test dose of primaquine and again the same course of events occurred.

DR. JAFFE: Thank you, Dr. Motulsky. We've speculated on this happening but have not yet had the opportunity to find such a patient.

DRUGS, ANESTHESIA AND ABNORMAL HEMOGLOBINS*

A. G. Motulsky and G. Stamatoyannopoulos
Departments of Medicine and Genetics
University of Washington
Seattle, Wash.

Introduction

Since hemoglobin is the main constituent of the red cell, it is not surprising that genetically determined alterations of this pigment predispose to red cell disease induced by various environmental agents. The role of red cell enzyme abnormalities in the pathogenesis of hemolytic anemia and methemoglobinemia has been discussed earlier in this Annal. Since red cell destruction and methemoglobinemia ultimately are associated with changes in hemoglobin, one might expect genetically altered hemoglobins to have similar consequences.

No other mammalian protein is as well understood from both the genetic and biochemical points of view as is hemoglobin. Adult hemoglobin synthesis is under the principal control of two nonlinked genes, one coding for the hemoglobin alpha and the other for the hemoglobin beta chain. The functional hemoglobin molecule is a tetramer comprised of two alpha and two beta chains; each chain is associated with a nonprotein heme group. The three dimensional structure of hemoglobin has been elucidated by the brilliant crystallographic work of Perutz and his group.[1] These results, and knowledge of the amino acid sequence of the hemoglobin chains has allowed the construction of three-dimensional models of hemoglobin.[2,3]

Most variant hemoglobins differ from the normal by a single amino acid substitution.[4,5] Understanding of the genetic code has revealed that all mutational amino acid substitutions in hemoglobins could be explained by single base pair changes in DNA codons.[6] Theoretically, every single one of the 141 amino acids of the alpha and of the 146 amino acids of the beta chain could be mutationally altered. Studies of the amino acid sequence of myoglobin and hemoglobin chains in different species have shown a remarkable tolerance for a wide variety of amino acid substitutions. Of the more than 140 amino acids in the myoglobin-hemoglobin chain, only 9 appear to be "invariant", i.e. they occupy structurally identical sites in all myoglobin-hemoglobin chains studied. Most amino acid replacements allow normal function of the molecule.[2,3]

Several classes of mutationally introduced alterations can be distinguished:

1. Mutations substituting amino acids of similar charge for each other. Such mutations are difficult to detect since electrophoretic differences usually do not exist. It has been estimated that over half of all mutations might not lead to alteration in charge.

2. Mutations causing differences in charge but no abnormalities in function. Most of the so-called abnormal hemoglobins detected by hemoglobin electrophoresis fall in this class. In a recent population survey on an unselected Danish and British population, 10 such hemoglobins were found among 8,000 people.[7]

3. Mutations causing molecular instability and interference with function. This class of hemoglobins is of interest to pharmacogenetics and will be dealt with in detail. Two hemoglobins (Hb Freiburg[8] and Hb Gun Hill[9]) classified

* Aided by grant GM 15253 of the National Institutes of Health.

in this category are produced by amino acid deletions rather than by amino acid substitutions. These two hemoglobins probably owe their origin to unequal crossover during meiosis.[8,9]

4. Mutations interfering with the three-dimensional stability of the molecule causing molecular lethality.[3] Since the gene products of such mutations are impossible to detect with current techniques, there is relatively little information about such mutations.

5. Lastly, thalassemias are genetically determined specific depressions of a given hemoglobin chain.[10] Beta-thalassemia is the most common form of thalassemia. The molecular mechanisms of most thalassemias remain unknown. Some thalassemias may owe their origin to molecular lethality as discussed in the previous paragraph. Hb H is an unstable hemoglobin and consists of four normal beta chains; this pigment is found in some cases of α-thalassemia.

Hemoglobins and Anesthesia

The exchange of a valine for a glutamic acid residue in the sixth N terminal position of the beta chain of Hb S[11] has remarkable consequences. During hypoxia, gelling and tactoid formation of Hb S take place and deform the red cell membrane into its characteristic sickled shape.[12] Murayama[13] has suggested that this phenomenon owes its origin to hydrophobic bonding between the N terminal valine residue and the mutationally introduced sixth valine residue. The valyl-valyl bond is said to present a projecting key on the molecule which fits a complementary site of the alpha chain of an adjacent Hb S molecule. Hb S molecules would align linearly, and by head-to-tail stacking produce a Hb S monofilament. In fact, sickled cells orient with their long axes perpendicular to magnetic lines of force while normal cells do not. Since the beta chains but not the alpha chains move closer together on oxygenation,[14,15] complementarity would be lost during oxygenation causing unsickling.

The severity of hypoxia required to produce sickling is proportional to the amount of hemoglobin S present in cells. In sickle trait heterozygotes, only 20–45% of the total pigment is Hb S, and hypoxia must be relatively severe before sickling will occur. In homozygotes for the sickling gene, practically all of the hemoglobin may be of the abnormal variety and a lesser degree of hypoxia will induce the above described changes.

Before, during, and after anesthesia hypoxia may occur. Over-heavy premedication, hypotension, anemia, visceral vessel dilatation with blood stagnation in high spinal analgesia, local stasis from positioning, respiratory depression and tissue depression by hypothermic anesthesia are contributory factors. Administration of ether-air anesthesia is always associated with hypoxemia.[16] Premedication by atropine causes a significant degree of hypoxemia.[17] Nunn and Payne[18] have shown that when a patient is allowed to breathe spontaneously during operation, postoperative hypoxemia occurs, even when minor surgery is performed; in such cases the arterial oxygen saturation falls rapidly after operation when the patient starts breathing room air and remains subnormal as long as twenty-four hours after operation. In one patient, an arterial oxygen tension of 39 mm Hg was recorded, i.e. a tension low enough to cause intravascular sickling. In their study, the mean postoperative arterial oxygen pressure corresponded to that found at an altitude of 10,000 feet. The importance of these findings is evident in view of the well-recognized tendency of sicklers to splenic infarction during high altitude flights in unpressurized aircraft.[19] Furthermore, Conway and Payne[20] have convincingly shown that even in controlled anesthesia, when oxygen at a concentration not greater than that in the atmosphere is administered, hypoxemia occurs during operation; low oxygen saturations are again found postoperatively in the arterial blood, even if respiration during anesthesia has been controlled by moderate hyperventilation. These data make a strong case for the routine postoperative administration of oxygen to all patients with hemoglobin S in their red cells, independently of the duration of the operation or the techniques used for anesthesia.

Sickled red cells cause increased blood viscosity.[21,22] Increased viscosity slows blood flow in small blood vessels causing further hypoxia and further sickling. Sickled cells may interlock with each other and form tumbleweed-type masses in blood vessels producing characteristic small vessel obstruction with symptoms of pains in the abdomen and around joints.[23] Acidosis[24-26] will further increase sickling and may be a factor in certain postanesthetic states. The spleen has a rather unique circulation with a very slow blood flow. Relative hypoxia and the slow circulation make for a vicious cycle which may lead to splenic infarction. Pulmonary infarcts have also been reported.[27,28] Complications [29,30] including acute red cell sequestration and even death[28,31] have been encountered in a number of patients subjected to general anesthesia. Various infarctive processes may be more common in nonanemic sickling states since viscosity on sickling increases with the square of the hematocrit.[22]

The clinical severity of the sickling hemoglobinopathies is related to the rate of increase of blood viscosity during deoxygenation which is largely dependent upon the Hb S concentration.[22] However, if other hemoglobins are present in red cells together with Hb S, modification of the sickling process may be striking. Measuring the rate of viscosity increase on deoxygenation and the minimum concentration of Hb S required for gelation, it appears that Hb D Punjab and Hb C interact more readily with Hb S in producing sickling than do Hb J and Hb A while Hb F is least reactive. Consequently, patients with Hb D-S and C-S combination often show symptoms while patients with Hb A-S and J-S are clinically unaffected unless challenged by fairly severe hypoxia. Patients carrying the genes of hereditary persistence of fetal hemoglobin and Hb S may have 70–80% Hb S in their red cells while the remaining pigment is Hb F and is distributed uniformly throughout their red cells. Red cell life-span in such patients is normal in spite of the high proportion of sickling hemoglobin, and there are no symptoms. In sickle-thalassemia disease where patients also may have 70–90% Hb S, Hb F is unevenly distributed and limited to a few red cells. Most erythrocytes contain mainly Hb S and readily undergo sickling and destruction.

It may be possible in the future to prevent the sickling state by molecular engineering so that drugs and chemicals are used to reverse a genetic lesion. Propane prevents the hydrophobic valyl-valyl bonding by forming hydrophobic bonds with the isopropyl groups of the valyl side chains and thereby blocks intermolecular valyl-valyl interactions.[13] This drug is too toxic for in vivo use, but other agents of this sort may be found. Kosower[32] has suggested that introduction of glutamic acid residues into Hb S might diminish gelling of Hb S and increase its solubility, and has, in fact, achieved these results in vitro by coupling the N-carboxy anhydride of glutamic acid to the N terminal end of the β chain of Hb S molecules. Other approaches such as induction of methemoglobin[33] which also prevents sickling interfere too drastically with the physiologic function of hemoglobin. Initially good results claimed for phenothiazines[34] were not confirmed.[35] Agents such as steroids[36] which appear to interfere with sickling by red cell membrane interaction appear less promising to use therapeutically than those which are based on molecular manipulations.

Unstable Hemoglobins

Unstable hemoglobins are hemoglobin variants which are abnormally labile in vitro as well as in vivo and therefore often associated with a hemolytic syndrome. In fact, most unstable hemoglobins described so far were detected because a patient presented either with chronic hemolytic anemia or with inclusion (Heinz) body anemia following splenectomy, or with acute hemolysis after drug administration. Ten unstable hemoglobins have been fully characterized, most of them within the last year. Their structural characterization is described in TABLE 1. The site in which the chemical lesion is located is shown in FIGURE 1. Various diagnostic and biochemical data are presented in TABLE 2. In addition to the listed variants, several other unstable hemoglobins have been detected in patients with hemolytic anemia.[40,60-64] However, in most cases, only electrophoretic characterization data are available. In Hb Ube I,[61] the abnormality was shown by hybridization to be located on the beta polypeptide chain; fingerprint study did not reveal an abnormal peptide pattern. The SH reactivity of cysteine in position 93 β was stated to be lost in this hemoglobin. However, this finding could be explained by conformational changes induced by the still unknown primary lesion in Hb Ube I. The abnormality in Hb St. Mary's probably resides in the "core" of the beta polypeptide chain.[40] It is likely that most, if not all, of the so-called "congenital Heinz body anemias" are caused by unstable hemoglobins. Hemoglobins with severe instability will be associated with the most severe hemolytic syndrome often making it difficult to demonstrate the presence of the abnormal pigment in such cases.

All patients with unstable hemoglobins have been heterozygotes. It is likely that the presence of these hemoglobins in the homozygote state would be incompatible with life.

Structural Characteristics

The structural data (TABLE 1) indicate that mutations in several sites of the polypeptide chain and different types of lesions may result in molecular instability. Examination of the lesions following the hemoglobin model of Perutz[2,3] indicates that several of the sites involved are of structural importance. In hemoglobins Köln and Sydney internal nonpolar residues which form stabilizing hydrophobic bonds with the porphyrin ring are replaced by residues which are also nonpolar but of different dimensions.[41] This replacement results in alterations in the tertiary structure of the beta chain and molecular instability. In the case of Hb Köln methionine in position 98β might displace the neighboring 97β histidine producing changes in its electric charge.[38] Alterations of the behavior of cysteine in position 93β and histidine in position 92β have also been suggested.[65] This type of replacement of internal nonpolar residues by other nonpolar amino acids of different dimensions may be a usual feature in the chemistry of unstable hemoglobins.[41] Replacements of internal nonpolar by polar residues may be lethal or cause extreme molecular instability, since the nonpolar internal residues together with nonpolar parts of the porphyrin ring are of crucial importance in determining the stability of the polypeptide chain.[3] Such an example of severe instability is found in Hb Hammersmith in which the invariant and nonpolar phenylalanine in position 42 β is replaced by the noncharged but polar serine.[44] Another molecular mechanism leading to instability is seen in Hb Genova,[42] in which proline

TABLE 1

UNSTABLE HEMOGLOBINS – STRUCTURAL DATA

Name and Reference	Chain	Residue No.	Amino Acid Substitution or Deletion	Structural Site Involved*	Significance of Structural Site*
Hb Zürich[37]	β	63	Histadine → Arginine	E7	Invariant.† Distal Histidine.
Hb Köln[38]	β	98	Valine → Methionine	FG5	Invariant in hemoglobins. Van der Waals bond with heme. Hydrogen bond with H23 tyrosine.
Hb Seattle[39, 40]	β	70	Alanine → Glutamic acid	E14‡	Surrounding of the heme group. (contact with the porphyrin ring?)
Hb Sydney[41]	β	67	Valine → Alanine	E11	Invariant with the exception of lamprey hemoglobin. Van der Waals bond with heme.
Hb Genova[42]	β	28	Leucine → Proline	B10	
Hb Tacoma[43]	β	30	Arginine → Serine	B12	Possible non polar contact between α_1 and β_1 chains.
Hb Hammersmith[44]	β	42	Phenylalanine → Serine	CD1	Invariant. Van der Waals bond with heme.
Hb Sinai[45] Seely[46]	α	47	Aspartic acid → Histidine	CD5	
Hb Freiburg[8]	β	23	Valine → 0	B5	
Hb Gun Hill[9]	β	93 to 97	(Cys-Asp-Lys-Leu-His) → 0	F9 to FG4	Region of chain-heme bond and of $\alpha_1\beta_2$ chains contact.

* Derived from Perutz's model (references 2 and 3) – see also FIGURE 1.

† The term invariant refers to the fact that this amino acid is found in structurally identical sites on myoglobins and various normal hemoglobin chains (α, β, γ, δ,) of all species that have been examined.

‡ It is possible that the substitutions aln→glu may affect residue 76 (E20). Structural considerations make this highly unlikely.

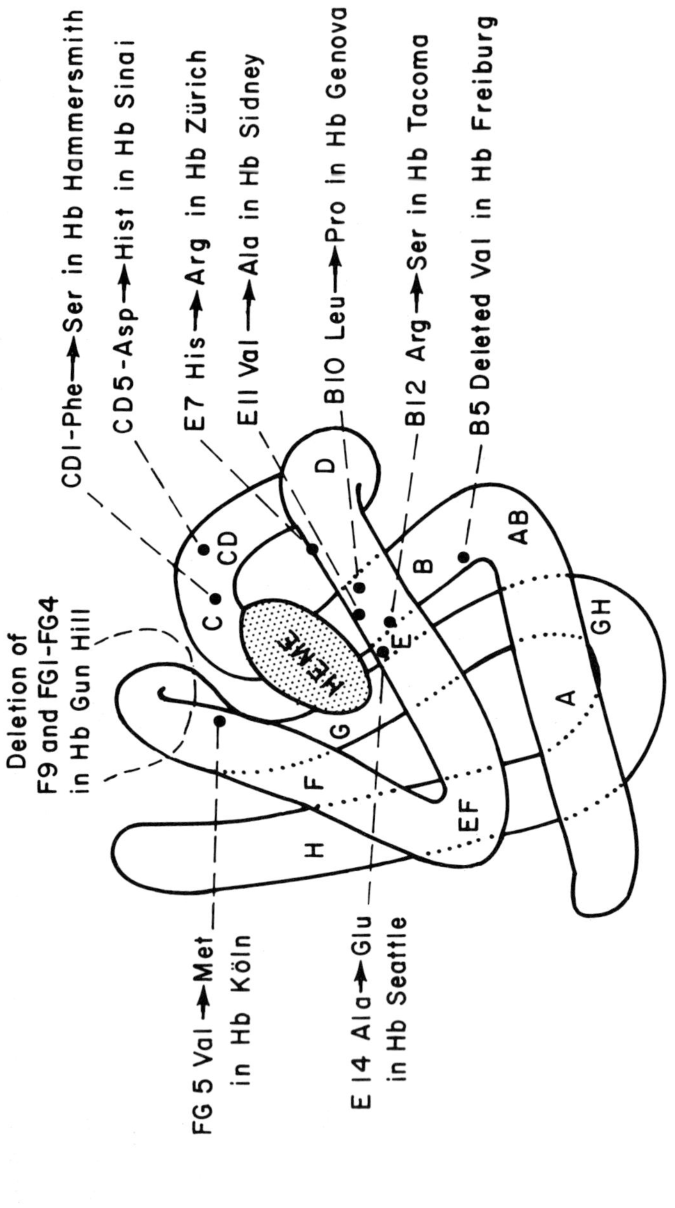

FIGURE 1. Schematic representation of the tertiary configuration of the hemoglobin chain, showing the sites and structural changes in the ten unstable hemoglobins described so far. All substitutions except for that producing Hb Sinai affect the β chain. The significance of the various structural sites is listed on TABLE 1. Possible explanations for instability of these hemoglobins are discussed in the text.

TABLE 2

UNSTABLE HEMOGLOBINS — DIAGNOSTIC CHARACTERISTICS

Name and References	Abnormal Hemoglobin: Electrophoretic Mobility at Alkaline pH	Abnormal Hemoglobin: Percentage	Percentage Hb A_2	Detection of Free α Chains in Hemolysate	Thermal Lability	Heinz bodies in Non-splenectomized Cases*	Accelerated Methemoglobin Formation after Incubation
Hb Zürich[47,48,49]	slow	20–36	2.6–2.9 (48) 3.4–5.4 (49)	not mentioned	yes	yes	yes
Hb Köln[50,51,52]	slow	10–15	normal	not mentioned	yes	yes	yes
Hb Seattle[39,40,53]	fast	43	2.5	yes	yes	yes	yes
Hb Sydney[41,54]	slow	30	not mentioned	yes	yes	yes	not tested
Hb Genova[42,55]	like A	25	normal	yes	yes	yes	not tested
Hb Tacoma[56]	fast	43	3.4–3.6	not mentioned	yes	not tested	no
Hb Hammersmith[44,57,58]	like A	30	3.2	not mentioned	yes	—	yes
Hb Freiburg[8]	slow	27–32	2.5–3.0	no	yes	—	Methemoglobin elevated in fresh blood
Hb Gun Hill[9,59]	slow	20	not mentioned	yes	yes	yes	not mentioned

* The usual "Heinz-body" or "Inclusion" tests using short incubation of whole blood with methyl violet or cresyl blue gives negative results in non-splenectomized patients with unstable hemoglobins. Exception: Cases with Hb Gun Hill[59] and one patient with Hb Köln.[51] In all other instances Heinz-bodies formation has been induced after incubation of blood for 24–48 hours or after challenge by redox compounds.

is found near the middle of the B helix of the polypeptide chain; this amino acid cannot enter the alpha helical sequence and its presence in the middle of a helical portion induces changes in the conformation of the B helix and subsequent molecular instability.

Deletions of structurally important regions of the polypeptide chain or of single amino acids would be another cause for unstable hemoglobins. In fact, both hemoglobins so far found to be due to deletions were also unstable. In Hb Gun Hill[9] structural sites of importance for hydrophobic bonding with the heme group as well as for the $\alpha_1\beta_2$ chains contact are deleted, while in Hb Freiburg[8] deletion of valine in position 23β was sufficient to produce molecular instability. The structural basis for instability in Hb Zürich is not clear. In Hb Tacoma, the fact that the replacement occurs in a site of $\alpha_1\beta_1$ contact may be of importance for the moderate instability observed. In hemoglobin Seattle the substitution involves either residue 70β or residue 76β.[39,40] The position of alanine 70β (E14) in the surroundings of the heme group makes it most probable as a site of substitution in this unstable hemoglobin. It is of interest that of the ten structurally characterized unstable hemoglobins, nine are beta polypeptide chain variants. In the only alpha chain variant described (Hb Sinai) only mild hemoglobin thermolability and mild hemolysis were found.[45]

Intraerythrocytic Precipitation

Because of molecular instability, unstable hemoglobins precipitate within red cells and are subsequently recognized with special staining as Heinz-bodies representing denatured globin. Heinz-bodies were found in the vast majority of cells in all splenectomized patients with unstable hemoglobins while in nonsplenectomized individuals they appear only after prolonged incubation of blood with brilliant cresyl blue or other redox agents (TABLE 2). An explanation for the absence of spontaneous Heinz-bodies in patients with intact spleens is that the precipitated unstable hemoglobin is removed from the red cells during their passage through the spleen. Preferential loss of the unstable hemoglobin in the spleen is suggested by the biosynthetic experiments in cases with Hb Zürich,[49] Gun Hill,[59] and an abnormal hemoglobin shown to be Hb Hammersmith.[58] These experiments indicate that the abnormal hemoglobin is synthesized at a rate at least equal to that of Hb A while its proportion in the peripheral blood is no more than 30%. The increase in the proportion of Hb A_2 measured in cases with hemoglobin Tacoma, St. Mary and in one series of patients with Hb Zürich[49] might only reflect a decrease in the proportion of the major hemoglobin fraction due to removal of the precipitated unstable abnormal pigment. Aggregation and precipitation of the labile beta chains (probably in vitro during handling of the hemolysates) results in excess of α chains which can be detected by electrophoresis in many cases with unstable hemoglobins.[40–42,59]

Methemoglobin Formation

A feature found in most unstable hemoglobins is the accumulation of red cell methemoglobin after prolonged incubation. In fresh-drawn blood, increased methemoglobin levels are found only in Hb Freiburg.[8] Hb Freiburg also has abnormal ferrihemoglobin spectra, and this hemoglobin was first considered as a variant of Hb M associated with hemolytic anemia.[66] The mechanisms which lead to increased oxidation of the unstable hemoglobins are not clear. The abnormality in most variants resides in the surroundings of the heme group (FIGURE

1), an area of great importance for the respiratory function of hemoglobin. Certain substitutions in three sites of this area (in E7: distal histidine, in F8: proximal histidine and in E11) favor the oxidized state of heme iron and are associated with chronic methemoglobinemia and cyanosis. These hemoglobins collectively are known as hemoglobins-M.[67] In two instances unstable hemoglobins and hemoglobins M were the result of replacements at the same structural sites: E7 (63β) distal histidine is replaced by arginine in Hb Zürich and by tyrosine in Hb M Saskatoon[68] while E11 (67β) valine is replaced by alanine in Hb Sydney and by glutamic acid in Hb M Milwaukee-1.[68] Instability in case of hemoglobins M has been postulated[40] but not yet documented.

The methemoglobin formation in hemoglobins M is fairly well explained by the "internal ligand" hypothesis.[68] This concept postulates direct bonding between the side chains of the substituted amino acid and heme iron. Such a molecular mechanism has not yet been postulated for the methemoglobin accumulation in unstable hemoglobins. At present, it is reasonable to consider methemoglobin accumulation in red cells containing unstable hemoglobins (with the exception of Hb Freiburg) as an acceleration of the normal oxidation of heme iron which is due to the alterations in the tertiary structure of the polypeptide chain. In Hb Köln, for example, it has been assumed[51] that the introduction of methionine near the entrance of the "pocket" formed by E and F helices may widen this region and permit entry of water; after deoxygenation, when iron is on the ferro-form, water could more easily occupy the position freed by oxygen, resulting in ferrihemoglobin formation. It is of interest that in Hb Tacoma in which the substitution is far from the heme surroundings, methemoglobin does not accumulate in the red cells after incubation.

Drugs and Unstable Hemoglobins

Several oxidant drugs induce erythrocyte destruction in individuals with deficiency of certain glycolytic enzymes (mainly Glucose-6-phosphate dehydrogenase deficiency) and also in normal persons when higher dosage of the oxidant drug is used.[69] Other drugs, like the nitrites, induce oxidation of hemoglobin without hemolysis. The exact mechanism of drug-induced hemolysis is not yet known; however, a probable series of events could be outlined as follows: oxidant drugs or compounds from their metabolism induce red cell peroxide generation.[70] Red cell glutathione peroxidase eliminates the produced peroxide; however, this reaction utilizes reduced glutathione and accumulates oxidized glutathione. In individuals with abnormalities in enzymes involving GSH or TPNH regeneration, GSH depletion after drug challenge takes place. It can be postulated, however, that GSH depletion will also occur in red cells with normal reduction systems when overwhelming oxidative mechanisms have been initiated by oxidant drugs, and the ability of the normal cell to regenerate GSH is surpassed. The accumulating peroxide, and probably other oxidation products, oxidize hemoglobin to methemoglobin. The next step leading to hemoglobin denaturation is not clear. A possible mechanism could be that GSSG combines with beta hemoglobin polypeptide chains, conformational changes in the Hb molecule are induced, the molecule becomes labile and precipitates within the red cell. The unstable hemoglobins are excellent candidates for oxidative denaturation after challenge by oxidant drugs for a variety of reasons: the inherent instability of the molecule, the tendency of these hemoglobins to oxidation, and the subnormal level of GSH in the red cells already detected in several individuals with unstable hemoglobin.[39,51,54,55,58] Studies of drug-induced hemolysis in unstable hemoglobins will be of great help in understanding the various steps of drug-induced red cell destruction in general.

So far, drug-induced hemolysis has been documented only in the case of Hb Zürich. Hemoglobin Zürich was first detected because two individuals in a Swiss family presented with acute, life-threatening hemolysis after administration of sulfonamides.[47] In a second family detected in Maryland, the hemolytic episodes were not as severe as in the Swiss cases.[49] Careful experiments using red cells of patients with Hb Zürich tagged with Cr^{51} and transfused to normal recipients have been performed by the Swiss investigators to test the susceptibility of erythrocytes in a number of drugs.[47] Sulfisomidine, sulfisoxazole, sulfamethoxypyridazine, sulfadimethoxine, sulfamerazine, and compounds of oxyquinolines (primaquine, etc.) caused fast destruction of red cells containing Hb Zürich. These same drugs are potentially hemolytic compounds for individuals with G6PD deficiency.[69] Experimentation of this sort to test drug sensitivity has not been done with the other unstable hemoglobins. Sulfonamide sensitivity was tested in Hb Sydney by giving one gram of Gantrisin orally and examining the blood four hours after administration for Heinz-bodies formation and rise of reticulocytes.[54] No changes were observed; however, such studies are inadequate for detection of a moderate degree of red cell destruction. In one patient with Hb Köln, hemoglobinuria occurred following a febrile episode during which analgesics had been received.[51] Accelerated red cell destruction is highly likely in this case. However, challenge of the red cells of this individual by one of the drugs received—phenacetine—did not induce red cell hemolysis.[51]

Unstable Hemoglobins in the Thalassemias (Hb α and Hb H)

Two abnormal hemoglobins found in thalassemias, Hb α and hemoglobin H (Hb β_4) are also characterized by molecular instability. Hb α represents alpha chain surplus, secondary to the severe beta chain deficiency in homozygous beta thalassemia.[71–73] Hb H (Hb β_4) represents beta chain surplus secondary to alpha chain deficiency in certain cases of alpha thalassemia. The most likely genetic mechanism for Hb H disease postulates the presence of two different alpha thalassemia genes—one causing severe, the other mild suppression—in such patients.[10] Both Hb α and Hb H have an abnormal quarternary structure since they consist of only one kind of polypeptide chain instead of showing the usual configuration of two pairs of nonidentical chains. While hemoglobin H is naturally found in the tetrameric form,[74] it is not yet known whether Hb α exists naturally as a tetramer. Other physicochemical characteristics of the two hemoglobins have been summarized by Benesch and Benesch[75] and Huehns *et al.*[76,77] In addition to their instability, other interesting properties are their abnormal oxygen equilibria resembling those of myoglobin, the absence of heme-heme interaction and the absence of a Bohr effect.[75,78,79] These findings render Hb α and Hb H valueless as respiratory pigments in blood.

Hb α is an exceedingly labile protein[76,77] which precipitates already within the erythroid precursors in the bone marrow and can be recognized as Heinz bodies in a large proportion of normoblasts in patients with homozygous beta thalassemia.[80] Precipitation of the unstable Hb α leads to in situ death of a large proportion of erythroid precursors—ineffective erythropoiesis.[71–73] Hb α intraerythrocytic precipitates are of further significance in causing the hemolytic syndrome in homozygous beta thalassemia either through damage of the erythrocyte membrane or by other as yet unrecognized mechanisms.

Compared to Hb α, the milder instability of Hb H permits better erythrocyte survival and subsequently, a clinical picture of milder disease; precipitation of Hb H in situ in the bone marrow red cell precursors is less apparent and ineffective erythropoiesis less severe than in homozygous beta thalassemia. Hemoglobin H in the red cell or in solution precipitates rapidly after oxidation.[18,82] Potentially oxidant drugs given to persons with Hb H disease may enhance hemolysis by inducing oxidation and intraerythrocytic precipitation of this unstable hemoglobin. In fact, Heinz-body formation has been achieved in vitro by challenging Hb H-containing red cells by sulfisoxazole in patients showing in vivo hemolytic episodes related to sulfisoxazole administration.[81] Hb H (β_4) shows most of the features of the unstable hemoglobins caused by single amino acid substitutions. Drug hemolysis induced by various oxidant drugs could be expected particularly in those patients with relatively large amounts of Hb H.

Note added in proof. After this paper was submitted for publication, two new unstable hemoglobins affecting the α chain have been reported. In Hb Torino, the internal nonpolar 43α (CDI) phenylalanine is substituted by nonpolar valine residue which, however, has different dimensions and lower efficiency in hydrophobic bonding.[83] In Hb Bibba, proline substitutes leucine at residue 136α, near the end of helix H.[84] Both hemoglobins Torino and Bibba are characterized by Heinz body formation and presence of increased methemoglobin in fresh blood (12.3% in Hb Bibba, 4.7% in Hb Torino). Drug sensitivity was definitely associated with presence of Hb Torino: the propositus had an acute hemolytic episode after treatment with a sulfonamide derivative and during that episode up to 60% of the circulated red blood cells contained precipitated hemoglobin.

Summary

Genetically altered hemoglobins are of pharmacogenetic interest in two general areas.

1. Red cells containing Hb S may be induced to take on a sickled shape under conditions of hypoxia. Intravascular sickling may have serious physiologic consequences. The most frequent iatrogenic cause of hypoxia is the anesthetic state. Recent studies suggest that hypoxia is frequently encountered after anesthesia. The various mechanisms favoring sickling and the possible role of drugs and chemicals in the prevention of sickling are discussed.

2. Red cells containing so-called unstable hemoglobins usually have a shortened life span and are particularly vulnerable to further destruction by oxidant drugs. Unstable hemoglobins fit into two categories: a. hemoglobins with amino acid substitutions or deletions affecting structurally important sites of a polypeptide chain; b. hemoglobins with abnormal quarternary structure such as Hb H (Hb β_4) or Hb α. The structure and various properties of the unstable hemoglobins are discussed with particular reference to possible deleterious drug action.

References

1. Perutz, M. F., M. G. Rossmann, A. F. Cullis, H. Muirhead, G. Will & A. C. T. North. 1960. Structure of haemoglobin. Nature **185:** 416.
2. Perutz, M. F. 1965. Structure and function of haemoglobin. I. A tentative atomic model of horse oxyhaemoglobin. J. Mol. Biol. **13:** 646.
3. Perutz, M. F., J. C. Kendrew & H. C. Watson. 1965. Structure and function of haemoglobin II. Some relations between polypeptide chain configuration and amino acid sequence. J. Mol. Biol. **13:** 669.
4. Ingram, V. M. 1963. The Hemoglobins in Genetics and Evolution. Columbia Univ. Press, N. Y.

5. BAGLIONI, C. 1963. Correlations between genetics and chemistry of human hemoglobins. *In*: Molecular Genetics. J. H. Taylor, Ed. : 405. Academic Press, N. Y.
6. BEALE, D. & H. LEHMANN. 1965. Abnormal haemoglobins and the genetic code. Nature **207:** 259.
7. SICK, K., D. BEALE, D. IRVINE, H. LEHMANN, P. T. GOODALL & S. MCDOUGALL. 1967. Haemoglobin G Copenhagen and Haemoglobin J Cambridge. Two new β chain variants of haemoglobin A. Biochim. Biophys. Acta **140:** 231.
8. JONES, R. T., B. BRIMHALL, T. H. J. HUISMAN, E. KLEIHAUER & K. BETKE. 1966. Hemoglobin Freiburg: Abnormal hemoglobin due to deletion of a single amino acid residue. Science **154:** 1024.
9. BRADLEY, T. B., R. C. WOHL & R. F. RIEDER. 1967. Hemoglobin Gun Hill: Deletion of five amino acid residues and impaired heme-globin binding. Science **157:** 1581.
10. MOTULSKY, A. G. 1964. Current concepts of the genetics of the thalassemias. Cold Spring Harbor Symp. on Quant. Biol. **29:** 399.
11. INGRAM, V. M. 1957. Gene mutations in human haemoglobin: The chemical difference between normal and sickle-cell haemoglobin. Nature **180:** 326.
12. HARRIS, J. W. 1959. The role of physical and chemical factors in the sickling phenomenon. *In* Progress in Haematology. L. Tocantins, Ed. **II:** 47. Grune & Stratton, N. Y.
13. MURAYAMA, M. 1966. Molecular mechanism of red cell sickling. Science **153:** 145.
14. MUIRHEAD, H. & M. F. PERUTZ. 1963. Structure of haemoglobin. A three-dimensional Fourier synthesis of reduced human haemoglobin at 5.5 Å resolution. Nature **199:** 633.
15. PERUTZ, M. F., W. BOLTON, R. DIAMOND, H. MUIRHEAD & H. C. WATSON. 1964. Structure of haemoglobin. An X-ray examination of reduced horse haemoglobin. Nature **203:** 687.
16. KULHIA, Y. 1961. Hypoxaemia in Ether Anesthesia. Helsinki.
17. TOMLIN, P. J., C. M. CONWAY & J. P. PAYNE. 1964. Hypoxaemia due to atropine. Lancet **1:** 14.
18. NUNN, J. F. & J. P. PAYNE. 1962. Hypoxaemia after general anaesthesia. Lancet **2:** 631.
19. ROTTER, R., W. L. LUTTGENS, W. L. PETERSON, A. E. STOCK & A. G. MOTULSKY. 1956. Splenic infarction in sicklemia during airplane flight: Pathogenesis, hemoglobin analysis and clinical features of six cases. Ann. Int. Med. **44:** 257.
20. CONWAY, C. M. & J. P. PAYNE. 1964. Hypoxaemia associated with anaesthesia and controlled respiration. Lancet **1:** 12.
21. HARRIS, J. W. 1950. Studies on the destruction of red blood cells. VIII. Molecular orientation in sickle-cell hemoglobin solutions. Proc. Soc. Exper. Biol. & Med. **75:** 197.
22. CHARACHE, S. & C. L. CONLEY. 1964. Rate of sickling of red cells during deoxygenation of blood from persons with various sickling disorders. Blood **24:** 25.
23. DIGGS, L. W. 1965. Sickle cell crises. Am. J. Clin. Path. **44:** 1.
24. LANGE, R. D., V. MINNICH & C. V. MOORE. 1951. Effect of oxygen tension and of pH on the sickling and mechanical fragility of erythrocytes from patients with sickle-cell anemia and the sickle-cell trait. J. Lab. Clin. Med. **37:** 789.
25. GREENBERG, M. S., E. H. KASS & W. B. CASTLE. 1957. Studies on the destruction of red blood cells. XII. Factors influencing the role of S hemoglobin in the pathologic physiology of sickle-cell anemia and related disorders. J. Clin. Invest. **36:** 833.
26. GREENBERG, M. S. & E. H. KASS. 1958. Studies on the destruction of red blood cells. XIII. Observations on the role of pH in the pathogenesis and treatment of painful crisis in sickle-cell disease. A.M.A. Arch. Int. Med. **101:** 355.
27. RAHIMTOOLA, S., C. J. GOOD & P. D. B. DAVIES. 1960. Pulmonary infarction in disorders associated with the sickle-cell trait. Thorax **15:** 320.
28. GILBERTSON, A. A. 1965. Anaesthesia in West African patients with sickle-cell anaemia, haemoglobin SC disease and sickle-cell trait. Brit. J. Anaesth. **37:** 614.
29. SHAPIRO, N. D. & M. F. POE. 1955. Sickle-cell disease: An anesthesiological problem. Anesthesiology **16:** 771.
30. LEWIN, P. & R. A. GOODELL. 1962. Postoperative blindness, with complete recovery, in a patient with sickle-cell anaemia. Brit. Med. J. **2:** 1373.
31. CILIBERTI, B. J., V. D. B. MAZZIA & L. C. MARK. 1962. Clinical anesthesia conference: Sickle-cell disease and anesthesia. N. Y. St. J. Med. **65:** 548.
32. KOSOWER, E. M., N. S. KOSOWER & P. C. LA COURSE. 1967. The solubilization of deoxyhemoglobin S. Proc. Nat. Acad. Sci. **57:** 39.
33. BEUTLER, E. & B. J. MIKUS. 1961. The effect of methemoglobin formation in sickle-cell disease. J. Clin. Invest. **40:** 1856.
34. HATHORN, M. & R. A. LEWIS. 1966. Inhibition of sickling by phenothiazines. Effect on red cell survival. Brit. J. Haemat. **12:** 195.

35. PEARSON, H. A. & W. D. NOYES. 1967. Failure of phenothiazines in sickle-cell anemia. J.A.M.A. **199:** 33.
36. ISAACS, W. A. & F. G. J. HAYHOE. 1967. Steroid hormones in sickle cell disease. Nature **215:** 1139.
37. MULLER, C. J. & S. KINGMA. 1961. Haemoglobin Zürich: $\alpha_2{}^A\beta_2{}^{63\ Arg.}$ Biochim. Biophys. Acta **50:** 595.
38. CARRELL, R. W., H. LEHMANN & H. E. HUTCHISON. 1966. Haemoglobin Köln (β-98 Valine→Methionine): An unstable protein causing inclusion-body anaemia. Nature **210:** 915.
39. HUEHNS, E. R., F. HECHT, J. HARTMAN & A. G. MOTULSKY. 1968. Hemoglobin Seattle ($\alpha_2{}^A\beta_2{}^{70\ or\ 76\ Glu}$) an unstable hemoglobin variant causing chronic hemolytic anemia in the heterozygous state. In press.
40. HUEHNS, E. R. & E. M. SHOOTER. 1965. Human Haemoglobins. J. Med. Genet. **2:** 48.
41. CARRELL, R. W., H. LEHMANN, P. A. LORKIN, E. RAIK & E. HUNTER. 1967. Haemoglobin Sydney: β67 (E11) Valine→Alanine: An emerging pattern of unstable haemoglobins. Nature **215:** 626.
42. SANSONE, G., R. W. CARRELL & H. LEHMANN. 1967. Haemoglobin Genova: β28 (B10) Leucine→Proline. Nature **214:** 877.
43. JONES, R. T., E. BAUER & B. BRIMHALL. Unpublished data.
44. DACIE, J. V., N. K. SHINTON, P. J. GAFFNEY, JR., R. W. CARRELL & H LEHMANN. 1967. Haemoglobin Hammersmith: [β42(CD1)phe→ser]. Nature **216:** 663.
45. CHARACHE, S. & A. M. MONDZAC. 1967. Hemoglobin Sinai ($\alpha_2{}^{47\ His}\beta_2$): an unstable hemoglobin causing occult hemolysis. Blood **30:** 879.
46. SCHNEIDER, R. G., S. UEDA, J. B. ALPERIN, B. BRIMHALL & R. T. JONES. 1968. Haemoglobin Sealy ($\alpha_2{}^{47\ His}\beta_2$) a new variant in a Jewish family. Am. J. Human Genet. **20:** 151.
47. FRICK, P. G., W. H. HITZIG & K. BETKE. 1962. Hemoglobin Zürich. I. A new hemoglobin anomaly associated with acute hemolytic episodes with inclusion bodies after sulfonamide therapy. Blood **20:** 261.
48. BACHMANN, F. & H. R. MARTI. 1962. Hemoglobin Zürich. II. Physicochemical properties of the abnormal hemoglobin. Blood **20:** 272.
49. RIEDER, R. F., W. H. ZINKHAM & N. A. HOLTZMAN. 1965. Hemoglobin Zürich. Clinical, chemical, and kinetic studies. Am. J. Med. **39:** 4.
50. HUTCHISON, H. E., P. H. PINKERTON, P. WATERS, A. S. DOUGLAS, H. LEHMANN & D. BEALE. 1964. Hereditary Heinz-body anemia, thrombocytopenia, and hemoglobinopathy (Hb Köln) in a Glasgow family. Brit. Med. J. **2:** 1099.
51. JONES, R. V., A. J. GRIMES, R. W. CARRELL & H. LEHMANN. 1967. Köln haemoglobinopathy. Further data and a comparison with other hereditary Heinz-body anaemias. Brit. J. Haemat. **13:** 394.
52. JACKSON, J. M., B. J. WAY & H. J. WOODLIFF. 1967. A West Australian family with a haemolytic disorder associated with haemoglobin Köln. Brit. J. Haemat. **13:** 474.
53. HUEHNS, E. R. 1965. Abnormal haemoglobins causing haemolytic anemia. Proc. Royal Soc. Med. **58:** 514.
54. RAIK, E., E. G. HUNTER & D. A. LINDSAY. 1967. Compensated hereditary haemolytic disease resulting from an unstable haemoglobin fraction. Med. J. Austr. **I:** 955.
55. SANSONE, G. & C. PIK. 1965. Familial haemolytic anaemia with erythrocyte inclusion bodies, bilifuscinuria and abnormal haemoglobin (Haemoglobin Galliera Genova). Brit. J. Haemat. **11:** 511.
56. BAUR, E. W. & A. G. MOTULSKY. 1965. Haemoglobin Tacoma. A beta-chain variant associated with increased Hb A_2. Humangenetik **1:** 621.
57. GRIMES, A. J. & A. MEISLER. 1962. Possible cause of Heinz bodies in congenital Heinz-body anemia. Nature **194:** 190.
58. GRIMES, A. J., A. MEISLER & J. V. DACIE. 1964. Congenital Heinz body anemia. Further evidence on the cause of Heinz-body production in red cells. Brit. J. Haemat. **10:** 281.
59. BRADLEY, T. B. & R. F. RIEDER. 1966. Hemoglobin Gun Hill, a beta chain abnormality associated with a hemolytic state. Blood **28:** 975.
60. SCOTT, J. L., A. HAUT, G. E. CARTWRIGHT & M. M. WINTROBE. 1960. Congenital hemolytic disease associated with red cell inclusion bodies, abnormal pigment metabolism, and an electrophoretic hemoglobin abnormality. Blood **16:** 1239.
61. SHIBATA, S., I. IUCHI, T. MIYAJI, S. UEDA & I. TAKEDA. 1963. Hemolytic disease associated with the production of abnormal hemoglobin and intraerythrocytic Heinz bodies. Acta Haem. Jap. **26:** 164.

62. Dacie, J. V., A. J. Grimes, A. Meisler, L. Steingold, E. H. Hemsted, G. H. Beaven & J. C. White. 1964. Hereditary Heinz-body anemia. A report of studies on five patients with mild anemia. Brit. J. Haemat. **10:** 388.
63. Goudemand, M., G. Biserte, D. Habay & D. Voisin. 1964. Hémoglobine anormale et anémie hémolytique familiale avec inclusions érythrocytaires et urines noires. Nouv. Rev. Franc. Hemat. **4:** 487.
64. Svensson, B. & L. Strand. 1967. A Swedish family with haemolytic anaemia, Heinz bodies and an abnormal hemoglobin. Scand. J. Haemat. **4:** 241.
65. Jacob, H. S., M. C. Brain & J. V. Dacie. 1967. Blockade of membrane and globin thiols in the pathogenesis of congenital Heinz-body hemolytic anemia (CHBHA) with dipyrroluria. J. Clin. Invest. **46:** 1073.
66. Betke, K., L. Heilmeyer, T. H. J. Huisman & E. Kleihauer. 1960. Abstracts of the IX Congress of Internatl. Soc. Hematol. Mexico City.
67. Heller, P. 1966. Hemoglobinopathic dysfunction of the red cell. Am. J. Med. **41:** 799.
68. Gerald, P. S. & M. L. Efron. 1961. Chemical studies of several varieties of haemoglobin M. Proc. Nat. Acad. Sci. **47:** 1758.
69. Beutler, E. 1966. Glucose-6-phosphate dehydrogenase deficiency. *In* Metabolic Basis of Inherited Disease. J. B. Stanbury, J. B. Wyngaarden & D. S. Frederickson, Eds. : 1061. McGraw-Hill, N. Y.
70. Cohen, G. & P. Hochstein. 1964. Generation of hydrogen peroxide in erythrocytes by hemolytic agents. Biochemistry **3:** 895.
71. Fessas, P. 1965. Forms of thalassemia. *In* Abnormal Hemoglobins in Africa, A Symposium. J. H. P. Jonxis, Ed : 71. Blackwell, Oxford.
72. Fessas, P. 1966. The disturbance of hemoglobin synthesis in thalassemia. *In* International Symposium on Comparative Hemoglobin Structure, Thessaloniki. D. J. Polychronakos, Ed. : 51. Triantaphylou, Thessaloniki.
73. Nathan, D. G. & R. B. Gunn. 1966. Thalassemia: The consequences of unbalanced hemoglobin synthesis. Am. J. Med. **41:** 815.
74. Jones, R. T., W. A. Schroeder, J. A. Balog & J. R. Vinograd. 1959. Gross structure of hemoglobin H. J. Amer. Chem. Soc. **81:** 3161.
75. Benesch, R. & R. E. Benesch. 1964. Properties of haemoglobin H and their significance in relation to function of haemoglobin. Nature **202:** 773.
76. Huehns, E. R., E. M. Shooter, N. Dance, G. H. Beaven & K. V. Shooter. 1961. Haemoglobin α^A. Nature **192:** 1057.
77. Huehns, E. R., N. Dance, E. M. Shooter & G. H. Beaven. 1962. The preparation and properties of haemoglobin α^A, a haemoglobin consisting of α^A polypeptide chains. J. Mol. Biol. **5:** 511.
78. Briehl, R. W. & H. M. Ranney. 1964. Oxygen equilibria of the subunits of hemoglobin. J. Clin. Invest. **43:** 1279.
79. Tyuma, I., R. E. Benesch & R. Benesch. 1966. The preparation and properties of the isolated α and β subunits of hemoglobin A. Biochemistry **5:** 2957.
80. Fessas, P. 1963. Inclusions of hemoblobin in erythroblasts and erythrocytes of thalassemia. Blood **21:** 21.
81. Rigas, D. A. & R. D. Koler. 1961. Decreased erythrocyte survival in hemoglobin H disease as a result of the abnormal properties of hemoglobin H: The benefit of splenectomy. Blood **18:** 1.
82. Gabuzda, T. G., M. T. Laforet & F. H. Gardner. 1967. Oxidative precipitation of hemoglobin H and its relation to reduced glutathione. J. Lab. Clin. Med. **70:** 581.
83. Beretta, A., V. Prato, E. Gallo & H. Lehmann. 1968. Haemoglobin Torino – α^{43} (CDl) Phenylalanine → Valine. Nature **217:** 1016.
84. Kleihauer, E. F., C. A. Raynolds, A. M. Dozy, J. B. Wilson, R. R. Moores, M. P. Berenson, C. S. Wright & T. H. J. Huisman. 1968. Hemoglobin Bibba ($\alpha_2{}^{136\mathrm{Pro}}\beta_2$), an unstable abnormal hemoglobin. Biochim. Biophys. Acta **154:** 220.

DISCUSSION OF THE PAPER

Dr. E. R. Jaffe (*Albert Einstein College of Medicine, N. Y.*): Since Dr. Motulsky helped me by adding supporting clinical information to my discussion, I would like to add a little information on Hemoglobin Gun Hill. I hope that Dr. Bradley will not be offended by my presentation of some of his studies, but the report has just appeared in Science.* Hemoglobin Gun Hill apparently has in-

* Science 1967, **157:** 1581–1583.

creased oxygen binding properties so that a tube of blood from the patient remains bright red in the refrigerator for several days, while normal blood becomes dark from formation of reduced hemoglobin. Although a Wright's stained smear of peripheral blood appears normal, the indices calculated from the hemoglobin concentration and the packed erythrocyte volume would suggest hypochromia because of loss of the heme group from the abnormal beta chain. This abnormal hemoglobin with deletion of five amino acids in the beta chain somewhere between residues 91 and 97 is associated with a well compensated hemolytic process and altered oxygen binding capacity. This hemoglobinopathy, therefore, is expressed with both an altered function and increased hemolysis.

ACETOPHENETIDIN-INDUCED METHEMOGLOBINEMIA*

N. T. Shahidi

Department of Pediatrics
University of Wisconsin
Madison, Wisc.

Introduction

Methemoglobinemia and hemolysis following the ingestion of some drugs have been the subject of extensive investigation. Most studies however, have been focused on the erythrocytes and little is known about the products of biotransformation of the drugs involved. Acetophenetidin, a well-known analgesic and antipyretic has often been incriminated in producing methemoglobinemia and hemolysis.[1–5] While in some cases an intrinsic erythrocyte defect has been demonstrated,[2] in others, there has been no valid explanation as to the mechanism of acetophenetidin toxicity and an overdosage has been advocated.[3] In addition to the hematological changes mentioned above, acetophenetidin may result in significant kidney damage known as "interstitial nephritis." This complication is usually associated with long-term acetophenetidin intake.

Recently, we had the opportunity to study the metabolism of acetophenetidin in a 16-year-old female who developed, on several occasions, severe methemoglobinemia and hemolysis following acetophenetidin intake. This report will comprise the result of our investigation on the patient and her family.

Clinical History and Initial Laboratory Investigation

The patient, a 17-year-old white female was admitted to the Children's Hospital in Zurich, Switzerland for the first time in November, 1963, because of recurrent abdominal pain and abnormal urinary findings. A diagnosis of pyelonephritis had been made but not confirmed. During the hospitalization, the patient was noted to be cyanotic, and examination of her blood revealed a methemoglobin concentration of 9% with the presence of occasional Heinz bodies in the peripheral blood. A history of a drug intake was denied by the patient. The symptoms subsided within a few days, and the patient was discharged to be readmitted again with similar findings. The cyanotic episodes associated with the Heinz bodies in the peripheral blood and methemoglobinemia occurred every 2–3 weeks. On several occasions, the methemoglobin reached 50% and the hemolysis was so severe that the patient required multiple blood transfusions.

To investigate the possibility of an enzyme deficiency, the activity of glucose-6-phosphate dehydrogenase, 6-phosphatogluconate dehydrogenase, diaphorase, glutathione reductase and the concentration of reduced glutathione within her red cells were measured. The results were all within normal range. The hemoglobin studies revealed no physico-chemical abnormalities. Thus, it became obvious that the factor or factors responsible for this oxidative hemolysis were extracorpuscular compounds and most likely were excreted in the urine. To verify this possibility, a simple test was devised. This consisted of incubating, at 37°C, normal washed erythrocytes with the patient's urine buffered to pH·7. Indeed, such incubation resulted in the production of 25% methemoglobin within three hours. When the same experiments were performed with neutral urine previously

* This investigation was supported in part by a grant from Swiss National Foundation and in part by grant AM11879–01 of the Department of Health, Education and Welfare.

hydrolized with β-glucuronidase, the methemoglobin formation was 65% within three hours. Normal urine or the urine collected from the patient during the remission period showed no significant oxidative properties.

During the period of methemoglobinemia, the patient's urine exhibited normal color. On standing at room temperature, however, it gradually darkened. The dark brown color appeared much faster if the pH of the urine was in the alkaline range. The urine yielded a deep violet color upon addition of a few drops of 10% ferric chloride solution. The addition of a few drops of a solution of 2% β-napthol in 1 N NaOH, following diazotization, gave an immediate intense deep red color.

In view of these findings, the possibility of a drug intake became obvious. After a meticulous search, it was finally discovered that the patient was secretly taking suppositories containing 500 mg acetophenetidin, 250 mg salycilate, and 20 mg codein phosphate. The estimated dose of acetophenetidin used during each crisis was 2 to 5 grams.

Extraction and Identification of Acetophenetidin Metabolites

To extract the acetophenetidin metabolites from the urine, a 24-hour urine (1,000 to 1,500 ml) collected during the period of methemoglobinemia was filtered and acidified with acetic acid to pH4. Deactivated charcoal was prepared with stearic acid as described by Dalgliesh.[6] The deactivated charcoal and acidified urine (2 g for 50 ml of urine) were thoroughly mixed and shaken for five minutes. The charcoal was collected on a Buchner funnel and was washed with 2 liters of water. The aromatic compounds were eluted with 7% aqueous phenol solution until the eluates were colorless. The eluates were pooled and dried at reduced pressure in a rotary evaporator. The dried residue was redissolved in 20 ml of water and evaporated again to dryness. The procedure was repeated several times until the phenol was evaporated. Finally, the dry residue was dissolved in 3 ml of water and was subjected to paper chromatography and electrophoresis.

Analytical Paper Chromatography. The samples were applied as spots on Whatman No. 1 paper strips 7 × 47 cm for one-way; and on 35 × 40 cm sheets for two-way runs. The chromatography was performed by the descending technique in equilibrated glass tanks (20 × 50 × 50 cm) at 20°C using the following solvent systems: (a) organic phase (upper layer) of $_n$-butanol-acetic acid-water (4:1:5); (b) $_n$-butanol-acetic acid-water (4:1:1); (c) isopropanol- 25% ammonia-water (20:1:2); (d) isopropanol- 25% ammonia-water (16:1:3); (e) benzene-propionic acid-water (2:2:1). The given Rf values refer to the center of gravity of the spots revealed by appropriate color reagents. The color reagents used were as follows:

A. Diazotized p-nitraniline was prepared and applied as suggested by Smith.[7]
B. Diazotized sulfanilic acid was prepared as described by Smith.[7]
C. β-Naphthol-coupling: The papers were first sprayed with a freshly prepared mixture of 5% sodium nitrite and 1 N HCl in the ratio of 1:3 (v/v), followed by a spray of 2% solution of β-naphthol in 1 N NaOH.
D. Ekman reagent: The papers were dipped into a freshly prepared mixture of 5 ml of 2 N HCl, 45 ml acetone, and 1 ml 5% aqueous sodium nitrite and subsequently dipped in 5% N-ethyl-2-naphthylamine in ethanol.
E. Nitrosonaphthol: The paper was dipped into a mixture of 90 ml of 0.1% α-nitroso-β-naphthol in ethanol and 10 ml concentrated HNO_3 and allow to damp-dry for 2–3 minutes and then heated for 3 minutes at 70°C.[8] The reagents were mixed immediately before use.

F. Ninhydrin: 3 drops of pyridin were added to 25 ml of 0.2% ninhydrin in acetone. The moistened papers were exposed for 5 minutes to 100°C.

G. Mercapturic acid: A first spray with 0.1 M-potassium dichromate in acetic acid was followed by a second with 0.1 M aqueous silver nitrate.

H. Ferric Chloride: Spray with 1% aqueous ferric chloride solution.

I. Silver Nitrate: Spray with 0.1 M $AgNO_3$ solution in 1% aqueous NH_4OH and allow to stand in daylight at room temperature.

Preparative Paper Electrophoresis. Crude metabolite mixtures were dissolved in 10 ml of 0.1 N formic acid and applied in 2 ml batches near the center lines of five sheets of 290×310×1 mm cartons of Schleicher and Schuell No. 2727. After moistening towards the center with 0.1 N formic acid, the electrophoresis was run at 300 v and 10 ma for two or three hours. The bands were located by means of a contact paper strip which was developed with the suitable color reagents. The bands were cut and eluted with water. The eluates from several paper electrophoreses were pooled and concentrated in a rotatory evaporator for repeat electrophoresis. Elementary analysis, melting points, mass spectra, U.V. spectra and proton resonance spectra (n.m.r.) were performed in the Department of Organic Chemistry at the University of Zurich, Switzerland.

The urinary acetophenetidin metabolites extracted by deactivated charcoal were best resolved on paper chromatograms run in solvents (a) and (c) for the first and second run, respectively. The paper chromatograms run in these solvents exhibited two intense fluorescent spots (purple and blue-purple) which reacted with ferric chloride in yielding a deep purple color. They were identified as salicylic and salicyluric acid. In some urine extract, a third fluorescent spot (white-blue) was also observed and was identified as gentisic acid. These are well-known metabolites of acetyl salicylic acid and will not be discussed here. The remainder of the compounds could not be readily identified. Their identification was achieved by their extraction, purification, and physicochemical analysis by procedures described above.

2-Hydroxy-$_p$-phenetidin-$_o$-glucuronide (2-OHPG): This highly polar metabolite could not be extracted in organic solvent. It was separated by means of deactivated charcoal adsorption method. It was detected on paper chromatogram using solvent systems (a) and (c) with R_f values of 0.45 and 0.11, respectively. The color reactions are shown on TABLE 1.

On electrophoresis in 0.1 N formic acid it migrated toward cathode and separated well from the other compounds. This latter procedure was selected for isolation and purification of this compound.

When the eluate from the repeat electrophoresis was concentrated to a volume of approximately 1 ml, some crystalline material appeared on the flask walls. The crystals and the mother liquor were removed from the flask and were placed in a centrifuge tube. After centrifugation, the mother liquor was removed and the crystals were washed twice with ½ ml of chilled distilled water. The crystals were dried in a vacuum over KOH. To recrystallize the compound, it was dissolved in 1 ml of Trifluoracetic acid. After evaporation of the solvent, the residue was dissolved in 1 ml of water. On addition of 3 drops of 2.5 N ammonia, the substance crystallized in microscopic needles. These were filtered, washed with water, and dried in a vacuum over KOH.

The hydrolysis of 2-OHPG was only possible with β-glucuronidase, for even 3 N HCl at 98°C for 2 hours could not split the glucuronide conjugation. Higher concentrations of the acid destroyed the compound.

2-Hydroxy-aceto-$_p$-phenetidin-$_o$-glucuronide (2-OHAPG): This compound was

TABLE 1

COLOR REACTION BY SOME OF THE ACETOPHENETIDIN METABOLITES DETECTED IN THE PATIENT'S URINE

Compound & Structure		UV	A	B	C	D	E	F	G	H
NAPA	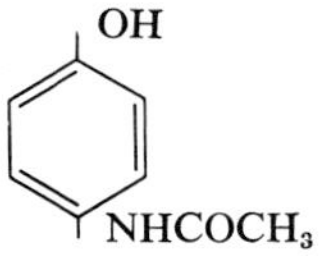	—	grey blue	orange red	—	—	—	—	—	very light blue haze
2–OHPS	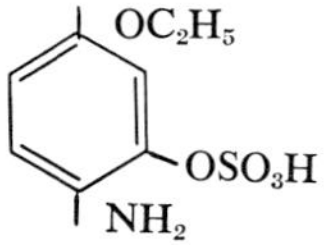	Weak yellow green	—	—	red	pink	—	—	—	—
2–OHPG	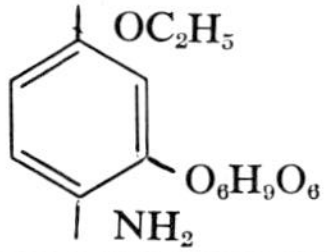	—	red brown	dark yellow	red	blue	—	—	—	—
2–OHAPG	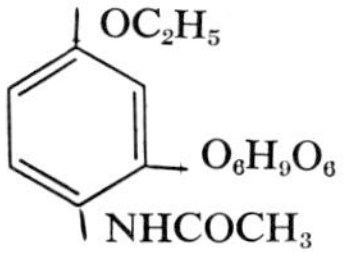	—	—	—	—	—	purple	—	—	—
S–2–OHAC	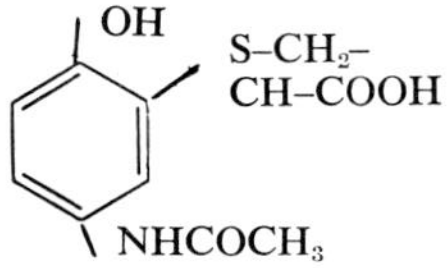	—	grey green	wine red	—	—	—	blue	yellow	—

detected on paper chromatogram using solvent systems (a) and (c). Its R_f values in these systems were 0.63 and 0.20, respectively. The color reaction E was used for its detection (TABLE 1). To isolate this compound, the concentrated solution obtained from a batch of charcoal extract was chromatographed preparatively for 15 hours using solvent (d). The band of $R_f=0.40$, detected with color reagent E, was cut and eluted with water. The eluates were concentrated and rechromatographed using solvent system (e). The substance in the band of $R_f=0.45$ was eluted with water and taken to dryness at reduced pressure.

2-Hydroxy-p-phenetidin sulfuric acid ester (2-OHPS): This compound in solvent system (a) and (c) exhibited R_f values 0.72 and 0.60, respectively, and was detected by color reagent D. This compound was best isolated by ethylacetate extraction from the urine at pH 3.5. The extract was concentrated and was subjected to preparative paper chromatography in solvent system (d). The band of metabolite (R_f 0.67) was detected by means of color reagent D on the control strip, and was eluted with water.

S-(2-hydroxy-5-acetamidophenyl)-cysteine: This metabolite in solvents (a) and (c) had R_f values of 0.36 and 0.10 respectively, and was developed with color reagent F. It was isolated by charcoal extraction and preparative paper electrophoresis in 0.1 N formic acid. The appropriate zone was detected by developing a control strip with color reagent F.

N-Acetyl-p-aminophenol (NAPA): This compound which is a well-known metabolite of acetophenetidin was located on paper chromatograms developed in solvents (a) and (c) (R_f values of 0.85 and 0.90, respectively) and located with color reagent A.

The In Vitro Methemoglobin Studies

Since 2-hydroxyphenetidin (2-OHP) is an *o*-aminophenol, its effects on the red cells were tested in vitro. To prepare 2-OHP, 30 mg of 2-OHPG were dissolved in 5 ml of 0.2 *M* sodium acetate buffer pH 5. Forty thousand Fishman units of beef liver β-glucuronidase were added to the solution. The mixture was placed in a 25 ml round flask with a long neck slightly narrowed in the middle. The mixture was frozen by placing the flask in a dry ice-aceton bath. After the solution had been frozen, the flask was removed from the bath and then attached to a high vacuum pump, and was allowed to thaw. The procedure was repeated until no further air bubbles were formed during the thawing step. Then, while still connected to the vacuum pump, the flask was sealed through the narrow portion of its neck with an oxygen torch. This procedure was found to be far superior to the nitrogen bubbling for satisfactory removal of oxygen. The sealed flask was placed in a water bath at 38°C for 48 hours, after which the flask was opened. The free 2-OHP was acetylated by a mixture of 3 ml of acetic anhydride and 3 ml of pyridin. The resulting 2-hydroxyacetophenetidin was extracted into ether and was crystallized. The crystals were added to 10 cc of 1 N HCl in a similar flask which was degassed as before. The flask was subsequently placed in a 98°C water bath for one hour. Following the evaporation of the HCl under vacuum in a rotary evaporator in a 70°C water bath, the crystalline 2-OHP was collected and was dried in a desiccator under nitrogen.

Red cells derived from fresh, defibrinated human blood were washed two times with 20 volumes of cold isotonic saline and were prepared as a 50% cell suspension in isotonic phosphate buffer pH 7.4 2-OHP was dissolved in the same buffer immediately prior to addition to the red cell suspension. 2-OHP and hemoglobin (as intact red cells), were placed in a flat bottom 10 ml vial in equimolar concentration.* The vials were subsequently covered with plastic caps and were placed in a Dubnoff metabolic shaker at 37°C. At the end of two hours, the methemoglobin measured by the method of Evelyn and Malloy[9] was found to be 33 percent. The preincubation methemoglobin concentration was 0.6 percent. Incubation studies were performed using synthetic 2-OHP, and yielded similar results.

The Fate of Acetophenetidin in the Patient

To assess the fate of acetophenetidin in the patient and to evaluate her sensitivity to this drug, the patient was given a single dose of 30 mg/kg orally. This resulted in an increase in methemoglobin concentration from 0.2% to 11.4% within six hours with the appearance of Heinz bodies in the peripheral blood (FIGURE 1). After administration of such a dose to seven controls, the methemoglobin concentration did not exceed 2.8 percent. To evaluate the extent of acetophenetidin deethylation in the patient, the total NAPA was measured in a 48-hour urine collection from the patient, using the method described by Brodie and Axelrod.[10] It was found that the patient excreted only 30% of the total dose as NAPA, while in normal controls the excretion of this compound was above 62% (TABLE 2).

To assess the magnitude of the excretion of 2-hydroxy derivatives of acetophenetidin in the patient's urine, one-tenth of total 24-hour urine, collected following a 30 mg/kg dose of acetophenetidin, was subjected to the charcoal adsorbtion method. The aromatic compounds were dried as described before and redissolved in 2 ml of water. Similar extractions were made from the

* 68 mg of hemoglobin as intact red cells per each micromole of 2–OHP.

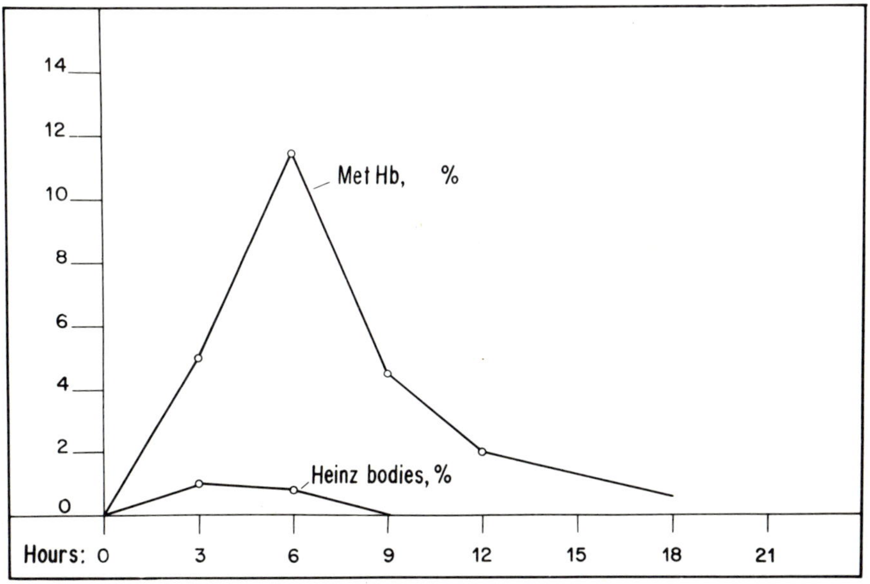

FIGURE 1. The methemoglobin concentration and Heinz bodies following the administration of 30 mg/kg of acetophenetidin to the patient.

TABLE 2

PERCENT MHB AND URINARY AP METABOLITES IN THE PATIENT AND SEVEN CONTROLS FOLLOWING AP INGESTION (30 MG/KG)

Subjects	Age	MHb % Before	MHb % Max. Rise After	2-OHAPG	2-OHPG	2-OHPS	NAPA Excretion %
Patient	17	0.2	11.4	++++	++++	++++	30
WB ♀	51	0.7	2.8	+	—	+	62
MH ♀	56	1.63	2.3	+	—	+	72
AK ♂	21	0.7	2.8	+	—	+	69
RB ♂	23	0.7	1.2	+	—	+	90
DF ♀	30	0.2	1.18	+	—	+	73
BR ♂	36	0.64	1.6	+	—	+	73
FR ♂	62	0	0.64	+	—	+	84

urine of seven healthy individuals given comparable doses. Fifty microliters of each urine extract was subjected to descending paper chromatography in solvent system (a) and the spots were detected with reagents D and E. It was observed that only the extract from the patient's urine contained 2-OHPG. 2-OHAPG and 2-OHPS, however, were present in the extracts from the urine of healthy individuals, but the concentration of these compounds, as judged by the size of the spots on paper chromatogram, was much greater in the extract from the patient's urine (TABLE 2). This procedure was repeated three times and each time similar results were obtained.

Pretreatment with Phenobarbital

Several investigators have pointed out that the treatment of animals with certain drugs, such as phenobarbital, stimulates the activity of drug-metabolizing enzymes in liver microsomes.[11,12] This adaptive increase of enzyme activity accelerates the biotransformation of drugs in vivo. To evaluate the effect of phenobarbital on the metabolism of acetophenetidin in this patient, she was given 400 mg of phenobarbital over a period of 72 hours. Shortly after the last dose, she was given 2 g of acetophenetidin. This resulted in a slightly higher methemoglobin and Heinz body formation (FIGURE 2). In addition, the patient developed severe neurological symptoms, including bilateral Babinski reflex. These symptoms subsided nine hours after the start of acetophenetidin intake. A normal control, similarly treated, developed neither methemoglobinemia nor neurological symptoms.

Family Studies

Five members of the patient's family were given similar dosages of acetophenetidin. The results, as shown on TABLE 3, revealed similar abnormalities in a 38-year-old sister whose methemoglobin rose from 0 to 5% within six hours, and excreted 49% of total dose as NAPA. The remaining members of the family did not show any significant methemoglobinemia and no 2-OHPG could be detected in their urine. The intensity of the spots of 2-OHAPG and 2-OHPS on the chromatogram were not as prominent as those from the patient and her 38-year-old sister.

DISCUSSION

The side effects of acetophenetidin have been the subject of a voluminous body of literature. In addition to the oxidative hemolysis mentioned above, the

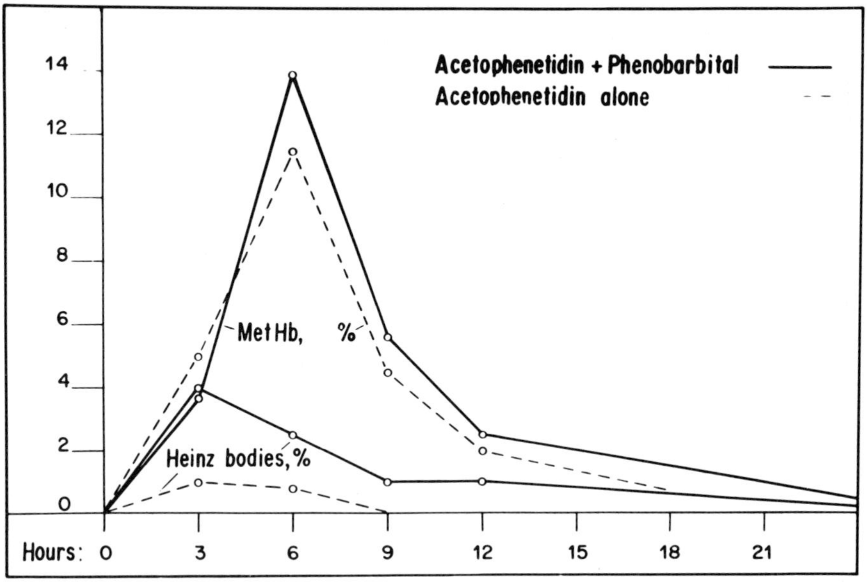

FIGURE 2. The methemoglobin concentration and Heinz bodies following the administration of 30 mg/kg of acetophenetidin to the patient with and without pretreatment with phenobarbital.

TABLE 3

PERCENT MHB AND URINARY AP METABOLITES IN THE PATIENT AND HER FAMILY FOLLOWING AP INGESTION (30 MG/KG)

Subjects	Age	MHb % Before	MHb % Max. Rise After	2-OHAPG	2-OHPG	2-OHPS	NAPA Excretion %
Patient	17	0.2	11.4	++++	++++	++++	30
Sister	51	0.4	0.4	+	−	+	72
Sister	38	0	5.4	++++	++++	++++	49
Brother	36	0.64	1.6	+	−	+	81
Father	62	1.1	1.9	+	−	+	68
Mother	61	0	0.64	+	−	+	60

occurrence of kidney damage, "interstitial nephritis" has been one of the most worrisome complications of prolonged acetophenetidin intake. Although explanations such as allergy to acetophenetidin have been advanced by some investigators,[4] It is generally believed that the oxidative hemolysis is most likely the result of biotransformation of this drug in vivo. Acetophenetidin in man was first studied by Brodie and Axelrod[13] who showed that the major part of this drug was deethylated in the organism and was excreted as free and conjugated NAPA (60–83% of a 2 g dose). A minor portion of this drug (approximately 0.1%) was found to be excreted in the deacetylated form as $_p$-phenetidin. These investigators were able to detect measurable amounts of $_p$-phenetidin in blood of dogs given acetophenetidin at the dosage of 75 mg/kg of body weight. They further found that the level of $_p$-phenetidin in the blood was proportional to the extent of methemoglobin formation. Since the incubation of $_p$-phenetidin with whole blood, in vitro, did not result in any methemoglobin formation, they postulated that a product of p-phenetidin must be the responsible factor. The possibility of N-hydroxylation of p-phenetidin resulting in the formation of p-ethoxyphenylhydroxylamine and its product of oxidation, nitrosophenetol, was investigated by Baader *et al.*[14] who found that injection of p-phenetidin in dogs at the dosage of 12 mg/kg resulted in a blood concentration of nitrosophenetol 0.25 γ ml. Baader *et al.*,[14] however, found no relationship between the concentration of blood nitrosophenetol and that of methemoglobin. From their studies, they concluded that other metabolites were probably involved in p-phenetidin induced methemoglobinemia.

Recently, Welch, Conney and Burns,[15] reported the occurrence of unknown primary aromatic amines in the urine of several species given acetophenetidin or NAPA. In contrast to the cat much less of this material appeared in the urine of dogs and only traces in human urine. It is of interest to note that the extent of excretion of these diazotizable amines, as found by Welch *et al.*, parallels the ability of acetophenetidin to cause methemoglobenimia in these species.[16]

Our preliminary studies[17] and the present investigation suggest the aromatic amines reported by Welch *et al.* are 2-OHPS and possibly 2-OHPG. The role of these aromatic amines in methemoglobin formation is further emphasized by in vitro studies using unconjugated 2-OHP which was found to be a potent methemoglobin former. This compound seems to be a normal metabolite of acetophenetidin, and is excreted as sulfate. In all individuals we have so far tested, this compound has been present. Similar observations have been previously made by Buch *et al.*,[18] who reported that normal individuals excreted as much as 8% of a 25 mg/kg dose of acetophenetidin as 2-OHPS within the first eight hours.

The excretion of 2-OHPG does not seem to occur normally and has not been previously reported. In ten healthy individuals tested by the above mentioned method we have not been able to detect this compound in the urine. The excretion of 2-OHPG, in addition to the 2-OHPS by the patient and her sister, may be the result of excessive formation of 2-OHP. Inadequate acetylation enhanced deacetylation or ring hydroxylation are other possible factors to be considered.

Whether deacetylation of the aromatic acetamido group occurs before or after hydroxylation is not certain. There are reasons to believe that deacetylation takes place after hydroxylation. Indeed, Bray, James, Thorpe and Wasdell[19] have shown that liver deacetylase in rabbit has much higher affinity for the ortho substituted aromatic acetamido compounds (such as 2-OHAP) than for para substituted ones (such as acetophenetidin itself).

Individual variation in drug metabolism as a cause of drug toxicity is well known. Individual variation in the metabolism of acetophenetidin is obviously another example. The occurrence of acetophenetidin induced kidney damage in two or more members of the same family has been reported by several investigators.[20-22] In one family described by Grimlund,[22] 6 of 11 siblings had interstitial nephritis. Recently, Prescott[23] has further emphasized this individual susceptibility by measuring the rate of excretion of tubular cell in the urine following acetophenetidin administration. It would be of particular interest to ascertain whether those individuals who show adverse hemotological reaction to acetophenetidin are candidates for interstitial nephritis. Our patient had definite signs of kidney damage. In this connection it is of interest to note that Nissen and Friis[24] observed a significant reduction in the erythrocyte survival following the administration of acetophenetidin to individuals who had acetophenetidin-induced kidney damage. When similar dosage of acetophenetidin was given to patients with renal insufficiency of other origin, no decrease in the red cell life-span was observed.

The treatment of the patient with phenobarbitol resulted in no improvement of acetophenetidin-induced hemotological reaction. Indeed, as judged by the extent of methemoglobin and Heinz body formation the pretreatment with phenobarbital had adverse effects. Similar observations have been recently made by Büch and associates[25] in rats receiving large doses of acetophenetidin.

In the course of identification of acetophenetidin metabolites, in addition to NAPA and aryl amines mentioned above, two other compounds were also identified. These were 2 hydroxyacetophenetidin and S-(2-hydroxy 5 acetamido phenyl) cystein (TABLE 1). From the available data[26,27] and the present study it appears that these two compounds are normal metabolites of acetophenetidin and are excreted in very small quantities. Because of acetylation of the aromatic amino group they are not redox compounds and consequently are unlikely to play a direct role in acetophenetidin-induced methemoglobinemia.

Summary

The administration of acetophenetidin (30 mg/kg in a single dose) may result, in some individuals, in significant increase in methemoglobin with formation of Heinz bodies in the peripheral blood. This susceptibility is not always associated with a deficiency of erythrocytes glucose-6-phosphate dehydrogenase. It has been thought that 2-hydroxyphenetidin an *o*-aminophenol, which is excreted as sulfate and glucuronide, may be responsible for methemoglobin formation. It was found that, by a semiquantitative method, sensitive individuals excreted more of the 2-hydroxy derivatives of acetophenetidin than did normal individuals. The exact reasons for this individual variation in the excretion of these compounds are not known. Inadequate deethylation may be a factor. The pretreatment with phenobarbital did not diminish acetophenetidin toxicity. Indeed, such a treatment resulted in higher methemoglobin and Heinz body formation.

Acknowledgment

The major part of this investigation was carried out by the author in Zurich, Switzerland, at the Children's Hospital. In this connection the author would like to particularly thank Professors W. H. Hitzig and A. Prader for their encouragement and collaboration. The author also wishes to thank Doctors H. Wyler, W. Fritzche, and Professors A. Dreiding and H. Langmann, from the Department of Organic Chemistry and Pharmacology, Zurich University, for their valuable help and advice in the identification of the compounds reported here.

References

1. Smith, P. K. 1958. Acetophenetidin. Interscience Publishers Inc. N. Y.
2. Houston, I. B. & A. M. Barlow. 1959. Lancet **II**: 1062.
3. Hutchinson, H. E., J. M. Jackson & P. Cassidy. 1962. Lancet **II**: 1022.
4. Lorentzen, J. & M. Schwartz. 1960. Acta Med. Scand. **168**: 461.
5. Whurmann, F. & B. Jasinksi. 1955. Dtsche. Med. Wschr. **80**: 1632.
6. Dalgliesh, C. E. 1955. J. Clin. Path. **8**: 73.
7. Smith, I. 1960. Chromatographic and Electrophoretic Techniques. Interscience Publishers Inc. N. Y.
8. Anger, V. 1961. Oestr. Chem. Ztg. **62**: 354.
9. Evelyn, K. A. & H. T. Malloy. 1938. J. Biol. Chem. **126**: 655.
10. Brodie, B. B. & J. Axelrod. 1948. J. Pharmacol. & Exptl. Ther. **94**: 22.

11. Remmer, H. 1959. Arch. Exp. Pharm. **235**: 279.
12. Conney, A. H., C. Davnon, R. Gastel & J. J. Burns. 1960. J. Pharmacol. Exp. Ther. **130**: 1.
13. Brodie, B. B. & J. Axelrod. 1949. J. Pharmacol. & Exptl. Ther. **97**: 58.
14. Baader, H., S. Girgis, M. Kiese, H. Menzel & L. Skrobot. 1961. Exp. Path. Pharmak. **241**: 317.
15. Welch, R. M., A. H. Conney & J. J. Burns. 1966. Biochem. Pharmacol. **15**: 521.
16. Lester, D. 1943. J. Pharmac. Exp. Ther. **77**: 154.
17. Shahidi, N. T., H. Wyler, W. H. Hitzig, A. Dreiding & A. Prader. 1966. Clin. Res. **24**: 327.
18. Büch, H., H. Hauser, K. Pfleger & W. Rudger. 1966. Arch. Exper. Path. & Pharmac. **253**: 25.
19. Bray, H. G., S. P. James, W. V. Thorpe & M. R. Wasdell. 1950. Biochem. J. **47**: 483.
20. Poli, M. 1955. Helv. Med. Acta **22**: 109.
21. Ask-Upmark, E. 1960. Br. Med. J. **2**: 823.
22. Grimlund, K. 1963. Acta Med. Scand. **174**: 3. Supp. 4 & 5.
23. Prescott, L. F. 1966. J. Pharm. Pharmac. **18**: 331.
24. Nissen, N. I. & T. Friis. 1962. Acta Med. Scand. **171**: 125.
25. Büch, H., W. Gerhards, K. Pfleger, W. Rudiger & W. Rummel. 1967. Biochem. Pharmacol. **16**: 1585.
26. Jagenburg, O. R. & K. Toczko. 1964. Biochem. J. **92**: 639.
27. Klutch, A., M. Hargenist & A. H. Conney. 1966. Med. Chem. **9**: 63.

PART II. HEREDITARY DISEASES OF PHARMACOGENETIC INTEREST

PHARMACOLOGIC AND GENETIC DETERMINANTS OF DISORDERED BILIRUBIN TRANSPORT AND METABOLISM IN THE LIVER*

Lawrence M. Gartner† and Irwin M. Arias

Departments of Pediatrics and Medicine
Albert Einstein College of Medicine
N. Y., N. Y.

Inheritable disorders of hepatic bilirubin uptake, conjugation and excretion have been described in both man and animals. Specific pharmacologic agents produce effects similar to the defects observed in these disorders. Studies of these inheritable disorders of bilirubin transport and metabolism and of pharmacologic effects on these processes has led to considerable understanding of the mechanisms of bilirubin uptake, conjugation and excretion by the liver.

Physiology and Biochemistry

Bilirubin is formed predominantly, although not exclusively, from senescent erythrocytes in reticuloendothelial tissue,[1] and is a lipid soluble tetrapyrrole which must be bound to albumin for transport in plasma at physiologic pH. Although one mole of albumin is theoretically capable of binding two moles of bilirubin, this capacity is rarely achieved.[2] Other plasma constituents (e.g. free fatty acids) and drugs (e.g. sulfonamides) compete with bilirubin for this binding.[3] When the capacity to bind bilirubin is exceeded, as occurs occasionally during the newborn period, the entrance of bilirubin into brain tissue is facilitated, resulting in bilirubin encephalopathy, called kernicterus.[4]

The transfer of unconjugated bilirubin from plasma into the liver cell is poorly understood, but may depend upon partial dissociation of bilirubin from albumin and facilitated diffusion across the sinusoidal membrane.[5] In addition, hepatic cytoplasm may contain a biological acceptor substance capable of binding bilirubin and facilitating its transport into the liver cell.[6] Within the hepatocyte, bilirubin is transported by an unknown mechanism to the endoplasmic reticulum[6] where each mole of bilirubin is conjugated with two moles of glucuronic acid in ester linkage.[5] Glucuronyl transferase is the enzyme, or family of enzymes, catalyzing the transfer of glucuronic acid from uridine diphosphate glucuronic acid to various amine, phenolic and carboxylic receptors, such as bilirubin. Although the conjugation of various substances with glucuronic acid has been demonstrated to occur in many organs of the body, the conjugation of bilirubin with glucuronic acid is performed predominantly in the liver. The question of whether a single enzyme or multiple enzymes are concerned with the formation of various glucuronides has not yet been resolved. The following examples illustrate the difficulties encountered in attempting to answer this question. (TABLE 1) The Gunn rat has chronic nonhemolytic unconjugated hyperbilirubinemia, and liver from this mutant animal is unable to form the glucuronide

* This work supported in part by a research grant from the National Institutes of Health (AM–02019).

† Career Development Awardee of the National Institute of Child Health and Human Development.

TABLE 1

HEPATIC GLUCURONYL TRANSFERASE ACTIVITY IN VITRO

	Bilirubin Glucuronide Formation	o-aminophenol Glucuronide Formation
Homozygous Gunn rat	absent	25% of normal
Crigler-Najjar (human)	absent	present (human normal unknown)
Hypophysectomized rat Thyroidectomized rat	normal	25% of normal
Newborn guinea pig:		
Day 1	20% of normal	10% of normal
Day 4	normal	30% of normal

of bilirubin either in vivo or in vitro.[7] It can, however, form the glucuronide of o-aminophenol to the extent of 25% of normal in vitro. The pattern of glucuronide formation in the human equivalent of the Gunn Rat, the Crigler-Najjar syndrome, is similar.[8] Liver from hypophysectomized of thyroidectomized rats forms bilirubin glucuronide to a normal extent in vitro but forms the glucuronide of o-aminophenol at a rate 25% of normal in vitro.[9] Liver from one-day-old guinea pigs forms both bilirubin and o-aminophenol glucuronide at markedly reduced rates, but liver from four-day-old guinea pigs forms bilirubin glucuronide at a normal rate while still demonstrating markedly deficient formation of o-aminophenol glucuronide.[10] Thus, in the genetically determined enzyme deficiency in the rat and the human, glucuronyl transferase activity for bilirubin is absent and for the phenolic compound is present but deficient, suggesting perhaps a single enzyme with differing affinities for the substrate. However, the situation with the hypophysectomized or thyroidectomized rats demonstrates a clear separation of ether and ester glucuronide formation, suggesting two distinct enzymes. The developmental pattern in the newborn guinea pig also suggests that there may be two distinct enzymes. N-Linked glucuronide formation, which has not been illustrated, is probably catalyzed by an enzyme separate from that for either ethereal or ester linked glucuronide formation.[11] Resolution of this problem of multiple transferases awaits complete solubilization and purification of the enzyme.

Bilrubin must be conjugated and rendered water soluble in order to be transported from the liver cell into bile. The site of this transport is not known but may occur at the canalicular membrane. It has also been postulated that transport into the lumen of the smooth endoplasmic reticulum (SER) may be the equivalent of excretion, with direct communication of the SER lumen with the bile canaliculus being postulated. Bilirubin glucuronide is believed to be excreted against a concentration gradient by an energy dependent transport system. In all animals in which this has been studied, including man, excretion from the liver cell is the rate limiting step in the overall transport of bilirubin from plasma into bile.[7,10] This capacity to transport bilirubin out of the liver cell, called excretory maximum, is different in each species and differs among strains of the same species. Within an inbred strain the maximal rate of excretion is reproducible. Other substances, such as sulfobromophthalein and indocyanine green are also excreted by the liver cell against a concentration gradient, but it is not clear whether these substances compete with bilirubin for excretion.

Hepatic Uptake of Bilirubin

Cornelius and Gronwall have described an inherited defect in the hepatic uptake of bilirubin, sulfobromophthalein (BSP), indocyanine green, rose bengal and phylloerythrin in Southdown sheep.[12] The disorder is detected when affected sheep develop photosensitive cutaneous eczema. The eczema results from the accumulation in the skin of phylloerythrin, a light activated metabolite of chlorophyll. The defect is probably inherited as an autosomal recessive. The mechanism of the defect is unknown. Histologically, the liver is normal.

The effect of drugs on hepatic uptake mechanisms has not been extensively studied, in part because adequate techniques for the quantitation of uptake by the liver are lacking. It was observed, however, that some patients receiving male fern extract for the treatment of fish tapeworm infestation developed hyperbilirubinemia. Purification of the fern extract resulted in isolation of flavispidic acid, which, when administered to rabbits produced retention of BSP, indocyanine green and unconjugated bilirubin, possibly by interfering with hepatic uptake mechanisms.[13]

Hepatic Conjugation of Bilirubin

Inherited defects in the conjugation of bilirubin are among the most dramatic clinical evidences of jaundice and the toxicity which may result from hyperbilirubinemia. Crigler and Najjar described six infants with severe jaundice from three related families; five of the infants developed kernicterus during the newborn period.[14] Of approximately 20 additional cases reported since that time, 14 of the infants have died during infancy as a direct result of kernicterus. Several additional children have developed kernicterus during later childhood or adolescence. In this disorder, which is probably inherited as an autosomal recessive,[15] severe unconjugated hyperbilirubinemia is noted during the first week of life and persists throughout life with serum bilirubin concentrations ranging from 14 to 45 mg percent. The formation of glucuronides of various administered substances such as menthol, corticosteroids, and salicylates is defective in the nonjaundiced parents and in some of the nonjaundiced siblings as compared with normal individuals. In the affected children themselves, the capacity to form these various glucuronide conjugates is even more severely limited. Although only two children with the syndrome have been studied to determine hepatic glucuronyl transferase activity in vitro using bilirubin as the substrate, in both cases no bilirubin glucuronide was formed.[8,16] In one of these, a child whom we studied, liver tissue was capable of forming the glucuronide conjugate of ortho-aminophenol, however. Thus, as would be expected from the studies performed in these children in vivo, there is some limited formation of ethereal conjugates, but no formation of the ester glucuronide conjugate of bilirubin.

The other form of chronic nonhemolytic unconjugated hyperbilirubinemia designated as a conjugating defect was described by Arias in 1962.[17] In this syndrome, the serum bilirubin concentrations remain less than 20 mg % and may range as low as 5 mg %, all of the accumulated bilirubin being in the unconjugated form. Kernicterus has been reported in only one such patient. The onset of jaundice may occur soon after birth, as in the Crigler-Najjar syndrome, or may be delayed until adolescence. Clinically it may be extremely difficult to differentiate this disorder from the Crigler-Najjar syndrome. However, examination of bile obtained from the gall-bladder at surgery in these individuals reveals abundant amounts of bilirubin glucuronide with a concentration of 50 to 100 mg per 100 ml. By contrast, gall-bladder bile obtained from patients with the Crigler-Najjar syndrome has a bilirubin concentration of less than 5 mg per 100 ml and is only faintly yellow. Patients with the milder form of the disorder form glucuronide conjugates of menthol and other substances at a reduced rate in vivo as compared with normal individuals. Some anicteric relatives of the jaundiced individuals will also demonstrate defective glucuronide formation, and the pattern of this defect suggests a dominant mode of transmission with variable penetrance. This is in contrast to the recessive pattern of transmission observed in the Crigler-Najjar syndrome. There is no evidence that the Crigler-Najjar syndrome and the milder disorder have occurred in the same family.

Chronic, nonhemolytic unconjugated hyperbilirubinemia inherited as an autosomal recessive trait was described in the Wistar strain of rats by Gunn in 1938.[18] In the past ten years these animals have been the subject of extensive investigation. In virtually all respects they are identical with the Crigler-Najjar syndrome, having nearly colorless bile containing almost no bilirubin and developing kernicterus during the newborn period. As noted previously, homogenates of liver from these rats are unable to form the glucuronide conjugate of bilirubin, but form the glucuronide conjugate of o-aminophenol, at a much reduced rate. The excretion of i.v. administered conjugated bilirubin is normal.

Although many drugs will interfere with the formation of various glucuronides in vitro,[19] few have been implicated in the production of jaundice in humans. The administration of the antibiotic novobiocin has been associated with a three-fold increase in the incidence of severe jaundice in newborn infants and has also resulted in the development of unconjugated hyperbilirubinemia in some adults.[20] Withdrawal of the drug results in prompt disappearance of jaundice. Although unconjugated hyperbilirubinemia could result from either a defect in hepatic uptake of bilirubin or from inhibition of glucuronyl transferase activity, it has been demonstrated that novobiocin is a noncompetitive inhibitor of glucuronyl transferase activity in vitro.[21]

Pharmacologic effects are generally considered only in relation to administration of a drug. In a broader sense, however, the maternal environment may be considered to exert a pharmacologic effect on the infant or fetus. The next two disorders are examples of this concept.

Approximately one percent of breast-fed newborn infants develop severe unconjugated hyperbilirubinemia which persists for three to 12 weeks. Artificially fed infants of these same mothers do not develop this syndrome. The temporal relation of breast-feeding to the severity of hyperbilirubinemia is noted when breast-feeding is interrupted in infants with this syndrome. The serum bilirubin concentration declines rapidly. With re-institution of nursing after five to seven days of artificial feeding, the serum bilirubin concentration increases.

Milk from mothers of these jaundiced infants inhibits glucuronyl transferase activity in vitro to a very significant degree, while milk from normal mothers is only very slightly inhibitory. These inhibitory milks contain pregnane-3-(α), 20(β)-diol, an isomer which has not previously been identified in humans. The usual isomer is pregnane-3-(α),20(α)-diol. The abnormal isomer has also been isolated from the urine of these same mothers obtained during the period of nursing, but not from urine obtained during pregnancy or following cessation of lactation.[22] This suggests that the inhibitory steroid is produced in the actively secreting mammary tissue. Administration of the inhibitory steroid, pregnane-3(α),20(β)-diol, to two normal infants resulted in the development of unconjugated hyperbilirubinemia, which promptly remitted when administration was discontinued.[23] There is no evidence, thus far, to suggest that secretion of this pregnanediol isomer in milk is related to either maternal drug ingestion or to genetically determined factors. Attempts are being made at the present time both in Greece and in Israel to evaluate two populations with high incidences of neonatal jaundice for the possible inheritence of breast-feeding jaundice.

The second syndrome, Transient Familial Neonnatal Hyperbilirubinemia, appears to have a similar etiologic basis, but is not related to breast-feeding.[24] Every infant of these mothers develops severe, unconjugated hyperbilirubinemia during the first few days of life, with jaundice persisting for approximately two weeks. Unlike the breast-feeding syndrome in which the infants remain healthy, many of the infants with the Transient Familial Neonatal Hyperibilirubinemia syndrome have developed kernicterus, probably because of higher serum bilirubin concentrations and the earlier period in life during which jaundice develops. The sera of both mothers and jaundiced infants contain very large amounts of an unidentified substance which inhibits glucuronyl transferase activity, in vitro. Inhibition of glucuronyl transferase activity gradually declines following delivery and becomes normal at approximately two weeks post-partum. It has been suggested that the inhibitory factor, perhaps a progestational steroid produced by the mother in large quantity during pregnancy, is transferred by the placenta to the fetus, resulting in interference with the infant's capacity to form the glucuronide of bilirubin. As in the breast-feeding jaundice syndrome, there is, as yet, no evidence to indicate that the mother has inherited the capacity to produce the inhibitor or that it is related to the administration of drugs.

Hepatic Excretion of Bilirubin

We can now turn to the defects in excretion of bilirubin from the liver. Two well known inherited disorders resulting in conjugated hyperbilirubinemia have been described – the Dubin-Johnson Syndrome[25] and the Rotor Syndrome.[26] Although very similar in many respects, they are probably distinct entities.[5] In both syndromes there is a reduced capacity to excrete sulfobromophthalein and conjugated bilirubin from the liver. The conjugation of bilirubin and sulfobromophthalein by liver from affected individuals is normal, as is the storage of BSP within the liver, suggesting that the defect is limited to the excretory transport system. Administration of radio-opaque dyes, such as iodopanoic acid, to patients with the Dubin-Johnson syndrome fails to result in radiologic visualization of the gall-bladder. In patients with the Rotor syndrome, the radio-opaque dye is excreted in sufficient concentration to permit visualization of the gall-bladder. The major point of differentiation in these patients is the accumulation of a black pigment in the liver of patients with the Dubin-Johnson syndrome, but not in those with the Rotor syndrome. Additional information concerning the Dubin-Johnson syndrome has derived from studies of a virtually identical syndrome observed in Corriedale sheep.[27,28] The hepatic pigment in both sheep and man accumulates in the controlobular areas of the liver, and electron microscopic studies suggest it is in lysosomes. Studies of the isolated pigment from sheep liver suggest that it is a melanin and may derive from polymerization of metabolites of epinephrine which accumulate in liver tissue as a result of the excretory defect.

The relationship of these two syndromes is not clear, and although there has been one family in which both the Dubin-Johnson and Rotor syndromes have occurred,[29] this may be entirely fortuitous. The limited data currently available suggests that the Rotor syndrome is transmitted with the characteristics of an autosomal dominant.[30] The Dubin-Johnson syndrome in both man and sheep is clearly inherited but the mode of transmission is still uncertain although probably an autosomal recessive.

The effect of drugs on the hepatic excretion of bilirubin and other substances, such as sulfobromophthalein, has come under considerable study in the past few years. The first agent to be studied was the plant alkaloid, icterogenin, a triterpene acid.[31] Administration of this alkaloid to rabbits and rats results in decreased excretion of intravenously administered conjugated bilirubin. Glucuronyl transferase activity is not affected by icterogenin, the defect being limited to the excretory mechanism. Because of the large reserve capacity for hepatic excretion of bilirubin in rodents, the animals do not develop hyperbilirubinemia.[32] The C-17 alkylated anabolic steroids, such as norethandrolone, have a very similar effect in rats.[32] Prolonged administration of norethandrolone to some human adults may produce detectable conjugated hyperbilirubinemia.[33] All patients treated with the C-17 alkylated anabolic steroids demonstrate a reduced capacity to excrete BSP, however. These alterations in hepatic excretory function are reversible following withdrawal of the drug. Enovid,® the annovulatory birth-control agent, also interferes with the capacity of the liver to excrete BSP.[34] Although not associated with the development of hyperbilirubinemia when administered to normal women, administration of Enovid, similar birth control agents, and progesterone to women with a history of recurrent jaundice of pregnancy may result in the development of conjugated hyperbilirubinemia. This suggests that some women who appear otherwise normal, may have a partial defect in the hepatic excretion of conjugated bilirubin from the liver. This partial defect may render them more susceptible to the effects of certain drugs and to pregnancy than is the case in normal women. Increased severity of hyperbilirubinemia during pregnancy also occurs in women with the Dubin-Johnson syndrome.

Phenobarbital and Hyperbilirubinemia

The effects of drugs and hormones on hepatic bilirubin transport and metabolism which we have discussed thus far have been to diminish the capacity of the liver to conjugate or transport bilirubin. However, in the past few years, largely through the work of a number of investigators studying the effect of various substances on the enhancement of drug-metabolizing enzymes by the liver, it has become apparent that certain polycyclic hydrocarbons, antihistamines and barbiturates are capable of increasing the capacity of hepatic microsomes to form glucuronides.[35-37] In 1966, Yaffe[38] and Crigler[39] each reported dramatic reduction of the serum bilirubin concentration in an infant with chronic, nonhemolytic unconjugated hyperbilirubinemia following three weeks of phenobarbital administration. The pretreatment serum bilirubin concentrations in the case reported by Yaffe[38] suggest that this is an example of the milder conjugating defect. It is more difficult to classify the case reported by Crigler,[39] but here too, the serum bilirubin concentrations were not as high as has been reported in most cases with the more severe syndrome. During the past year, with Dr. Michael I. Cohen, we have had the opportunity to study the effect of phenobarbital administration on the serum bilirubin concentration in an infant with the Crigler-Najjar syndrome. Exploratory laparotomy prior to phenobarbital administration revealed that gall-bladder bile had a bilirubin concentration of only 5 mg per 100 ml, and liver tissue obtained at surgery revealed a virtually complete inability to form the glucuronide of bilirubin in vitro.

Serum bilirubin concentrations ranged from 19.8 to 32 mg per 100 ml during the control period. Administration of phenobarbital for 100 days in a dose of 10 mg per kg per day did not lower the serum bilirubin concentration. The lowest concentration achieved during the study period was 20 mg per 100 ml. On the 95th day of phenobarbital administration, the capacity of the infant's liver tissue to form the glucuronide of bilirubin was again estimated in vitro. The result was the same as in the pretreatment period; glucuronyl transferase activity was absent. The failure of phenobarbital to influence both the serum bilirubin concentration and the glucuronyl transferase activity suggests that the defect in the classical Crigler-Najjar syndrome is such that that genetic information necessary for the synthesis of the glucuronyl transferase enzyme is completely absent and, therefore, cannot be stimulated by phenobarbital. In those infants demonstrating a decrease in serum bilirubin concentration following phenobarbital administration there may be only a partial defect. However, the possibility of a qualitatively different defect in the infants with the milder disorder must also be considered, especially in view of the different pattern of inheritance. Phenobarbital could also stimulate other pathways for the disposal of unconjugated bilirubin, such as the formation of colorless dipyrrole metabolites.

We have also studied the effect of phenobarbital administration on rats with chronic nonhemolytic unconjugated hyperbilirubinemia – Gunn rats.[40] Phenobarbital in increasing dosage was administered intraperitoneally to three groups of jaundiced rats for 12 weeks. The serum bilirubin concentrations remained unchanged throughout this period. Hepatic glucuronyl transferase activity, using bilirubin as substrate, was completely absent in the rats following 12 weeks of treatment.

These studies of the effect of phenobarbital suggest that a pharmacologic agent may be useful in differentiating two types of inherited disorders which present with a similar clinical appearance. The failure or success of pharmacologic agents to alter genetically determined enzymatic defects may shed light on the mechanisms underlying the abnormality and offer a significant means of therapy.

References

1. Arias, I. M. The formation of bile pigment. Handbook of Physiology. Williams and Wilkins Co. Baltimore, Md.
2. Ostrow, J. D. & R. Schmid. 1956. Bilirubin-protein linkages in serum and their relation to the van den Bergh reaction. J. Clin. Invest. **35:** 537.
3. Schmid, R., I. Diamond, L. Hammaker & C. B. Gundersen. 1965. Interaction of bilirubin with albumin. Nature **206:** 1041.
4. Johnson, L., M. L. Garcia, E. Figueroa & F. Sarmiento. 1961. Kernicterus in rats lacking glucuronyl transferase II. Factors which alter bilirubin concentration and frequency of kernicterus. Am. J. Dis. Child. **101:** 322.
5. Arias, I. M. 1966. Hepatic aspects of bilirubin metabolism. Ann. Rev. Med. **17:** 257.
6. Bernstein, L. H., J. Ben Ezzer, L. M. Gartner & I. M. Arias. 1966. Hepatic intracellular distribution of tritium-labelled unconjugated and conjugated bilirubin in normal and Gunn rats. J. Clin. Invest. **45:** 1194.
7. Arias, I. M., L. Johnson & S. Wolfson. 1961. Biliary excretion of injected conjugated and unconjugated bilirubin by normal and Gunn rats. Am. J. Physiol. **200:** 1091.
8. Gartner, L. M. Unpublished data.
9. Gartner, L. M. 1967. The hormonal regulation of hepatic bilirubin excretion. *In* Bilirubin Metabolism Eds. I. A. D. Bouchier & B. H. Billing. Blackwell Scientific Publications, Oxford, Eng. 175.
10. Gartner, L. M. & I. M. Arias. 1967. The transfer of bilirubin from blood to bile in the neonatal guinea pig. Manuscript submitted for publication.
11. Arias, I. M. 1961. Etheral and N-linked glucuronide formation by normal and Gunn rats *In Vitro* and *In Vivo*. Biochem. Biophys. Res. Comm. **6:** 81.

12. Cornelius, C. E. & R. R. Gronwall. 1965. A mutation in Southdown sheep affecting the hepatic uptake of sulfobromophthalein (BSP), indocyanine green, rose bengal, sodium cholate and phylloerythrin from blood. Federation Proc. **24:** 144.
13. Nosslin, B. & E. H. Morgan. 1965. The effect of phloroglucinol derivatives from male fern on dye excretion by the liver in the rabbit and rat. J. Lab. Clin. Med. **65:** 891.
14. Crigler, J. F. & V. A. Najjar. 1952. Congenital familial nonhemolytic jaundice with kernicterus. Pediatrics **10:** 169.
15. Childs, B., J. B. Sidbury & C. J. Migeon. 1959. Glucuronic acid conjugation by patients with familial non-hemolytic jaundice and their relatives. Pediatrics **23:** 903.
16. Szabo, L., Z. Kovacs & P. B. Ebrey. 1962. Crigler-Najjar Syndrome. Acta Pediat. Hung. **3:** 49.
17. Arias, I. M. 1962. Chronic unconjugated hyperbilirubinemia without overt signs of hemolysis in adolescents and adults. J. Clin. Invest. **41:** 2233.
18. Gunn, C. K. 1938. Hereditary acholuric jaundice. J. Hered. **29:** 137.
19. Lathe, G. H. & M. Walker. 1958. Inhibition of bilirubin conjugation in rat liver slices by human pregnancy and neonatal serum and steroids. Quart. J. Exper. Physiol. **43:** 257.
20. Hargreaves, T. & T. B. Holton. 1962. Jaundice of the newborn due to novobiocin. Lancet **I:** 839.
21. Hsia, D. Y. Y., R. M. Dowben & S. Riabov. 1963. Inhibitors of glucuronyl transferase in the newborn. Ann. N. Y. Acad. Sci. **111:** 326.
22. Rosenfeld, R. S., I. M. Arias, L. M. Gartner, T. F. Gallagher & L. Hellman. 1967. Pregnane-3(α),20(β)-diol: An unusual urinary metabolite associated with neonatal jaundice. J. Clin. Endocrin. and Metab. **27:** 1705.
23. Gartner, L. M. & I. M. Arias. 1964. Production of unconjugated hyperbilirubinemia in full-term newborn infants following ingestion of pregnane-3(α),20(β)-diol. Nature **203:** 1292.
24. Arias, I. M., S. Wolfson, J. F. Lucey & R. McKay, Jr. 1965. Transient familial neonatal hyperbilirubinemia. J. Clin. Invest. **44:** 1442.
25. Dubin, I. N. & F. B. Johnson. 1954. Chronic idiopathic jaundice with unidentified pigment in liver cells: new clinico-pathologic entity with report of 12 cases. Medicine **33:** 155.
26. Schiff, L. & B. H. Billing. 1959. Congenital defects in bilirubin metabolism as seen in the adult. Gastroenterology **37:** 595.
27. Arias, I. M., L. H. Bernstein, R. Toffler, C. E. Cornelius, A. Novikoff & E. Essner. 1964. Black liver disease in Corriedale sheep: A new mutation affecting hepatic excretory function. J. Clin. Invest. **43:** 1249.
28. Cornelius, C. E., I. M. Arias & B. I. Osburn. 1965. Hepatic pigmentation with photosensitivity: A syndrome in Corriedale sheep resembling Dubin-Johnson syndrome in man. J. Am. Vet. Med. Assoc. **146:** 709.
29. Arias, I. M. 1961. Studies of chronic familial non-hemolytic jaundice with conjugated bilirubin in serum with and without an unidentified pigment in the liver cells. Am. J. Med. **31:** 510.
30. Rotor, A. B., L. Manahan & A. Florentin. 1948. Familial non-hemolytic jaundice with direct Van den Bergh reaction. Acta Med. Phillipina **5:** 37.
31. Heikel, T., B. C. Knight, C. Rimington, H. D. Ritchie & E. J. Williams. 1960. Studies on biliary excretion in the rabbit. I. The effect of icterogenin and rehmannic acid on bile flow and the excretion of bilirubin, phylloerythrin coproporphyrin, alkaline phosphatase and bromsulphalein. Proc. Royal Soc. London, B, **153:** 47.
32. Arias, I. M. 1963. Effect of a plant acid (Icterogenin) and certain anabolic steroids on the hepatic metabolism of bilirubin and sulfobromophthalein (BSP). Ann. N. Y. Acad. Sci. **104:** 1014.
33. Scherb, J., M. Kirschner & I. M. Arias. 1963. Studies of hepatic excretory function. The effect of 17α-ethyl-19-nortestosterone on sulfobromophalein sodium (BSP) metabolism in man. J. Clin. Invest. **42:** 404.
34. Kleiner, G., L. Kresch & I. M. Arias. 1965. Studies of hepatic excretory function II. The effect of 17α-ethynl-17-β-hydroxy 5(10)-estren-3-one and theynylestradiol 3 methyl ether on sulfobromophthalein sodium (BSP) metabolism in women of child-bearing age. New Eng. J. Med. **273:** 420.
35. Burns, J. J., A. H. Conney & R. Koster. 1963. Stimulatory effect of chronic drug administration on drug-metabolizing enzymes in liver microsomes. Ann. N. Y. Acad. Sci. **104:** 881.

36. Arias, I. M., L. M. Gartner & S. Wolfson. 1963. Effect of various drugs and chemicals on hepatic glucuronide formation in newborn rats. Proc. Soc. Exper. Biol. Med. **112:** 1037.

37. Catz, C. & S. J. Yaffe. 1962. Pharmacological modification of bilirubin conjugation in newborn. Am. J. Dis. Child. **104:** 516.

38. Yaffe, S. J., G. Levy, T. Matsuzawa & T. Baliah. 1966. Enhancement of glucuronide-conjugating capacity in a hyperbilirubinemia infant due to apparent enzyme induction by phenobarbital. New Eng. J. Med. **275:** 1461.

39. Crigler, J. F., Jr. & N. I. Gold. 1966. Sodium phenobarbital-induced decrease in serum bilirubin in an infant with congenital nonhemolytic jaundice and kernicterus. J. Clin Invest. **45:** 998.

40. De Leon, A., L. M. Gartner & I. M. Arias. 1967. The effect of phenobarbital on hyperbilirubinemia in glucuronyl transferase deficient rats. J. Lab. and Clin Med. **70:** 273.

EXPERIMENTAL HEPATIC PORPHYRIA: STUDIES WITH STEROIDS OF PHYSIOLOGICAL ORIGIN IN MAN

Attallah Kappas and S. Granick
The Rockefeller University, N. Y., N. Y.

Introduction

This report describes the ability of steroids derived from sources physiological to man, to stimulate the activity of the porphyrin and heme biosynthetic pathway in liver cells. This new biological action of natural steroids is considered to have possible relevance to the normal cellular control of heme formation,[1-3] and to the mechanism of the periodic exacerbations which characterize the natural history of the hereditary form of hepatic porphyria.[4,5]

The porphyrin and heme biosynthetic pathway is summarized in FIGURE 1. The initial and terminal reactions depicted take place in the mitochondria; the intermediate reactions occur in the cytoplasm. The mitochondrial enzyme ALA-synthetase which condenses glycine and activated succinate to form δ-aminolevulinic acid, controls the rate limiting step in this pathway; and it has been suggested that over-all regulation of porphyrin and heme biosynthesis resides in a repressor-operator control on the activity of the structural gene which codes for this enzyme.[1,2]

This synthetic pathway is normally regulated at a low level in the liver since heme requirements for cytochromes and other heme-proteins are small. In hereditary hepatic porphyria, however, the control mechanism for heme synthesis is defective. Such patients have abnormally high levels of ALA-synthetase in the liver and excrete excessive amounts of intermediates in this biosynthetic pathway in the urine. Patients carrying the genetic lesion of this disease are also extremely sensitive to small amounts of certain drugs which may provoke severe chemical and symptomatic exacerbations of the disease. These drugs have been shown to act by stimulating the de novo formation of ALA-synthetase in liver cells.

The majority of the episodic relapses which characterize the clinical course of hepatic porphyria occur spontaneously however and not in clear relation to drug ingestion. This suggests that there might be endogenous substances which like drugs act as inducing agents in genetically susceptible subjects. The chemical nature of these endogenous inducing substances is not known, although clinical observations suggest that one class of such agents may be endocrine in origin and specifically steroidal in type. These observations include: the high female preponderance of acute intermittent hepatic porphyria despite its inheritance as an autosomal dominant trait; the almost exclusive occurrence of the disease at post-pubertal ages, the direct relation of attacks of porphyria to specific phases of the menstrual cycle or to pregnancy in some women; and the symptomatic and chemical exacerbations of the disease which have been evoked by the administration of natural and synthetic hormones, including those steroid mixtures used for contraceptive purposes.[6-10]

Methods

The present study was therefore undertaken to examine the possibility that natural steroids were capable of inducing porphyrin synthesis in liver cells. We used, in this study, an in vitro liver cell culture technique in which porphyrin production is known to be greatly enhanced by drugs and foreign chemicals

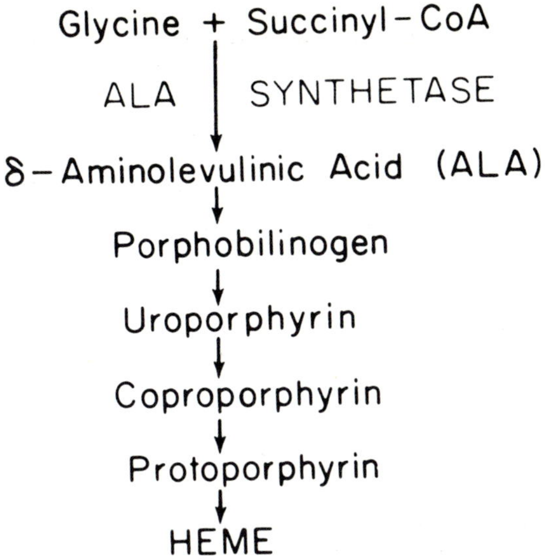

FIGURE 1. Summary of the heme biosynthetic chain. The enzyme, δ-amenolevulinic acid (ALA) synthetase controls the rate limiting step in this pathway.

which provoke hepatic porphyria in humans and in experimental animals. This culture technique has been described in detail previously.[11] It consists, briefly, in growing chick embryo liver cells in vials containing coverslips on which they form a monolayer of colonies. Steroid and other chemical additions to the vials are made one day after the cultures are started. Approximately 20–24 hours later the excess porphyrins which have been induced in the cells may be extracted and determined chemically, or may be estimated semi-quantitatively in the fluorescence microscope; the latter technique was used exclusively in this study.

Results and Discussion

Utilizing this culture technique, a variety of steroid hormones, intermediates and metabolites was examined for porphyrin-inducing activity. A number of these natural compounds were shown to have inducing action equal to or exceeding that which characterizes the most potent porphyria-inducing drugs previously described.

These potent inducing steroids are listed in TABLE 1. They are not primary endocrine secretions but are metabolites derived from the biotransformation of several adreno-cortical and gonadal hormones, as well as intermediates in the steroid biosynthetic pathway. They evoke a maximal induction response in concentrations of approximately 10^{-5} M, and may show detectable inducing action in concentrations as low as 10^{-8} M. Since the fluorescence method used depends on the accumulation of excessive amounts of porphyrins in the cells, these steroids are probably active in concentrations even lower than those studied.

Steroid-induction of porphyrin synthesis resembles in its rate of onset and course of development the induction response evoked by drugs. The inducing effects of steroids and drugs are additive if they are incorporated in the medium in sub-optimal amounts; they are not additive, nor is the latent period

TABLE 1

STEROIDS WITH STRONG PORPHYRIN-INDUCING ACTIVITY IN LIVER CELL CULTURE*

Etiocholanolone	Pregnandiol
Etiocholandiol	Pregnanolone
Etiocholandione	Pregnandione
II = O Etiocholanolone	Pregnantriol
Etiocholanolone-3β	II = O Pregnanolone

* A complete list of inducing streoids which have been studied is found in Reference 2.

shortened if they are added to the culture in optimal amounts. This suggests to us that steroids and drugs probably act at the same cellular site; or on the same rate-limiting process. The acidic steroids, or bile acids, derived from cholesterol degradation have no inducing action; C21 hydroxylated hormones such as cortisol and aldosterone are also inactive. Estradiol and related estrogens, including those synthetics used in contraceptive mixtures have weak but consistent inducing action, as do the hormonal precursors of the metabolites listed in TABLE 1, such as progesterone and testosterone.

FIGURE 2 shows, in conventional and stereochemical representations, the basic nuclear structures of the two main series of metabolites derived from steroid hormone biotransformations in man. These series are distinguished by the orientation of the hydrogen atom which is inserted at C5 during reduction of the double bond in the A ring of the hormone, and the resultant effect this has on the form of the A:B ring junction. It is of interest that all of the potent porphyrin-inducing steroids we have identified share the basic steroid nucleus characteristic of 5β-H compounds – that is metabolites in which the A:B ring junction is highly angulated. The 5α-H epimers of these inducing compounds, which have a planar or flat ring junction like the precursor hormones have weak or little activity. Recently we have shown that these 5β-H steroids also stimulate hemoglobin synthesis in the cultured embryonic erythroid cells of the chick blastoderm,[3] a preparation in which 5α-H steroids as well as precursor hormones are also only weakly active or inert. The special ability of the 5β-H structural configuration to confer inducing activity extends to other pharmacological actions of these steroids as well since 5β-H metabolites are known to have powerful hemolytic and inflammatory properties, to be potent anesthetic agents and to provoke consistent and intense pyrogenic reactions in man.[12] The mechanism by which this steroid transformation confers biological potency to metabolites which is distinct from that possessed by precursor hormones is not known, but is a problem of considerable interest to endocrinology and pharmacology.

The inducing steroid metabolites listed in TABLE 1, normally do not remain in the free form in the body, but usually undergo rapid conjugation with glucuronic acid in the liver and are excreted. It was of interest therefore to examine the effects of such conjugation on their porphyrin-inducing action. As shown in TABLE 2, the glucuronidation process entirely abolishes the activity of even potent inducing compounds like pregnandiol and etiocholanolone. We infer from these results that probably all steroid glucuronides formed in vivo are devoid of porphyrin-inducing action.

The glucose-glucuronic acid pathway via UDP, is intimately involved in conjugation mechanisms for drugs and a number of physiological substances, such as the steroids. The possibility that porphyrin-induction by free steroids could also be blocked by components of this cycle, was therefore studied. As shown in

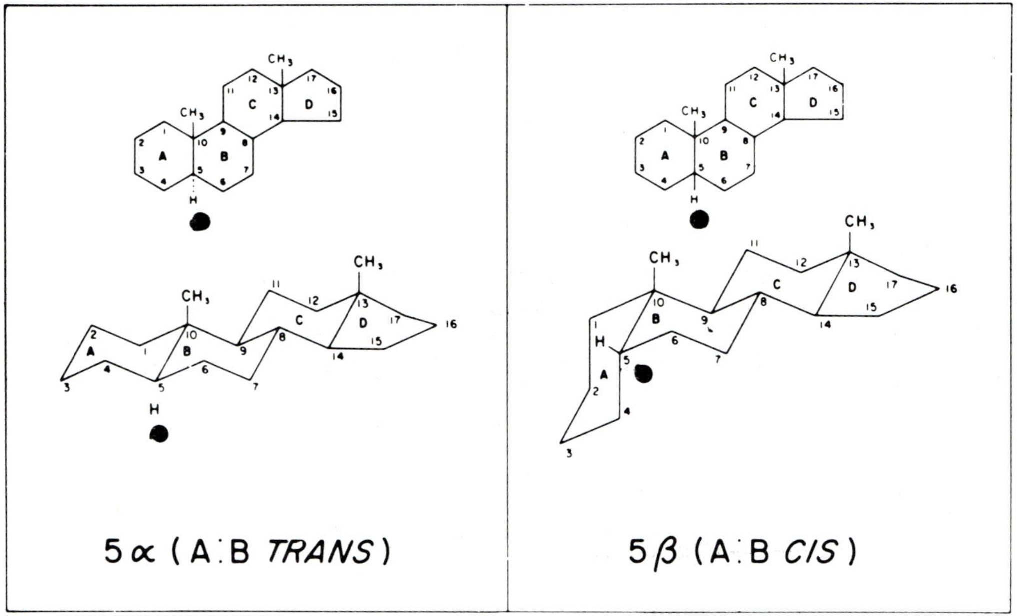

FIGURE 2. Conventional and stereochemical representations of the basic nuclear structures characteristic of 5α-H and 5β-H steroid metabolites. In these models, for purposes of simplification, only the orientations of the methyl groups at C10 and C13, and the hydrogen atom at C5 (shown by the solid dot) are indicated. The striking difference in the nature of the A:B ring junctions in these two series of metabolites is evident.

TABLE 3, uridine diphosphoglucuronic acid (UDPGA) and only this component of the cycle was able to block the induction response evoked by steroids. UDPGA is the immediate donor of glucuronic acid in conjugation reactions catalyzed by UDP-glucuronyl transferase (s). By analogy with its ability to stimulate conjugation reactions of other substrates which undergo glucuronidation, its ability to block porphyrin-induction by steroids is considered to reflect the enhanced conversion of the active free steroids to their inactive conjugates. The large amounts of UDPGA required to block steroid-induction probably reflect the relative impermeability of the cells to the nucleotide and its rapid intra-cellular hydrolysis by microsomal pyrophosphorylase.

Glucose has previously been shown to inhibit the porphyria induced by certain chemicals in animals, and high carbohydrate diets also are known to diminish porphyrin production in human porphyria.[13–15] The inhibitory influence of UDPGA on steroid-induction of porphyrin synthesis which we have demonstrated in these studies raises the possibility that these effects described in animals and man may be accounted for, in part, or perhaps in whole, by conversion of administered glucose to UDPGA which then facilitates glucuronidation—and thus inactivation—of exogenous or endogenous inducing substances.

Drugs which provoke hepatic porphyria act by stimulating the de novo production of ALA-synthetase in liver cells, and this drug effect can be blocked by inhibitors of nucleic acid and protein synthesis. As shown in TABLE 4, such agents also block the induction response evoked by steroids. Drug induction of porphyria is also blocked by heme and other metalloporphyrins which, in liver cells, appear to control the formation of ALA-synthetase by the mechanism of end-product repression. As shown in TABLE 5, these metalloporphyrins, including iron-protoporphyrin or heme, similarly compete with steroids to block their inducing action in the liver. These data extend the similarities in modes of action of porphyria-

TABLE 2

THE EFFECT OF GLUCURONIDATION ON THE PORPHYRIN-INDUCING ACTIVITY OF NATURAL STERIODS

Pregnandiol – strong inducer	Pregnandiol glucuronide – inactive
Androsterone – weak inducer	Androsterone glucuronide – inactive
Etiocholanolone – strong inducer	Etiocholanolone glucuronide – inactive
Dehydroepiandrosterone – weak inducer	Dehydroepiandrosterone glucuronide – inactive
Epiandrosterone – weak inducer	Epiandrosterone glucuronide – inactive

TABLE 3

THE EFFECTS OF COMPONENTS OF THE GLUCOSE-GLUCURONIC ACID (UDP) CYCLE ON STEROID INDUCTION OF PROPHYRIN SYNTHESIS IN LIVER CELL CULTURE

Additions to the culture medium	Effects on prophyrin synthesis
Glucose	100–1000 μg/ml no inhibition
Glucose-6-phosphate	100–1000 μg/ml no inhibition
Glucose-1-phosphate	100–1000 μg/ml no inhibition
Uridine triphosphate	100–1000 μg/ml no inhibition
Uridine diphosphate	100–1000 μg/ml no inhibition
Uridine diphosphoglucose	100–1000 μg/ml no inhibition
Glucuronic acid	100–1000 μg/ml no inhibition
Uridine diphosphoglucuronic acid	100– 250 μg/ml 25– 50% inhibition
	500–1000 μg/ml 50–100% inhibition

TABLE 4

THE EFFECTS OF INHIBITORS OF NUCLEIC ACID AND PROTEIN SYNTHESIS ON STEROID-INDUCTION OF PROPHYRINS

Additions to the culture medium		Effects on prophyrin synthesis
Actinomycin D	0.01 – 0.05 μg/ml	50–100% inhibition
Mitomycin C	0.5 – 2.0 μg/ml	25– 75% inhibition
Puromycin	1.0 – 5.0 μg/ml	50–100% inhibition
Acetoxycycloheximide	0.005– 0.010 μg/ml	50–100% inhibition
p-Fluorophenylalanine	20.0 –80.0 μg/ml	25–100% inhibition

TABLE 5

EFFECTS OF METALLOPORPHYRINS ON THE INDUCTION OF PORPHYRINS BY STEROIDS

Additions to the culture medium		Effects on prophyrin synthesis
F_e-protoporphyrin	1.5 μg/ml	50% inhibition
	4.5 μg/ml	75% inhibition
Mn-protoporphyrin	4.5 μg/ml	75% inhibition
Zn-protoporphyrin	4.5 μg/ml	75% inhibition

inducing drugs and natural steroids, and are consistent with the view that the latter compounds stimulate porphyrin formation in liver by inducing ALA-synthetase the rate-limiting enzyme in this biosynthetic pathway. Recent unpublished studies from this laboratory in which direct estimation of this enzyme activity has been made in whole animal preparations confirm this view.

It is suggested as a working hypothesis that inducing steroids control formation of ALA-synthetase by the mechanism depicted in FIGURE 3. Control of porphyrin and heme synthesis in the liver is considered to reside in a repressor-operator mechanism which regulates the activity of the structural gene (G_1) which codes for the limiting enzyme ALA-synthetase (E_1). All other enzymes (E_2–E_7) in the heme biosynthetic chain are present normally in nonlimiting amounts. The repressor comprises an aporepressor protein to which a co-repressor, heme, is bound. The repressor is inactivated by chemicals such as porphyria-inducing drugs, or steroids of appropriate structure, which compete with heme for its binding site on the apoprotein. Inactivation of the repressor leads to "derepression" of the structural gene for ALA-synthetase, enhanced formation of this rate-limiting enzyme, and increased production of heme as well as of the intermediate porphyrins and precursors in this biosynthetic pathway. The concentration of active steroid-inducers in the hepatic cell would depend on the rate of their conversion by UDP-glucuronyltransferase to the inactive glucuronides and the rate of hydrolysis of the glucuronides back to the active free form by β-glucuronidase.

The role of steroids as endogenous provocative agents in hereditary hepatic porphyria would be contingent on the quantity of unconjugated steroid-inducers which gained access to the inducing site (s) in the liver. Thus, any process such as starvation or glucose restriction which impaired glucuronidation of steroids might lead to the accumulation of free steroids in liver cells, in concentration sufficient to stimulate further production of ALA-synthetase in subjects carrying the genetic lesion of hepatic porphyria. Excessive production of inhibitors of UDP-glucuronyltransferase could also lead to the accumulation of high concentrations of inducing-steroids in liver cells. In this respect it is of interest that certain porphyrin-

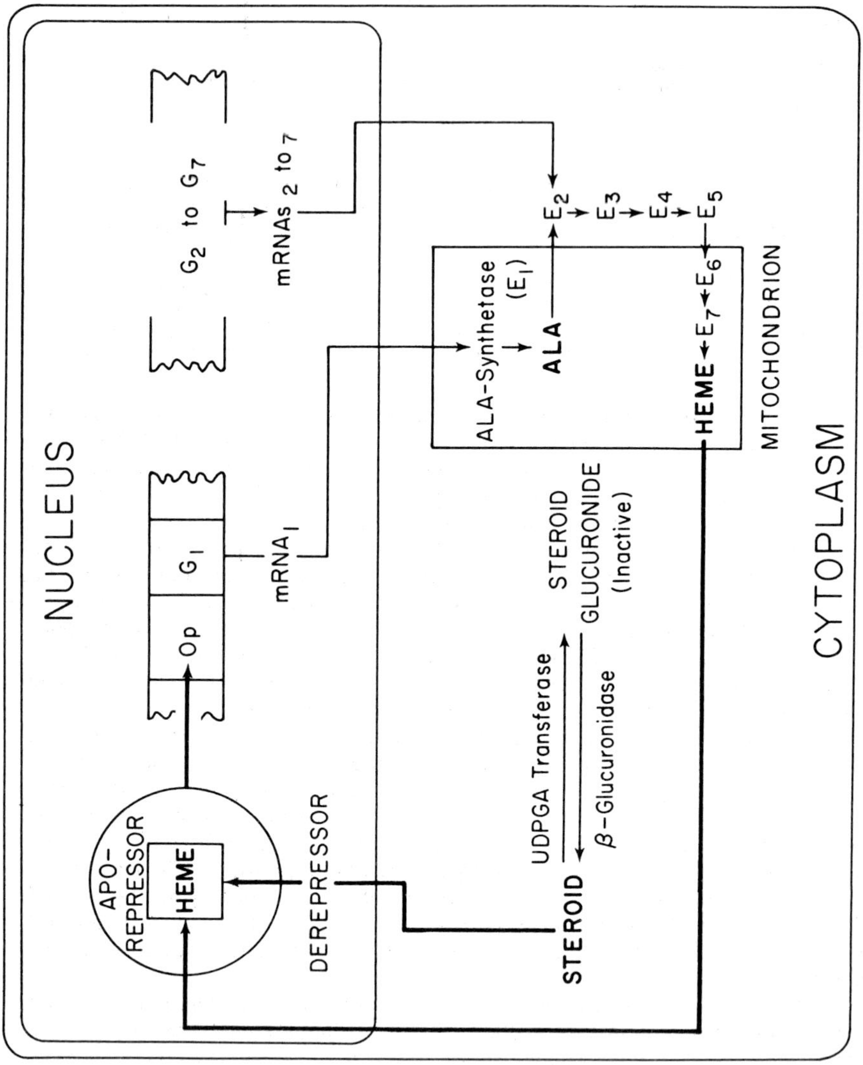

FIGURE 3. Schema depicting a proposed mechanism for steroid control of heme biosynthesis. The details of the schema are discussed in the text.

inducing steroids themselves, such as pregnandiol, are known to inhibit the activity of UDP-glucuronyltransferase.[16–18] This raises the theoretic possibility of a vicious cycle in which such steroids having initially accumulated in liver cells in sufficient concentration, would inhibit UDP-glucuronyltransferase, leading to further inhibition of steroid glucuronidation which would further increase the concentration of free steroid-inducers, etc. Patients carrying the genetic defect for hepatic porphyria would be especially susceptible to the action of endogenous steroids postulated here. However, in normal subjects contraceptive steroid mixtures may enhance porphyrin-precursor excretion and drug or chemical-induced porphyria may be evoked in normal man, and normal experimental animals under appropriate conditions. It is considered possible therefore that the inducing effect of endogenous steroids might also be reflected in the porphyrinurias which characterize certain patients with acquired types of liver disease, such as cirrhosis, in whom steroid conjugation is known to be impaired and in whom elevated levels of ALA-synthetase have recently been demonstrated.[19]

The hypothetical nature of the schema depicted in FIGURE 3, is emphasized. It does not uniquely explain the data reported and other interpretations of them can be made. As a working hypothesis, however, this model may be a useful formulation to consider in examining the mechanism of this new steroid action. Moreover, there is substantial clinical evidence which suggests the deleterious interplay of endocrine factors in the pathogenesis of hereditary hepatic porphyria. The data reported here, define a class of agents and mode of action by which this endocrine-genetic interplay may be effected in some patients.

References

1. GRANICK, S. & A. KAPPAS. 1967. Proc. Natl. Acad. Sci. **57**: 1463.
2. GRANICK, S. & A. KAPPAS. 1967. J. Biol. Chem. **242**: 4587.
3. LEVERE, R. D., A. KAPPAS & S. GRANICK. 1967. Proc. Natl. Acad. Sci. **58**: 985.
4. KAPPAS, A. & S. GRANICK. 1968. J. Biol. Chem. **243**: 346.
5. KAPPAS, A. & S. GRANICK. 1967. Trans. Assoc. Amer. Physicians **80**: 323.
6. LEVIT, E. J., J. H. NODINE & W. H. PERLOFF. 1957. Am. J. Med. **22**: 831.
7. WELLAND, F. H., E. S. HELLMAN, A. COLLINS & G. W. HUNTER, JR. & D. P. TSCHUDY. 1964. Metabolism **13**: 251.
8. ZIMMERMAN, T. S., J. M. MCMILLAN & C. J. WATSON. 1966. Arch. Int. Med. **118**: 229.
9. KOTTRA, J. & A. KAPPAS. 1967. Ann. Rev. Med. **18**: 325.
10. KOSKELO, P., A. EISALO & I. TOIVONEN. 1966. Brit. Med. J. **1**: 652.
11. GRANICK, S. 1966. J. Biol. Chem. **241**: 1359.
12. KAPPAS, A. & R. H. PALMER. 1963. Pharmacological Rev. **15**: 123.
13. TSCHUDY, D. P., F. H. WELLAND, A. COLLINS & G. HUNTER, JR. 1964. Metabolism **13**: 396.
14. DE MATTEIS, F. 1964. Biochem. & Biophysic. Acta **82**: 641.
15. WELLAND, F. H., E. S. HELLMAN, E. M. GADDIS, A. COLLINS & G. HUNTER, JR. 1964. Metabolism **13**: 232.
16. LATHE, G. H. & M. WALKER. 1968. Quart. J. Exper. Physiol. **43**: 257.
17. ARIAS, I., L. M. GARTNER, S. SEIFTER & M. FURMAN. 1964. J. Clin. Invest. **43**: 2037.
18. HSIA, D., R. DOWBEN, R. SHAW & A. GROSSMAN. 1960. Nature **187**: 603.
19. LEVERE, R. D. 1967. Biochem. Med. **1**: 92.

CLINICAL ASPECTS OF DRUG REACTIONS IN HEREDITARY HEPATIC PORPHYRIA

Donald P. Tschudy
Metabolism Branch, National Cancer Institute
National Institutes of Health, Bethesda, Md.

It was first demonstrated by Schmid, Schwartz and Watson[1] that the chemical abnormalities of the various types of porphyria originated in either the bone marrow or liver. This led to the classification of these diseases into two major groups–erythropoietic and hepatic. The erythropoietic type can now be clearly divided further into two types: (a) congenital erythropoietic porphyria and (b) erythropoietic protoporphyria. The latter disorder was only recently recognized as a type of porphyria because it is the only form of porphyria in which increased urinary excretion of porphyrins or porphyrin precursors is not seen.[2] Further classification of the hepatic porphyrias is more difficult because there is some degree of overlap in the biochemical and clinical findings in this group. Until the specific enzymatic defects characteristic of each form of these diseases have been elucidated, the problem of subdivision of the hepatic porphyrias will not be completely resolved. The similar classifications of Watson[3] and Eales[4] subdivide the hepatic porphyrias into three main groups which have been given various names in the past:

A. Acute intermittent porphyria, Swedish genetic porphyria, pyrrolporphyria (dominant).

B. Porphyria variegata, mixed porphyria, South African genetic porphyria, porphyria cutanea tarda hereditaria, protocoproporphyria (dominant).

C. Porphyria cutanea tarda, symptomatic porphyria, urocoproporphyria, constitutional porphyria, porphyria cutanea tarda symptomatica.

It is in the first two of the above listed types of hepatic porphyria where ingestion of certain drugs can be dangerous. While both of these disorders may have episodes of acute neurologic dysfunction which produce similar clinical manifestations, they differ in several other respects. In acute porphyria: a) skin lesions do not occur, b) there is little or no increase of fecal copro- or protoporphyrin, and c) porphyria precursor excretion is usually significantly increased in the quiescent phase as well as during the acute attacks in most adults. In variegate porphyria: a) skin lesions occur in the patient or in other members of the patient's family, b) the fecal protoporphyrin is usually increased, and c) porphyrin precursor excretion is considerably increased during the acute attack, but often returns to normal or near normal during quiescence.[5] Unfortunately, there are some patients who do not fit neatly into these categories.

Both of these diseases are inborn errors of metabolism in which the symptomatic episodes of neurologic dysfunction may be precipitated by drugs, infections, endocrine factors,[6] and starvation.[7,8]

Because they produce abnormalities of porphyrin metabolism in animals which resemble those seen in some of the human porphyrias, certain drugs and other synthetic compounds are proving to be of value in attempts to elucidate the biochemcial defects in these diseases. Drugs or hormones which are known to precipitate clinical attacks in these diseases include barbiturates,[9] sulfonamides,[9] griseofulvin,[10] diphenylhydantoin,[11] estrogen,[12] and possibly ergot and alcohol. While these drugs can produce changes in porphyrin metabolism in experimental systems,[13] it is still not clear how these changes in liver are related to the episodes of damage to the nervous system. Some patients have greatly increased excretion of porphyrin precursors for years while remaining asymptomatic.

During acute attacks, damage may occur in any area of the nervous system. Autonomic neuropathy has been demonstrated histologically and is thought to be the explanation of the abdominal pain, constipation, tachycardia, hypertension or postural hypotension and sweating which may be seen during acute attacks. Imbalance in the autonomic innervation of the gut leads to areas of spasm which produce abdominal pain. This may be misdiagnosed as appendicitis, renal or gall bladder colic, intestinal obstruction, etc., resulting in needless surgery. This explanation of the abdominal pain is supported not only by histologic evidence, but also by pharmacologic evidence in that ganglionic blocking agents alleviate the abdominal pain. Much of the effectiveness of chlorpromazine in relieving the abdominal pain of porphyria is undoubtedly related to its ganglionic blocking action.

Peripheral neuropathy may exist as either sensory or motor neuropathy. Pain in the legs and back is common and may precede the onset of motor paralysis, or may occur intermittently or chronically without motor involvement. Less commonly, pain occurs in the arms or chest. In severe attacks, motor involvement may be both extensive and rapidly progressive. Some patients develop complete quadriplegia, aphonia, respiratory paralysis, dysphagia, and cranial nerve palsies over periods of 48 to 72 hours. Evidence of involvement of the spinal cord or cere-

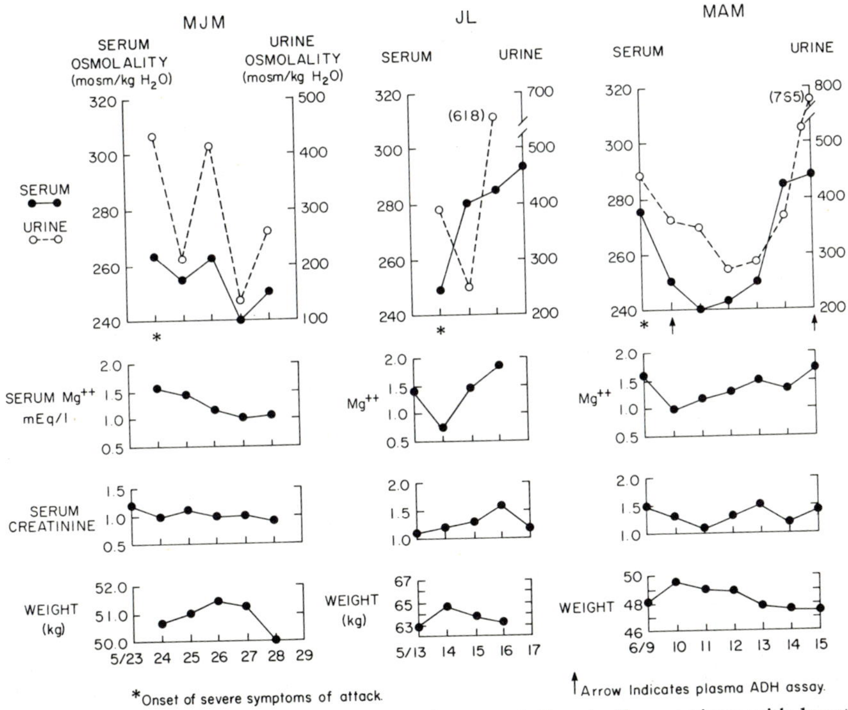

FIGURE 1. Parameters of water and electrolyte metabolism in three patients with hepatic porphyria studied from the onset of symptoms of an acute attack.

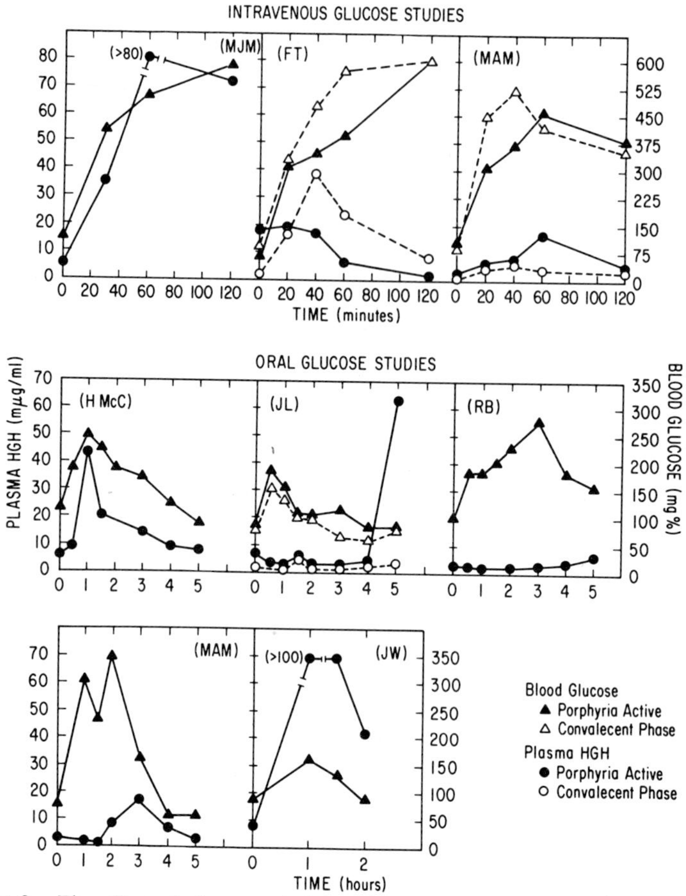

FIGURE 2. The effect of glucose administration on plasma levels of growth hormone in patients with hepatic porphyria.

bellum may be masked on physical examination by the peripheral neuropathy. Death may result from bulbar involvement.

The psychiatric manifestations of these disorders include both neuroses and psychoses. In one study, 1.1% of 2,500 consecutive admissions to a mental hospital had a positive Watson-Schwartz test.[14] The psychoses may be of the schizophrenic or manic-depressive types. In some patients, the onset of an attack may be ushered in by hallucinations, confusion, agitation or seizures—manifestations of an "organic brain syndrome." This situation undoubtedly results at times from water intoxication secondary to the syndrome of inappropriate release of antidiuretic hormone.

The first suggestion of hypothalmic involvement in acute porphyria was made[15] when some of the episodes of hyponatremia seen in this disorder were attributed to this syndrome.[15,16] An excess of antidiuretic material was later demonstrated in the urine of a patient with this disease.[17] Histological evidence of hypothalmic

TABLE 1

ADRENAL FUNCTION STUDIES IN ACUTE INTERMITTENT PORPHYRIA

		Dexamethasone Suppression Tests				Methopyrapone (SU4885) Tests				
Patient	Duration of Test (days)	Urine* 17 Hydroxycorticoids, mg/24 hrs		Blood† 8 AM plasma 17 hydroxy-corticoids	Route of Adminis-tration	mcg/24 hrs‡ (urine)		mcg/100 ml§ (plasma)		Clinical Activity of Disease (1-4+)
		Control	Minimum			Control	Maximum	Control	Maximum	
MJM	2	7.0	1.0	11.1						0
J Le		8.7	—	4.8						1+
MAM	3	7.2	4.6	10.7	IV			10.7	26.4	3+
MAM	2	11.6	4.0							1+
J La	3	6.9	1.9		oral	6.8	17.8			1+
FT	2	6.0	2.9							2+
RB	3	9.7	4.8		oral	8.0	27.1			2+
CA	3	6.7	3.3							1+
NM	3	8.1	4.1							1+
MT	3	5.7	2.7		oral	5.7	14.3			0

* Test performed as described by Liddle, *et al.*[54]

† Patients received 1.0 mg dexamethasone at 11 PM prior to 8 AM sample.[33,55]

‡ Patients received 750 mg methopyrapone orally every 4 hr for 6 doses.[51,52]

§ Patient received 1.5 g methopyrapone i.v. over a 4 hr period.[53]

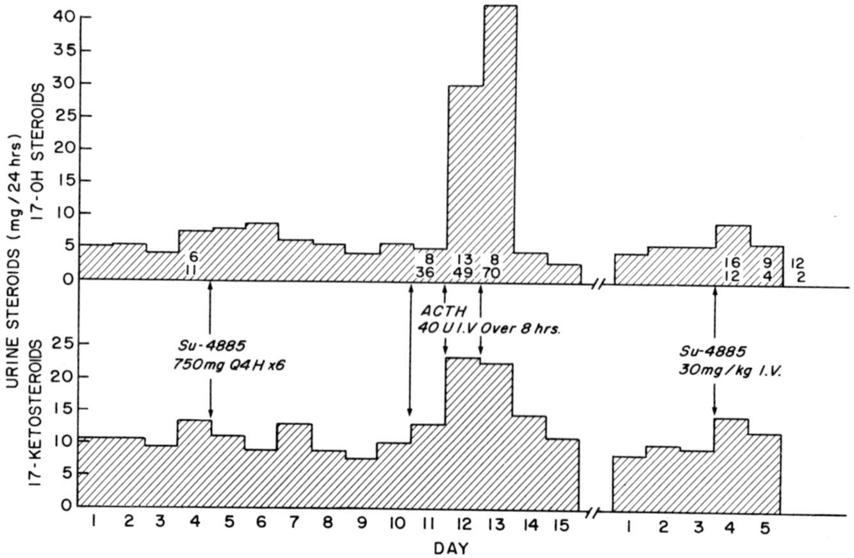

FIGURE 3. The effect of methopyrapone (SU 4885) and ACTH on 17-keto- and 17-hydroxysteroids in a symptomatic adult male patient with acute intermittent porphyria. Urinary steroid excretion values are plotted in the bar graphs. Plasma 17-hydroxycorticoids are indicated as the numbers in the upper bar graphs. The upper number represents the 8 AM and the lower number the 4 PM value. The first study with methopyrapone was performed by administration of 750 mg of the compound every 4 hours for 6 doses.[51,52] The later study with this compound was performed after intravenous administration of 30 mg/kg.[53]

damage has now provided definitive proof that this portion of the nervous system may be involved by the disease process.[18] A destructive lesion involving the median eminence and the fibers of the supraoptic and paraventricular nuclei was evident in a patient who died of acute porphyria. The pathogenesis of the syndrome of inappropriate release of antidiuretic hormone (ADH) in porphyria can be postulated as follows. Damage of the fibers of the supraoptic and paraventricular nuclei caused by the disease process allows leakage of ADH into the circulation. This leakage cannot be shut off by decreased osmolality of the plasma. The sequence of events which follows may be identical to that seen in normal individuals given injections of exogenous ADH.[19,20] Hyponatremia results from both water retention and from increased urinary sodium loss. However, the increased urinary sodium loss only occurs when there is an increased body fluid volume.[21] Maintenance of sufficient water intake during Pitressin® administration is associated with an initial decrease of urine volume and excessive sodium excretion which continue for a few days, after which a new equilibrium state occurs with lower serum osmolality. In several patients a profound decline of serum sodium to levels below 100 mEq/L has occurred during acute attacks of porphyria. Since the water intoxication which can result from this syndrome may cause seizures and hallucinations or other manifestations of an "organic brain syndrome" it is important to recognize and treat this complication. Water restriction is usually adequate therapy for this problem.

Another complication sometimes seen in this syndrome is hypomagnesemic tetany.[15,17] Hypomagnesemia is not produced in normal volunteers by magnesium restriction for considerable periods of time, but its occurrence with this syndrome is probably explained by the fact that ADH augments magnesium excretion by the kidney.[22]

Examples of the abnormal findings which are thought to result from excessive circulating levels of ADH are presented in FIGURE 1.* These three patients were studied from the onset of symptoms of an attack of acute intermittent porphyria. In all three there was decreased serum osmolality, hypomagnesemia, and weight gain. Assays of circulating ADH performed in patient No. 3 of FIGURE 1[23] provided further evidence for the existence of the syndrome in this patient.

The degree to which excessive ADH will be accompanied by decreased serum osmolality is a function of water intake. During acute attacks, patients sometimes develop nausea and vomiting which may curtail their fluid intake sufficiently to prevent a marked decrease of serum osmolality and water intoxication. Intravenous administration of excessive amounts of dextrose and water in this situation may lead to the full-blown syndrome. While the fact that evidence for excessive ADH can often be found in patients with active porphyria suggests that hypothalamic damage occurs frequently in this disease, it should be emphasized that hyponatremia can sometimes result from the vomiting or less commonly observed diarrhea of symptomatic episodes. With administration of excessive intravenous dextrose in water, a decline of serum osmolality can thus also occur in the absence of excessive ADH.

* Data of M. G. Perlroth and D. P. Tschudy.

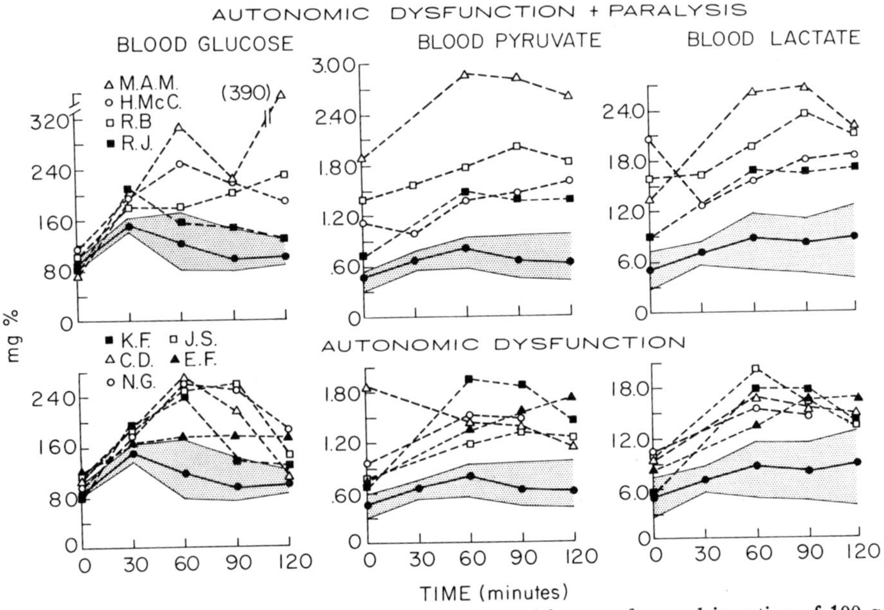

FIGURE 4. The curves of blood glucose, pyruvate and lactate after oral ingestion of 100 g glucose by patients with acute intermittent porphyria. The solid lines represent the mean values from a group of normal controls and the shaded area represents the range of this group. The upper set of graphs is from patients who experienced both autonomic dysfunction and paralysis. The lower set is from a group who were less severely afflicted by the disease in that they had evidence of only autonomic neuropathy.

The pathologic lesion observed in the hypothalamus of the patient who died from acute intermittent porphyria involved the median eminence. Since this is an area where releasing factors for anterior pituitary hormones are known to occur,[24–26] it was suspected that perhaps abnormalities of the control of the secretion of these hormones might occur in this disease. The first hormone studied in this regard was growth hormone, and the above suspicions were fully confirmed.[27] When normal adults are given a glucose load, growth hormone levels in the blood fall to virtually immeasurable levels (< 1 mμg/ml) over a three hour period, followed by a rebound between three and four hours, which again returns to baseline by six hours.[28] As seen in FIGURE 2, there was a normal response of circulating growth hormone levels in only one of the first seven patients with acute intermittent porphyria studied after glucose loading. The only other normal response in the 11 studies performed on these seven patients was in J. L. during convalescence. During her symptomatic period, there was a greater than normal rebound of plasma growth hormone level five hours after glucose administration. In six of the other eight studies, an increase of plasma growth hormone occurred as blood glucose levels rose. The increase was sometimes to very high levels. This response is the opposite of that seen in normals. In all three patients studied during both the active phase of their disease and during convalescence, abnormalities of growth hormone response to glucose persisted in the convalescent phase. However, the degree of abnormality was somewhat less in two of the three patients during convalescence. These studies demonstrate that "inappropriate release of growth hormone" occurs frequently in acute intermittent porphyria and further substantiate the concept that altered hypothalamic function occurs frequently in

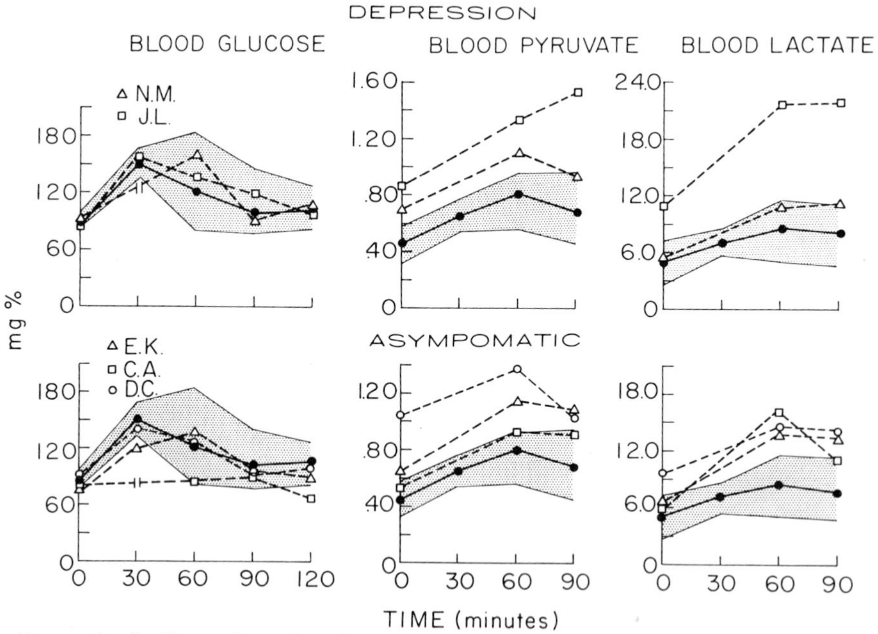

FIGURE 5. Studies performed as those described in FIGURE 4. The upper set of graphs is from patients with only mental depression and the lower set is from patients with latent porphyria who had never been ill with the disease.

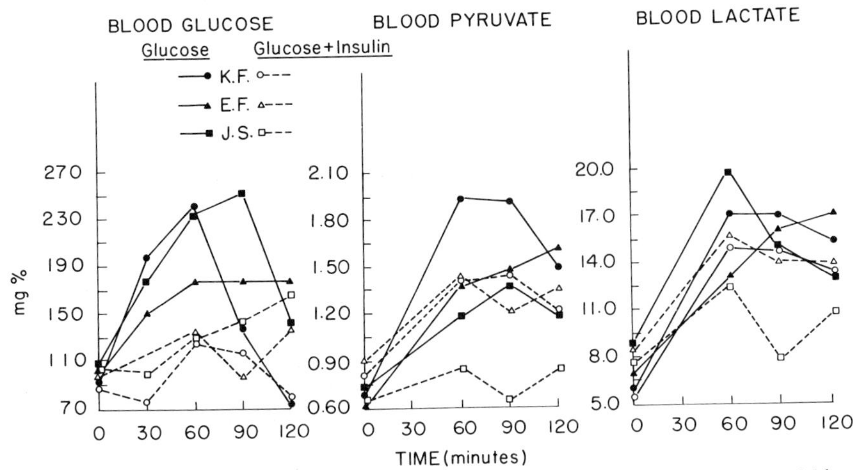

FIGURE 6. The effect of insulin administration (0.1 unit/kg i.v.) on the curves of blood glucose, pyruvate and lactate after oral ingestion of 100 g glucose by three patients with acute intermittent porphyria. The solid lines are the values after glucose administration and the dotted lines are those after insulin was administered concomitantly with glucose.

this disease. A similar paradoxical hypersecretion of growth hormone during hyperglycemia has also been observed in newborn infants,[29] acromegaly, a child with an optic glioma[30,31] and in breast cancer.[32]

It has been suggested that stress can cause elevation of plasma growth hormone levels. During the stress of abdominal surgery, mild elevations of plasma growth hormone up to the range of 10 mμg/ml have been observed.[28] These stress-induced increases of growth hormone differ from the findings in porphyria in two respects. First, the stress-induced increases of plasma growth hormone were lower than the peak values in the porphyrics; and second, glucose administration caused the appropriate decline of the circulating growth hormone in the patients where stress had increased its level. These findings make it unlikely that the paradoxical secretion of growth hormone observed in the porphyric patients is caused by stress.

The next pituitary hormone studied was ACTH. Since circulating levels of this hormone could not be assayed directly, measurements of steroids were made which only secondarily reflect changes in ACTH levels. These may be far less accurate indications of changes in ACTH levels than direct measurements of ACTH itself. The responsiveness of the adrenal-pituitary axis was studied by means of dexamethasone suppression tests and methopyrapone (SU 4885) administration as shown in TABLE 1.* Approximately half the porphyric patients studied by dexamethasone administration suppressed to the borderline level of 17-hydroxycorticoid excretion seen in normals.[33] It is well known that stress can raise the threshold to feedback inhibition of ACTH secretion.[34,35] Nugent[33] studied plasma 17-hydroxycorticoid suppression in acutely ill nonporphyric patients and found responses similar to those seen in the porphyric patients presented in TABLE 1. These findings, therefore, cannot be interpreted as evidence of a syndrome of "inappropriate release of ACTH" in acute intermittent porphyria.

* Data of M. G. Perlroth, A. Waxman and D. P. Tschudy.

In all of the patients in TABLE 1 who were given methopyrapone (SU 4885) a normal rise of urinary or serum 17-hydroxycorticoids was seen, indicating a normal ability to secrete ACTH. However, one other patient who was studied later because of a question of adrenal insufficiency during an acute attack of the disease was found to have impaired ability to secrete ACTH after methopyrapone administration, as seen in FIGURE 3.* Adrenal steroid secretion was normal after exogenous ACTH. While the data in FIGURE 3 do not allow a differentiation between a pituitary or hypothalamic lesion as the cause of the defective ACTH secretion, it is possible that this man had a lesion in the hypothalamus involving the control of the releasing factor for ACTH.

Carbohydrate metabolism has been studied in patients with acute porphyria for two reasons. First, the inappropriate release of growth hormone following a glucose load might impair glucose utilization in these patients. Secondly, it has been demonstrated that the excessive porphyrin precursor excretion of experimental porphyria[13,36–39] and acute intermittent porphyria[40,41] results from a markedly increased level of hepatic δ-aminolevulinic acid synthetase (ALA synthetase), the first and rate-controlling enzyme of porphyrin biosynthesis. The induction of this enzyme in liver is blocked by carbohydrate administration[38] and studies of the effects of diet on porphyrin precursor excretion in acute intermittent porphyria indicate that the genetically mediated induction in man is also blocked by carbohydrate.[42] Since carbohydrate utilization exercises a regulatory influence over the level of hepatic ALA synthetase, it is possible that an abnormality of this regulatory mechanism could be related to the induction of hepatic ALA synthetase in acute intermittent porphyria.

As seen in FIGURE 4,† all patients with paralysis and/or autonomic neuropathy had a markedly abnormal glucose tolerance test. In all of this group of patients, blood lactate and pyruvate rose to levels well above those seen in normals. These findings differ from those of non-insulin secreting diabetics who have a normal or less than normal rise of blood pyruvate or lactate following a glucose load.[43–45] Asymptomatic patients with acute intermittent porphyria had a normal glucose tolerance test (FIGURE 5) and only slight elevation of pyruvate and lactate. Thiamine administration had no effect on the abnormal curves of glucose or pyruvate, but insulin, when given along with the glucose load, tended to move the curves of glucose, pyruvate and lactate toward normal (FIGURE 6). This tendency to lowering of pyruvate and lactate levels in the porphyric patients when insulin and glucose are given together again differs from the findings seen in insulin-requiring diabetics. In the latter group, an increase of blood pyruvate occurs after insulin and glucose when compared with glucose alone. This occurs because glucose will raise the blood pyruvate level when it is able to enter the cell under the influence of insulin.[45]

The decreased glucose tolerance and increased blood pyruvate and lactate levels after glucose ingestion were seen in some porphyric patients who had a normal growth hormone response to glucose. Therefore, the "inappropriate release of growth hormone" cannot be the sole explanation of the abnormal glucose metabolism seen in these patients. Since the degree of abnormal carbohydrate metabolism appears to correlate fairly well with the clinical activity of the disease, it is possible that these findings might result from stress. Certain steroids[46–48] and epinephrine[46] are known to produce changes in carbohydrate metabolism similar to those seen above. The baseline 17-hydroxysteroid values on the ten patients

* Data of A. Waxman and D. P. Tschudy.

† Data of A. Waxman and D. P. Tschudy.

presented in TABLE 1 and other studies of 17-ketosteroids have thus far not detected any evidence of increased steroid production in these patients. However, a highly active steroid present in small amounts might not be evident as an increase of a major steroid fraction.

A number of other chemical findings in patients with acute porphyria include increased serum protein bound iodine,[49] hypercholesterolemia[49,50] and BSP retention.[1,49] The manner in which all of these diverse biochemical changes are related to what is presumed to be a single mutation remains a mystery. The solution of this mystery will undoubtedly have implications which extend far beyond porphyria.

References

1. SCHMID, R., S. SCHWARTZ & C. J. WATSON. 1954. Arch. Int. Med. **93:** 167.
2. MAGNUS, I. A., A. JARRETT, I. A. J. PRANKERD & C. RIMINGTON. 1961. Lancet **2:** 448.
3. WATSON, C. J. 1960. New Eng. J. Med. **263:** 1205.
4. EALES, L. 1963. S. Afr. J. Lab. Clin. Med. **9:** 151.
5. DEAN, G. 1963. S. Afr. J. Lab. Clin. Med. **9:** 145.
6. GOLDBERG, A. & C. RIMINGTON. 1962. Diseases of Prophyrin Metabolism. Charles C. Thomas Co. Springfield, Ill.
7. KNUDSEN, K. B., M. SPARBERG & F. LECOQ. 1967. New Eng. J. Med. **277:** 350.
8. PERLROTH, M. G. & D. P. TSCHUDY. Unpublished observations.
9. SCHMID, R. 1966. The porphyrias. *In* The Metabolic Basis of Inherited Disease. McGraw-Hill, N. Y.
10. BERMAN, A. & R. L. FRANKLIN. 1965. J. Amer. Med. Assoc. **192:** 1005.
11. GRETTER, T. E., P. K. DANNER, D. W. NIBBELINK, D. GREEN & A. L. SAHS. 1963. Trans. Amer. Neurol. Assoc. **88:** 176.
12. ZIMMERMAN, T. S., J. M. MCMILLIN & C. J. WATSON. 1966. Arch. Int. Med. **118:** 229.
13. GRANICK, S. 1966. J. Biol. Chem. **241:** 1359.
14. KAEBLING, R., J. CRAIG & B. PASAMANICK. 1961. Arch. Gen. Psychiatry **5:** 494.
15. HELLMAN, E. S., D. P. TSCHUDY & F. C. BARTTER. 1962. Amer. J. Med. **32:** 734.
16. LUDWIG, G. D. & M. GOLDBERG. 1963. Ann. N. Y. Acad. Sc. **104:** 710.
17. NIELSEN, B. & N. A. THORN. 1965. Amer. J. Med. **38:** 345.
18. PERLROTH, M. G., D. P. TSCHUDY, H. S. MARVER, C. W. BERARD, R. F. ZIEGEL, M. RECHCIGL & A. COLLINS. 1966. Am. J. Med. **41:** 149.
19. WESTON, R. E., I. B. HANENSON, J. GROSSMAN, G. A. BENDASCO & M. WOLFMAN. 1953. J. Clin. Invest. **32:** 611.
20. JAENIKE, J. R. & G. WATERHOUSE. 1959. Clin. Res. **7:** 272.
21. LEAF, A., F. C. BARTTER, R. F. SANTOS & O. WRONG. 1953. J. Clin. Invest. **32:** 686.
22. NIELSEN, B. 1964. Acta Endocrin. **45:** 151.
23. PERLROTH, M. G., D. P. TSCHUDY & J. DINGMAN. Unpublished data.
24. HALASZ, B. & L. PUPP. 1965. Endocrinology **77:** 553.
25. VERNIKOS-DANELLIS, J. 1964. Endocrinology **75:** 514.
26. MCCANN, S. M. 1962. Am. J. Physiol. **202:** 395.
27. PERLROTH, M. G., D. P. TSCHUDY, A. WAXMAN & W. D. ODELL. 1967. Metabolism **16:** 87.
28. GLICK, S. M., J. ROTH, R. S. YALOW & S. A. BERSON. 1965. Recent Progress Horm. Res. **21:** 241.
29. CORNBLATH, M., M. L. PARKER, S. H. REISNER, A. E. FORBES & W. H. DAUGHADAY. 1965. J. Clin. End. & Metab. **25:** 209.
30. ROTH, J., S. M. GLICK, R. S. YALOW & S. A. BERSON. 1963. Metabolism **12:** 577.
31. BECK, P., D. S. SCHALCH, M. L. PARKER, D. M. KIPNIS & W. H. DAUGHADAY. 1965. J. Lab. Clin. Med. **66:** 366.
32. SAMAAN, N., O. H. PEARSON, D. GONZALEZ & O. LLERENA. 1966. J. Lab. Clin. Med. **68:** 1011.
33. NUGENT, C. A., T. NICHOLS & F. H. TYLER. 1965. Arch. Int. Med. **116:** 172.
34. GOLD, E. M., J. R. KENT & P. H. FORSHAM. 1961. Ann. Int. Med. **54:** 175.
35. YATES, F. E. & J. H. URQUHART. 1962. Physiol. Rev. **42:** 359.
36. GRANICK, S. & G. URATA. 1963. J. Biol. Chem. **238:** 821.
37. TSCHUDY, D. P., F. H. WELLAND, A. COLLINS & G. HUNTER, JR. 1964. Metabolism **13:** 396.
38. TSCHUDY, D. P., H. S. MARVER & A. COLLINS. 1965. Biochem. Biophys. Res. Comm. **21:** 480.

39. Narisawa, K. & G. Kikuchi. 1965. Biochim. Biophys. Acta **99:** 580.
40. Tschudy, D. P., M. G. Perlroth, H. S. Marver, A. Collins, G. Hunter, Jr. & M. Rechcigl, Jr. 1965. Proc. Nat. Acad. Sc. **53:** 841.
41. Nakao, K., O. Wada, T. Kitamura, K. Uono & G. Urata. 1966. Nature **210:** 838.
42. Welland, F. H., E. S. Hellman, E. M. Gaddis, A. Collins, G. W. Hunter, Jr. & D. P. Tschudy. 1964. Metabolism **13:** 232.
43. Smith, M. J. H. & K. W. Taylor. 1956. Brit. Med. J. **ii:** 1035.
44. Butterfield, W. J. H. & R. H. S. Thompson. 1957. Clin. Sc. **16:** 679.
45. Anderson, J. & V. Marks. 1962. Lancet **i:** 1159.
46. Weil, R. 1965. Acta Endocrin. Suppl. **98:** 1.
47. Wynn, V. & J. W. Doar. 1966. Lancet **i:** 715.
48. Hennes, A. R., B. L. Wajchenberg, S. S. Fajans & J. W. Conn. 1957. Metabolism **6:** 339.
49. Hellman, E. S., D. P. Tschudy, J. Robbins & J. E. Rall. 1963. J. Clin. End. & Metab. **23:** 1185.
50. Taddeini, L., K. L. Nordstrom & C. J. Watson. 1964. Metabolism **13:** 691.
51. Oppenheimer, J. H., L. V. Fisher & J. W. Jailer. 1961. J. Clin. Endocr. & Metab. **21:** 1023.
52. Liddle, G. W., D. Island, E. M. Lance & A. P. Harris. 1958. J. Clin. Endocr. & Metab. **18:** 906.
53. Gold, E. M., J. R. Kent & P. H. Forsham. 1961. Ann. Int. Med. **54:** 175.
54. Liddle, G. W. 1960. J. Clin. Endocr. & Metab. **20:** 1539.
55. Pavlatos, F. C., R. P. Smilo & P. F. Forsham. 1965. Clin. Res. **13:** 133.

GENETIC FACTORS RELATED TO GLAUCOMA*†

Mansour F. Armaly

Department of Ophthalmology
University of Iowa
Iowa City, Iowa

Introduction

The anti-inflammatory glucocorticoids were shown to produce an increase in intraocular pressure when applied topically to the eye,[1-3] or when administered systemically.[4] This hypertensive response was similar to that appearing spontaneously in open angle glaucoma in that it was virtually symptomless and could reach clinically significant levels that lead to glaucomatous destruction of visual function.[5,6] In this presentation I shall briefly describe the characteristics of this response and summarize the results of a series of studies that demonstrated its genetic nature and its role in the determination of important ocular parameters such as ocular pressure and aqueous outflow facility, as well as disease states that include open angle glaucoma, post-traumatic glaucoma and diabetes.

The Characteristics of the Response in the Normal Eye

The characteristics of the response in the clinically normal eye appear in FIGURE 1. Following the topical application 0.1% ophthalmic solution of dexamethasone 21-diphosphate to the right eye (OD); the intraocular pressure (P_A) as measured by the applanation tonometer[7] showed a progressive increase in the treated eye only. This ocular hypertension increased with the duration of drug application. The mechanism of the ocular hypertension is evident in the simultaneous reduction in aqueous outflow facility (C) as measured by tonography.[7] The reversible nature of this response was clearly demonstrated by discontinuing the drug application to the right eye and starting it to the left eye (OS); complete recovery of pretreatment values of outflow facility and of applanation pressure occurred a week after cessation of the drug application. Furthermore, the left eye of the same individual demonstrated, on treatment, a hypertensive response identical in course and in magnitude with that of the right eye. FIGURE 2 demonstrates a greater magnitude of the response in another individual. In the treated eye, the pressure rise and the reduction in outflow facility increased with the duration of drug application and did not reach maximum level after four weeks of treatment. Furthermore, the reversible nature of the response and its equality in the two eyes of the same individual were similarly demonstrated.

Additional studies[8] demonstrated clearly that in the same individual the magnitude of the steroid-induced pressure rise depended upon the concentration of the drug, the frequency of application, and the duration of application. Keeping these factors constant, the magnitude of the response exhibited marked individual variation.[9] It was also observed that high responders tended to occur in families, suggesting a familial incidence and the heritable nature of the response.[10,11] In order to investigate the heterogeneity of the response and develop a phenotypic yardstick, a randomly selected sample of 80 individuals with normal eyes was

* This investigation was supported in part by Research Grants NB-03636 and NB-01689 from the National Institute of Neurological Diseases and Blindness, United States Public Health Service, Bethesda, Md.

† This paper was presented at the conference by Dr. Roger Sayegh.

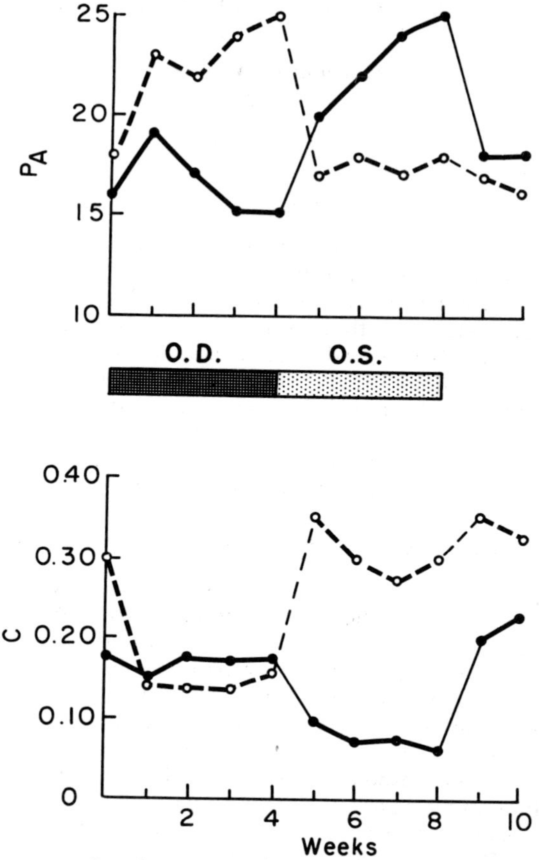

FIGURE 1. The course of applanation pressure (upper tracing) and tonographic C values (lower tracing) in the right (open circle) and in the left (solid circle) eye, during dexamethasone application. The duration of drug application to the right eye is indicated by the solid horizontal bar and that of the left eye by the stippled horizontal bar. Drug application consisted of three times daily application of eye drops using 0.1% ophthalmic solution of dexamethasone-21-diphosphate. Ocular pressure (P_A) appears in mm Hg on the ordinate of the upper tracing and tonographic outflow facility, (C) appears in cubic mm/mm Hg/minute on the ordinate of the lower tracing. The abscissa or both tracings indicates time in weeks.

studied in a standard manner. Dexamethasone 21-diphosphate 0.1% ophthalmic solution was applied to the right eye three times daily for four weeks. Ocular pressure (P_A) was monitored at weekly intervals. The change in ocular pressure (ΔP_A) after four weeks of drug application was used as a measure of the response and its frequency distribution appears in FIGURE 3. The distribution deviates from that of a single Gaussian distribution, and the deviation is significant at the 1% level of confidence. Thus the hypothesis that the random sample behaves as a single homogeneous group that demonstrates a single level of response had to be rejected. Significant heterogeneity existed indicating the presence of more than one level of response.

By inspection of the bar graph in FIGURE 3, it was postulated that at least three levels of response exist: a low level which is limited to responses less than a rise of 6 mm Hg; an intermediate level which included a pressure rise of 6 to 15 mm Hg; and a high level which included a pressure rise greater than 15 mm Hg. Examination of the data in these groups revealed that each forms a single Gaussian distribution.[9] Thus similar treatment of different individuals showed significantly different levels of response. Additional studies showed the magnitude of the response to be constant for the same individual on repeated testing.[6]

The Genetic Determination of the Response

Keeping in mind the familial factor alluded to previously, the hypothesis was proposed that the response is genetically determined by a pair of alleles, P^L for low pressure rise and P^H for high pressure rise and that the three levels of response described above are phenotypes for the three possible gene combinations; the low level P^LP^L, the intermediate level P^LP^H and the high level

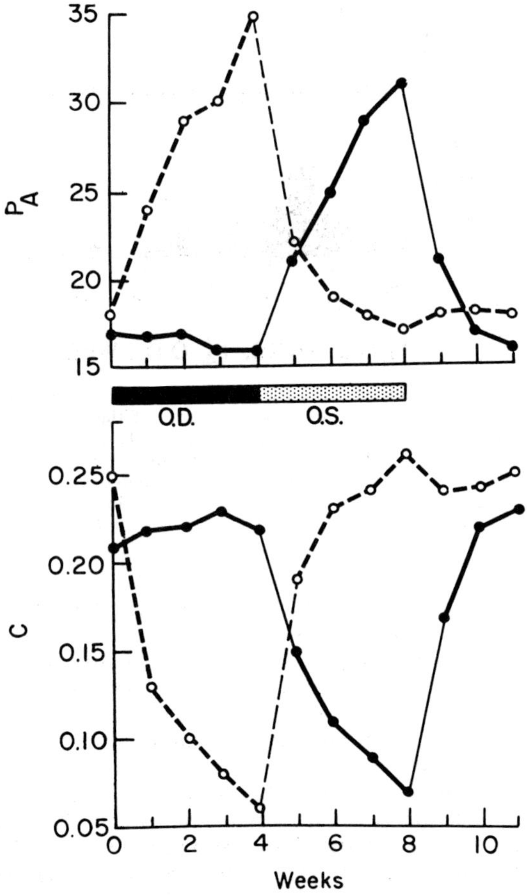

FIGURE 2. The effect of dexamethasone on ocular pressure and on aqueous outflow facility. Key is similar to that of FIGURE 1.

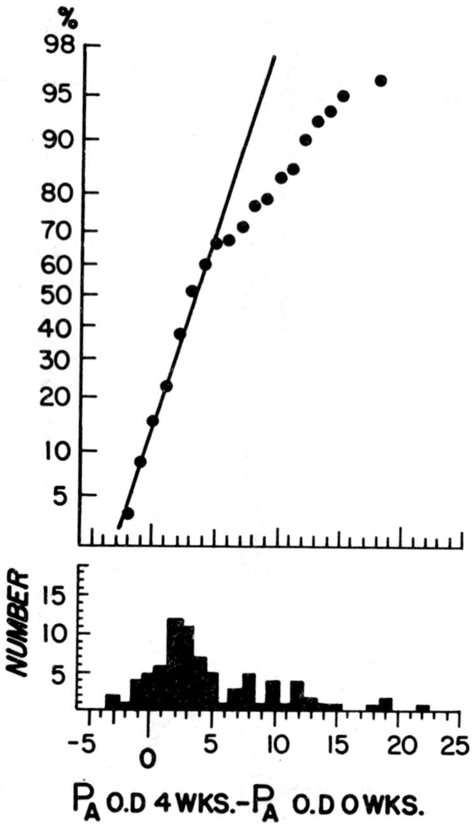

FIGURE 3. Bar graph (lower set) and the cumulative percent frequency plot (upper set) of the distribution of the change in applanation pressure of the right eye after four weeks of dexamethasone application. Abscissa scale is the same for the two sets. Note the deviation of the right-hand side of the distribution points from the line, describing perfectly the left-hand side of the distribution. This deviation occurs around 66 percent and corresponds to a score of 6 mm Hg in the bar graph. Note the apparent separation into two normal curves at 6 mm Hg in the bar graph and the impressive discontinuity between 15 and 18 mm Hg.

$P^H P^H$ (TABLE 1). The relative frequency of the different phenotypes in the random sample is consistent with this hypothesis.

I then investigated the possible existence of qualitative differences among the responses of the different phenotypes. FIGURE 4 shows the mean ocular pressure of the treated eye before and at weekly intervals during the four weeks of drug application in the different groups. It is apparent that quantitative as well as qualtative differences exist in the behavior of the three groups. Group I with the low level response showed that the maximum effect is attained after two weeks of drug application and that further increase in duration of application does not increase the magnitude of the response. On the other hand, the remainder of the sample (group II) demonstrated a progressive increase of pressure with duration of drug application which did not reach maximum effect at the end of four weeks. Furthermore the one with the intermediate level

TABLE 1

EXPLANATION OF GENOTYPE CLASSIFICATION FOR FIRST PERSONS TESTED

Phenotype of Pressure Rise	Low	Intermediate	High
Limits of pressure rise in mm Hg	5 or less	6–15	16 or more
Mean pressure rise in mm Hg	1.96	10.0	19.5
Standard deviation in mm Hg	± 2.00	± 2.5	*
Genotype	P^LP^L	P^LP^H	P^HP^H
Number of individuals	53	23	4
Percent of individuals	66%	29%	5%

* Range in sample 18–22 mm Hg.

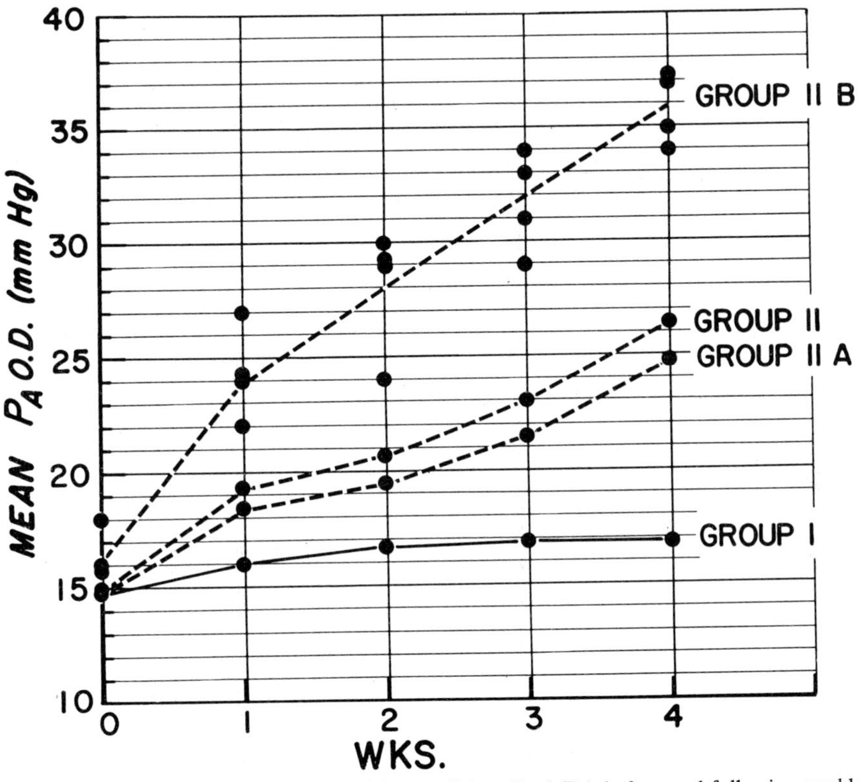

FIGURE 4. Mean applanation in the right eye (Mean P_A O.D.) before and following weekly intervals of drug application in group I, group II, group II-A, and group II-B. Note attainment of maximum pressure rise in group I by the third week and that there was no further increase following an additional fourth week of drug application. In contrast, note the different course of pressure rise in groups II, II-A and II-B. The pressure rise is still occurring with increasing duration of drug application in these groups, and does not show significant reduction in rate within this interval.

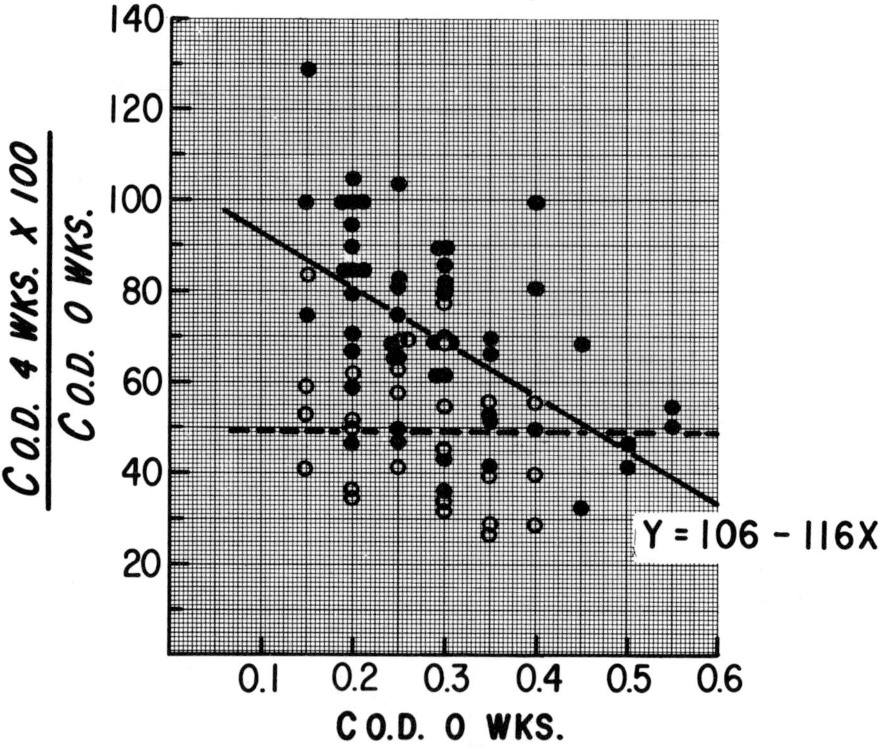

FIGURE 5. Scatter diagram and regression line of the ratio of aqueous outflow facility in the right eye after four weeks of drug application to that before drug application (ordinate C_{OD}-4 weeks/C_{OD}-0 weeks) and aqueous outflow facility in the right eye before treatment C_{OD}-0 weeks (abscissa of group I, solid circles and solid lines and of group II, open circles and interrupted line).

(group II-A) showed quantitative differences from that with the high level (group II-B) throughout the entire period of drug application.

If now we examine the change in outflow facility after four weeks in groups I and II we find a behavior suggestive of a difference in the mechanism or reduction of outflow facility. In group I (the low level response) the ratio of final to initial facility was significantly and inversely related to the initial facility (FIGURE 5); the percent reduction increased with initial facility whereas in the remainder of the sample the ratio was independent of initial facility. This difference indicates that different mechanisms are involved in reducing outflow facility in the two groups, one which is related to initial facility and another which is independent of it. Thus the group containing the P^{H} gene behaved qualitatively and quantitatively differently from that with $P^{L}P^{L}$, and the quantitative difference between $P^{L}P^{H}$ and $P^{H}P^{H}$ is in keeping with a dosage effect.

Having formulated the genetic hypothesis and devised a certain quantitative yardstick of converting the pressure response to genotype, it became important and feasible to test the genetic hypothesis in family units.[12] In this fashion both parents and all their available offspring were tested, using the above limits. The pressure rise after four weeks automatically assigned each individual to a genotype, which was then tested in the family unit for consistency of prediction.

FIGURE 6 shows that a family in which both parents demonstrated a low level of response had all their offspring demonstrate the same level as was to be expected. FIGURE 7 shows that when both parents are of the intermediate level or the heterozygous genotype, their offspring demonstrate segregation: the three phenotypes are seen and their relative frequency is consistent with the genetic model.

TABLE 2 shows a sample of family units where both parents had P^LP^L genotype. Only one of the 41 offspring was outside the phenotypic limit of P^LP^L and even then, his pressure rise was only 6 mm Hg. TABLE 3 shows family units wherein the parents' genotypes were P^HP^H and P^LP^H. Among their 15 offspring none demonstrated P^LP^L; they were almost equally divided between P^LP^H and P^HP^H. The results are in excellent agreement with the genetic model. TABLE 4 shows families where both parents had the genotype P^LP^H. The 19 offspring showed segregation into the three genotypes in the expected frequency, 5, 10 and 4; again demonstrating the excellent agreement with the genetic model.

No sex effect, could be discerned in any of the studies conducted to date.

The Response In Glaucoma

Having demonstrated and confirmed the genetic nature of the response it was then important to investigate spontaneous open angle glaucoma.[10,13] FIGURE 8 demonstrates the important feature of the response in medically controlled glaucoma. In the first situation glaucoma therapy was discontinued on one eye and the pressure was allowed to reach a steady glaucomatous level; dexamethasone was then applied and the pressure showed a very marked brisk rise, reaching 40 mm Hg after two weeks of application. On cessation, the

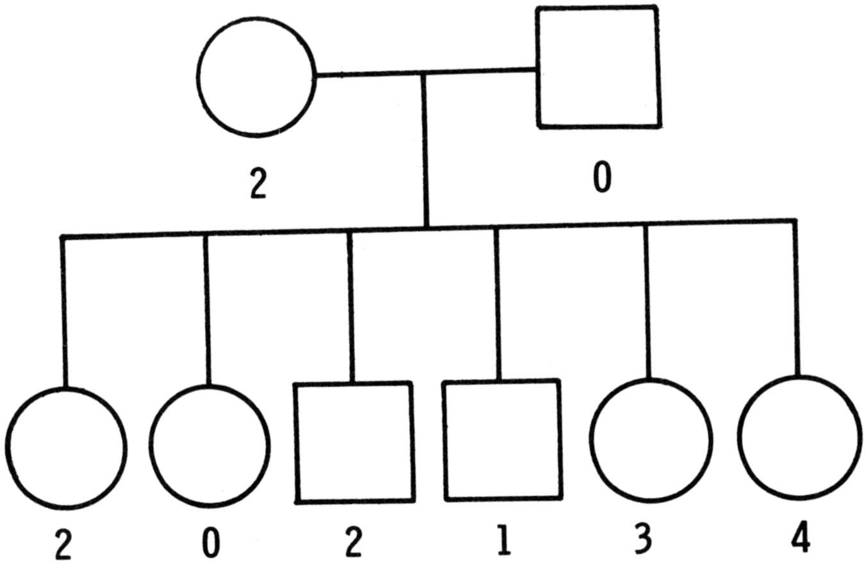

FIGURE 6. The response of parents and offspring of family No. 13. The magnitude of pressure rise after four weeks of topical application O.D. dexamethasone 0.1%, three times daily, appears below each symbol. Circle = females, square = males, open symbol indicates P^LP^L.

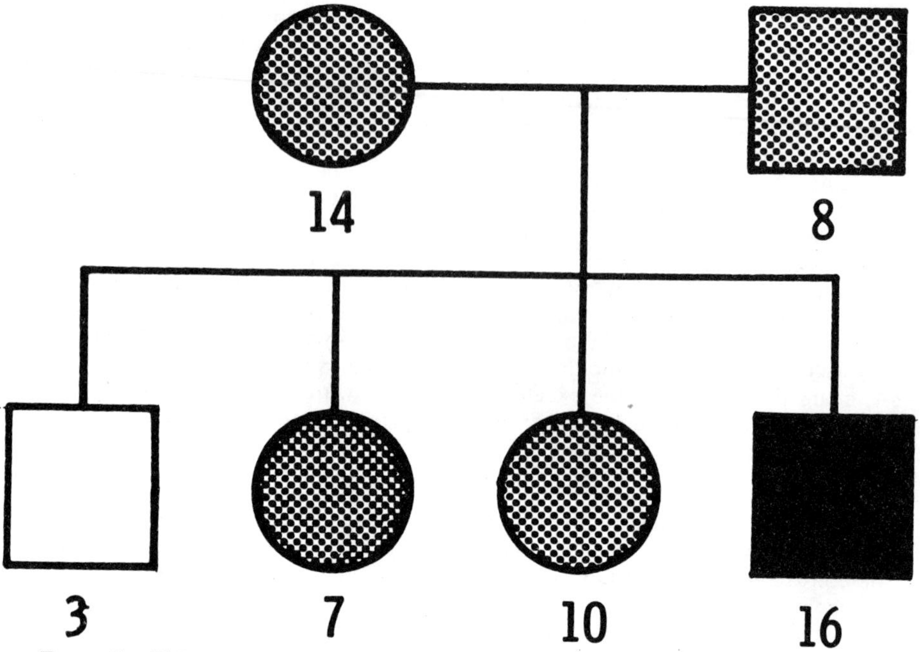

FIGURE 7. The response of parents and offspring of family No. 9. The magnitude of pressure rise after four weeks of topical application of dexamethasone 0.1% three times daily appears below each symbol. The key is the same as in FIGURE 6. Stippling = P^LP^H, Solid = P^HP^H.

TABLE 2

RESPONSE OF OFFSPRING OF $P^LP^L \times P^LP^L$ PARENTS

Family Number	Number of Offspring Tested	P^LP^L $\Delta P_A < 6$ mm Hg	P^LP^H ΔP_A 6-15 mm Hg	P^HP^H $\Delta P_A > 15$ mm Hg
1	7	7	0	0
2	9	8	1	0
3	5	5	0	0
12	3	3	0	0
13	6	6	0	0
14	7	7	0	0
17	4	4	0	0
Total	41	40	1	0

pressure recovered the control level demonstrating its reversible nature. In the second situation, glaucoma therapy was maintained in both eyes and the pressure was kept under control; then in addition, dexamethasone was applied to one eye only. The dexamethasone-induced pressure rise proceeded to occur with the same magnitude and rate in spite of the presence of the hypotensive medication for glaucoma. Thus the high level of hypertension in glaucoma occurred in spite of the simultaneous use of what otherwise would have been adequate hypotensive therapy.

TABLE 3

RESPONSE OF OFFSPRING OF $P^LP^H \times P^LP^H$ PARENTS

Family Number	Number of Offspring Tested	P^LP^L ΔP_A <6 mm Hg	P^LP^H ΔP_A 6-15 mm Hg	P^HP^H ΔP_A >15 mm Hg
9	4	1	2	1
10	6	2	3	1
15	3	1	1	1
18	6	1	4	1
Total	19	5	10	4

TABLE 4

RESPONSE OF OFFSPRING OF $P^HP^H \times P^LP^H$ PARENTS

Family Number	Number of Offspring Tested	P^LP^L ΔP_A <6 mm Hg	P^LP^H ΔP_A 6-15 mm Hg	P^HP^H ΔP_A >15 mm Hg
11	5	0	2	3
16	3	0	1	2
19	7	0	4	3
Total	15	0	7	8

I next studied a sample of open angle hypertensive glaucoma and found that the distribution of response levels was markedly different from that of the random sample (FIGURE 9). There was a marked reduction in P^LP^L and a great increase in P^HP^H. It is important to point out that the three response levels existed in open angle glaucoma and in so doing negated the hypothesis of identity between P^HP^H and glaucoma.

A similar frequency was found in low tension glaucoma (TABLE 5). This category is characterized by the typical visual loss of glaucoma and by the optic nerve changes, yet it fails to demonstrate a high ocular pressure. The similarity between the frequency of the different levels of the steroid response in this group and in hypertensive open angle glaucoma is the first independent evidence which demonstrates a common factor between these otherwise different categories. A more surprising finding was the similar increase in frequency of high response in the uninvolved eye of individuals that develop unilateral post-traumatic glaucoma.

A comparison of these selected glaucomas and the random sample (TABLE 5) shows clearly that the glaucomas have a greater frequency of P^H (P^LP^H, P^HP^H) and a great reduction in P^LP^L. Thus, while P^HP^H is not identical with glaucoma the presence of the P^H gene must be intimately related to the development of the types of glaucoma enumerated above.

There remained the need to show in each of these groups, that the findings reflected genetic factors. Family units were thus studied and in each case the response of the individual was accounted for by the responses of his parents and first degree relatives. TABLE 6 demonstrates that offspring of patients with hypertensive glaucoma validate their genotypic classification. Similar results were obtained in offspring of patients with low tension glaucoma (TABLE 7). Thus the hypothesis is offered that the allele pair P^L, P^H is one of the determinants of the types of glaucoma specified above.

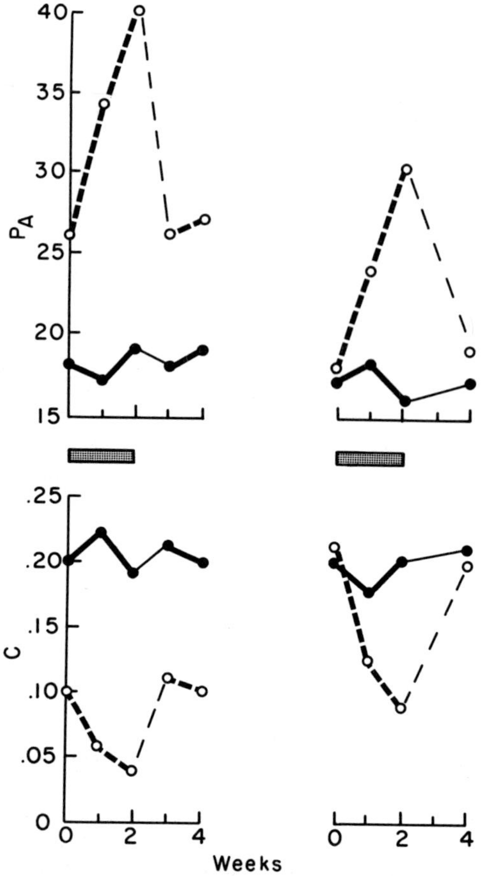

FIGURE 8. The course of applanation pressure (upper tracing) and tonographic C value (lower tracing) of the right eye (open circle) and left eye (solid circle) during the application of 0.1% dexamethasone drops, three times daily, to right eye in a patient with bilateral hypertensive open-angle glaucoma. Left-hand side shows the effect after hypotensive therapy had been discontinued in the right eye. Right-hand side shows the effect when dexamethasone was applied in addition to hypotensive therapy (pilocarpine 2% four times daily). The left eye in both conditions was treated with pilocarpine 2% four times daily. Beginning and duration of dexamethasone application is indicated by the solid horizontal bar. P_A represents applanation pressure in millimeters of Hg and C, tonographic outflow facility, in cu mm/mm of Hg/minute.

The Response and Normal Aqueous Dynamics

I have demonstrated in independent population studies[14] that the ocular pressure level is a genetically determined variable controlled by polygenic multifactorial type of inheritance. The question arises as to wether the allele pair P^L, P^H is one of the determinants of the normal ocular pressure level. TABLE 8 shows clearly that that is indeed the case. The mean ocular pressure that prevailed in individuals with normal eyes prior to the steroid testing was significantly related to their genotypic classification with respect to P^L, P^H. The mean ocular pressure was significantly lower for P^LP^L than it was for P^HP^H,

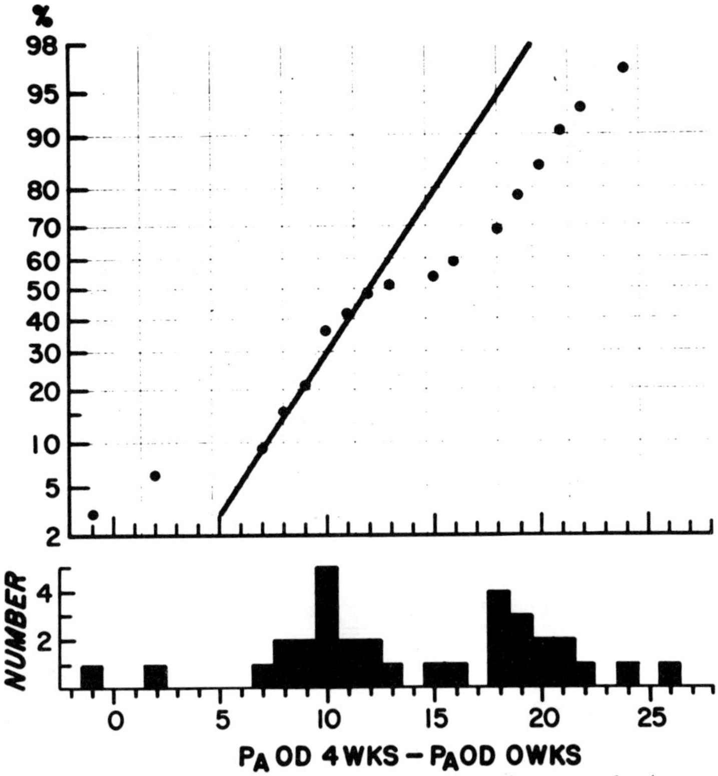

FIGURE 9. Bar graph (lower set) and the cumulative percent frequency plot (upper set) of the distribution of the change in applanation pressure of the right eye after four weeks of dexamethasone application in 33 patients with open-angle glaucoma. The change in applanation pressure appears on the abscissa in each set.

TABLE 5

DEXAMETHASONE HYPERTENSION IN DIFFERENT CLINICAL CATEGORIES

Category	Number of Subjects Tested	Percent Frequency of Genotypes		
		$P^LP^L \triangle P_A < 6$ mm Hg	$P^LP^H \triangle P_A$ 6-15 mm Hg	$P^HP^H \triangle P_A > 15$ mm Hg
Random sample	80	66%	29%	5%
Open-Angle hypertensive Glaucoma	33	6%	48%	44%
Low tension glaucoma	15	7%	53%	40%
Normal eye in recessed Angle glaucoma	15	—	53%	47%
Normal eye in angle Recession without Glaucoma	4	75%	25%	—

TABLE 6

GENOTYPES OF OFFSPRING OF PATIENTS WITH OPEN ANGLE HYPERTENSIVE GLAUCOMA

Family Number	Genotype of Patient and of Spouse	Genotypes of Offspring		
		P^LP^L	P^LP^H	P^HP^H
1	$P^LP^L \times P^LP^H$	3	1	—
2	$P^LP^L \times P^LP^H$	2	2	1
3	$P^LP^L \times P^LP^H$	2	2	—
4	$P^LP^L \times P^LP^H$	2	1	—
5	$P^LP^L \times P^LP^H$	4	3	—
6	$P^LP^L \times P^HP^H$	1	4	—
7	$P^LP^L \times P^HP^H$	—	4	1
8	$P^LP^H \times P^HP^H$	1	1	1
9	$P^LP^H \times P^LP^H$	—	2	1
10	$P^LP^H \times P^LP^H$	—	2	—

TABLE 7

GENOTYPES OF OFFSPRING OF PATIENTS WITH OPEN ANGLE GLAUCOMA WITHOUT HYPERTENSION

Family Number	Genotype of Patient and of Spouse	Genotype of Offspring		
		P^LP^L	P^LP^H	P^HP^H
11	$P^LP^L \times P^HP^H$	—	3	1
12	$P^LP^H \times P^LP^L$	3	1	—
13	$P^LP^H \times P^LP^H$	1	2	—
14	$P^LP^L \times P^LP^H$	2	3	1

TABLE 8

NORMAL OCULAR PRESSURE AND OUTFLOW FACILITY IN DIFFERENT GENOTYPES

	Number of Subjects	Mean P ± S.D.M.	Mean C ± S.D.M.
P^LP^L	169	15.0 ±0.23	0.29 ±0.008
P^HP^H	44	16.8 ±0.30	0.22 ±0.010

indicating that this allele pair is involved in the determination of normal ocular pressure level. Also, the facility of aqueous outflow demonstrated a similar relationship indicating that this allele pair is similarly involved in the determination of normal aqueous outflow facility.

The Response, Eosinopenia and Glucose Tolerance Test

I next searched for a systemic effect that might be tied to this allele pair. The magnitude of the eosinopenic response to systemically administered dexamethasone was investigated and found to be independent of this allele pair.[15] I examined the glycemic and glycosuric responses to glucose loading in normal individuals who were not diabetic and differed only in their steroid response. The results were startling. A greater glycemia and glycosuria occurred when P^H was present (TABLE 9). Taking the median glycemic level for P^LP^L, as a reference, the proportion exceeding the median in P^LP^H and in P^HP^H was significantly greater (TABLE 10). Thus P^L, P^H is one of the determinants of

TABLE 9

THE RESULTS OF GLUCOSE TOLERANCE TEST (G.T.T.) IN DIFFERENT GENOTYPES

Genotype	Number of Individuals	Glycemia* During G.T.T.									Glycosuria during G.T.T.	Fasting Glucose >100 mg /100 ml
		200-249	250-299	300-349	350-399	400-449	450-499	500-549	550-599	600-649		
P^LP^L	14	4	5	2	2	–	–	–	–	–	1	0
P^LP^H	25	4	6	9	5	–	–	–	–	1	3	3
P^HP^H	10	–	2	3	1	1	1	1	–	1	3	3

* Sum of Glucose Plasma Concentration (mg/100 ml) at 30, 60, and 90 minutes of G.T.T.

TABLE 10

THE DISTRIBUTION OF INDIVIDUALS WITH DIFFERENT GENOTYPES WITH REFERENCE TO THE MEDIAN GLYCEMIC LEVEL OF P^LP^L

Genotype	Median Glycemia for P^LP^L	Number of Individuals Below Median	Number of Individuals Above Median	Total Number Tested
P^LP^L	264 mg/100 ml	7	7	14
P^LP^H	264 mg/100 ml	7	18	25
P^HP^H	264 mg/100 ml	1	9	10

glycemia and glycosuria following glucose loading and in this fashion one of the determinants of diabetes.

In conclusion, an undesirable ocular side effect of topically applied glucocorticoids was demonstrated to be genetically determined. It was also shown to be intimately involved in the determination of important normal parameters as well as disease states. These were normal ocular pressure, normal aqueous outflow facility and glycemic and glycosuric responses to glucose loading, open angle hypertensive glaucoma, open angle low tension glaucoma and post-traumatic glaucoma.

References

1. FRANCOIS, J. 1954. Cortisone et tension oculaire. Ann. Oculist (Paris) **187:** 805.
2. ARMALY, M. F. 1963. Effect of corticosteroids on intraocular pressure and fluid dynamics: I. The effect of dexamethasone in the normal eye. Arch. Ophth. **70:** 482.
3. BECKER, B. & D. W. MILLS. 1963. Corticosteroids and intraocular pressure. Arch. Ophth. **70:** 500.
4. BERNSTEIN, H. N. & B. SCHWARTZ. 1962. Effects of long-term systemic streoids on ocular pressure and tonographic values. Arch. Ophth. **68:** 742.
5. GOLDMANN, H. 1962. Cortisone glaucoma. Arch. Ophth. **68:** 621.
6. ARMALY, M. F. 1964. Effect of corticosteroids on intraocular pressure and fluid dynamics: III. Changes in visual function and pupil size during topical dexamethasone application. Arch. Ophth. **71:** 636.
7. BECKER, B. & R. SHAFFER. 1965. Diagnosis and Therapy of the Glaucomas. 2nd Ed. C. V. Mosby, Ed. St. Louis, Mo.
8. ARMALY, M. F. 1966. Dexamethasone ocular hypertension in the clinically normal eye: II. The untreated eye, outflow facility, and concentration. Arch. Ophth. **75:** 776.
9. ARMALY, M. F. 1965. Statistical attributes of the steroid hypertensive response in the clinically normal eye: I. The demonstration of three levels of response. Inves. Ophth. **4**(2): 187.
10. ARMALY, M. F. 1963. Effect of corticosteroids on intraocular pressure and fluid dynamics: II. The effect of dexamethasone in the glaucomatous eye. Arch. Ophth. **70:** 492.
11. BECKER, B. & K. A. HAHN. 1964. Topical corticosteroids and heredity in primary open-angle glaucoma. Am. J. Ophth. **57:** 543.
12. ARMALY, M. F. 1966. The heritable nature of dexamethasone-induced ocular hypertension. Arch. Ophth. **75:** 32.
13. ARMALY, M. F. 1967. Inheritance of dexamethasone hypertension and glaucoma. Arch. Ophth. **77:** 747.
14. ARMALY, M. F. 1967. The genetic determination of ocular pressure in the normal eye. Arch. Ophth. **78:** 187.
15. ARMALY, M. F. 1967. Dexamethasone ocular hypertension and eosinopenia and glucose tolerance test. Arch. Ophth. **78:** 193.

DISCUSSION OF THE PAPER

DR. J. C. SAUNDERS (*Riverhouse, Upper Nyack, N.Y.*): Dr. Armaly is to be congratulated in obtaining data to support his hypothesis that open angle glaucoma and diabetes are determined by polygenetic factors. I would like to ask if Dr. Armaly obtained any data to indicate that thyroid disturbances might be associated with glaucoma since triiodothyroine by subconjuctival injection on conscious rabbits caused a decrease in ocular pressure? We found on a series of 100 patients with pressure greater than 5mm Hg above normal levels that 56 had open angle glaucoma and 8 patients had narrow angle glaucoma. Did you test your series of patients for PTC (phenylthiourea) tasting? In the primary glaucoma we observed that 30 patients with open angle glaucoma were nontasters of PTC and only 2 patients of the narrow angle glaucoma were nontasters. Since the nontasters in a random population sample is 25 percent this provides tempting data for speculation.

In addition to the data presented by Dr. Armaly, I would like to know if he has other support of the probable genetic relationship of glaucoma to diabetes and if he has data to indicate a probable genetic relationship to hypothyroidism and to nontasters of PTC? I think it is well known that when two or more traits appear together, more often than not, it is likely they are on the same chromosome and close together. When cross-over occurs in meiosis the traits remain on the one chromosome in more than 50 percent of crossovers. Does the grouping together of glaucoma, diabetes, hypothyroidism and nontasters of PTC fit a genetic hypothesis of polygenetic type of determination? Would he be willing to speculate on any relationship between the thyroid and adrenergic system and that to glaucoma?

DR. ARMALY: Dr. Saunders' comments are indeed most relevant and in fact involve the natural extension of the present investigation. Studies designed to identify the possible components with which glaucoma may be grouped in a genetic association are currently in progress. Unfortunately, it is premature to draw any conclusions from them. However, some relevant information is already available in the literature. Becker, *et al.*, (1964), found that PTC nontasters occur more frequently in open angle glaucoma than in the general population and significantly less frequently in angle closure glaucoma. McLenachan and Davies, (1965), and Becker, Kolker, and Ballin, (1966), reported significant association between thyroid dysfunction and open angle glaucoma. This latter however could not be confirmed by Cheng and Perkins, (1967).

I am currently pursuing this aspect by attempting to collect all data relevant to these conditions in the same individual and in family groups with a hope that a more definitive conclusion can be made in this respect.

References

BECKER, B. & W. R. MORTON. 1964. Phenyl thiourea taste testing and glaucoma. A.M.A. Arch. Ophthal. **72:** 323.

MCLENACHAN, J. & D. M. DAVIES. 1965. Glaucoma and the thyroid. Brit. J. Ophthal. **49:** 441.

BECKER, B., A. E. KOLKER & N. BALLIN. 1966. Thyroid function and glaucoma. Amer. J. Ophthal. **61:** 997.

CHENG, H. & E. S. PERKINS. 1967. Thyroid disease and glaucoma. Brit. J. Ophthal. **51:** 547.

ALTERED DRUG RESPONSE IN FAMILIAL DYSAUTONOMIA

Joseph Dancis*

Department of Pediatrics, New York University School of Medicine, N. Y.

Familial dysautonomia is an inherited disease, restricted to Jewish children with protean manifestations which appear to be neurogenic in origin. Manifestations often begin in infancy with difficulty in swallowing, failure to thrive, and absence of overflow tears. This is followed by slow achievement of developmental milestones such as sitting, walking, talking. Recurrent pneumonia is common. Periodic crises with vomiting, abdominal pain and sometimes fever plague many children. There is emotional lability, often associated with flushing and sweating. Sensitivity to pain is reduced, and the risks of surgery are increased. The lifespan is shortened.[1]

Because of the prominence of symptoms referable to the autonomic nervous system, the response to infused norepinephrine was measured.[2] The patient with dysautonomia displayed an exaggerated hypertensive response (FIGURE 1). It was noted that the bradycardia that commonly accompanies norepinephrine-induced hypertension was not evident. This suggested that a parasympathetic insufficiency may have contributed to the exaggerated response.

Methacholine was infused into a group of dysautonomic subjects.[3] Again, there was a more severe response than in normal subjects. The blood pressure fell to lower levels without the usual increase in pulse rate. The vagal signs—cough, borborygmi with abdominal cramps, sweating – appeared at lower infusion rates and were more intense. An incidental but significant observation was the return towards normal of some of the manifestations that are characteristic of dysautonomia. In two subjects the patellar jerks returned and remained for hours; in two others, the histamine flare could be elicited. This will be discussed further. Overflow tears were commonly seen, an observation previously reported by others.

In further pursuit of the question of autonomic imbalance, the pupillary response to a series of locally-instilled pharmacologic agents was investigated.[4] The most significant of these were epinephrine 0.1% and methacholine 2.5%. There was no response to the former, but the latter induced miosis in 16 of 18 subjects. This response is characteristic of parasympathetic denervation.

As a minor digression, it is worth noting that the diagnosis of dysautonomia can be made with considerable confidence by an ophthalmological examination. The characteristic tetrad is alacrima, corneal hypesthesia, exodeviation and the miotic response to 2.5% methacholine.

The normal response to intradermal histamine 1:1000 is well known. There is immediate pain radiating from the site of injection, followed shortly by a wheal and flare. In the dysautonomic, the radiating pain and flare, both attributable to the axon reflex, are absent.[5]

In an attempt to further explore the sensory deficiencies, the respiratory response to hypercapnia and hypoxia were measured.[6] When the ambient concentration of CO_2 was increased, the compensatory increase in ventilation was not as effective as in the normal, and the arterial pCO_2 increased (FIGURE 2). The response to hypoxia was dramatic. In addition to an abrupt fall in oxygen saturation, the dysautonomic subject developed alarming symptoms. This con-

* Career Investigator, The National Institute of Child Health and Human Development. Aided by a grant from the National Foundation.

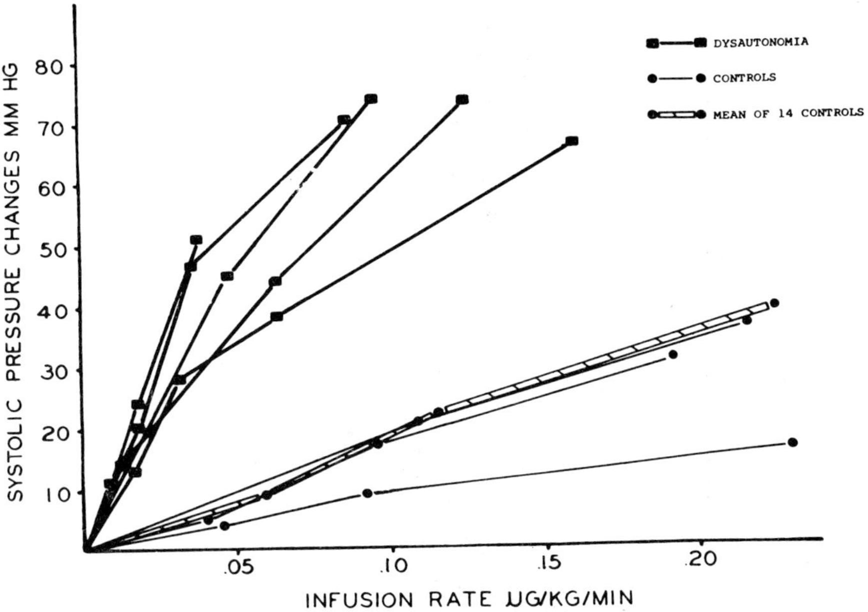

FIGURE 1. Change in systolic blood pressures during infusion with 1-norepinephrine (mean of 14 controls calculated from data of Goldenberg *et al.* Am. J. Med. **5**: 792–806, 1948). Reproduced with permission of The New England Journal of Medicine.

trasted sharply with the benign course in normal individuals.

Another sensory defect is that of taste discrimination.[7] This is associated with an absence of the fungiform papillae and taste buds, an almost pathognomic sign of dysautonomia.[8] The development of taste buds has been related to neurogenic stimuli. Fungiform papillae may be similarly dependent.

A recent observation, that may appear paradoxical in view of the clinical symptomatology, is the high catecholamine content in the adrenals obtained at autopsy from patients with dysautonomia[9] (TABLE 1). The relatively low content of the adrenals commonly found at autopsy has been attributed to adrenal

TABLE 1

CATECHOLAMINE CONCENTRATIONS IN THE ADRENAL GLANDS OF 6 NONDYSAUTONOMIC AND 3 DYSAUTONOMIC CHILDREN*

Subject	Age	Cause of Death	Epinephrine Concentration μg/gm	Norepinephrine Concentration μg/gm
N.N.	2 days	Respiratory distress	12	28
J.P.	4 mo	Meningitis	146†	—
A.S.	5 mo	Aortic surgery	56	38
B.L.	1 yr	Hydrocephalus	50	38
A.P.	2 yr	Measles & pneumonia	32	0
M.Z.	3 yr	Cystic fibrosis & pneumonia	68	24
O.R.	1 yr	Dysautonomia – seizures with apnea	671	321
B.G.	5 yr	Dysautonomia – measles, pneumonia	336	157
J.C.	11 yr	Dysautonomia – pneumonia	1367	130

* Reproduced with permission of the New England Journal of Medicine.

† Total catecholamines.

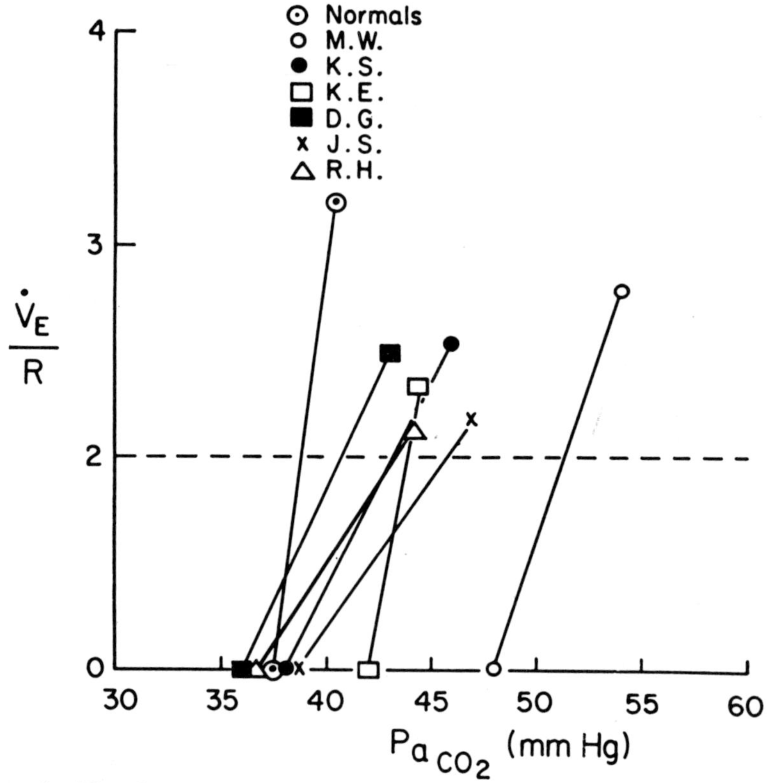

FIGURE 2. The relation between arterial pCO_2 (Pa_{CO_2}) and the increase in minute ventilation. The average of the results in five control subjects is presented as one line; the dysautonomic responses are presented individually. The greater slope in dysautonomia indicates that a greater change in Pa_{CO_2}, is necessary to produce a corresponding increase in minute ventilation. From Smith and Dancis: J. of Pediatrics **63**: 889–894, 1963, The C. V. Mosby Company, St. Louis, Mo.

exhaustion associated with dying. This would suggest that the dysautonomic has difficulty in releasing catecholamines, and that this may be the explanation for the high HVA:VMA ratio[10] and the postural hypotension.

It is evident that the pharmacological approach to familial dysautonomia has proved particularly rewarding. Diagnostic tests have been developed. We have gained insights into the mechanisms of the disease that have permitted a more rational approach to therapy. However, the fundamental defect, assuming that there is one, remains elusive.

References

1. RILEY, C. M. 1957. Familial dysautonomia. Adv. in Pediatrics **9**: 157–190.
2. SMITH, A. A. & J. DANCIS. 1964. Exaggerated response to infused norepinephrine in familial dysautonomia. New Eng. J. Med. **270**: 704–707.
3. SMITH, A. A., J. I. HIRSCH & J. DANCIS. 1965. Response to infused methacholine in familial dysautonomia. Pediatrics **36**: 225–230.
4. SMITH, A. A., J. DANCIS & G. BREININ. 1965. Ocular responses to autonomic drugs in familial dysautonomia. Invest. Ophth. **4**: 358–361.

5. Smith, A. A. & J. Dancis. 1963. Response to intradermal histamine in familial dysautonomia: diagnostic test. J. Pediat. **63:** 889–894.
6. Filler, J., A. A. Smith, S. Stone & J. Dancis. 1965. Respiratory control in familial dysautonomia. J. Pediat. **66:** 509–516.
7. Smith, A. A. & J. Dancis. 1964. Taste discrimination in familial dysautonomia. Pediatrics **33:** 441–443.
8. Smith, A. A., A. Farbman & J. Dancis. 1965. Absence of taste-bud papillae in familial dysautonomia. Science **147:** 1040.
9. Smith, A. A. & J. Dancis. 1967. Catecholamine release in familial dysautonomia. New Eng. J. Med. **277:** 61–64.
10. Smith, A. A., T. Taylor & S. B. Wortis. 1963. Abnormal catechloamine metabolism in familial dysautonomia. New Eng. J. Med. **268:** 705–707.

INHERITED FORMS OF DIABETES INSIPIDUS AND DIAGNOSTIC DRUG APPLICATIONS

Richard Relkin
Kingsbrook Medical Center, Brooklyn, N. Y.

The excretion of persistently large volumes of sugar-free urine having low osmolality characterizes the clinical entity diabetes insipidus (DI).

While the subject of inherited forms of DI usually brings to mind those cases which have been termed nephrogenic, cases of idiopathic DI have occurred in families. In these latter instances the inheritance has been described variously as autosomal dominant,[1] with incomplete female penetrance,[2] and sex-linked recessive.[3] A loss of nerve cells in the supraoptic and paraventricular nuclei of the hypothalamus was noted in a few of the sparse reports of pathology in the inherited idiopathic type of DI.[4] The hereditary hypothalamic DI found in the Brattleboro strain of rats seems to represent the animal counterpart of this human situation.[5] As the use of almost any drug may result in the formation of antibodies, it was recently suggested that such loss of nerve cells in the hypothalamus may actually have been the result of an antigen-antibody reaction between these cells and anti-antidiuretic hormone antibodies formed against the exogenous antidiuretic hormone (ADH) the patients had been receiving.[6] In other words, the hypothalamic changes may have been secondary to the treatment of DI, and not the cause.

ADH in the human is the octapeptide 8-arginine vasopressin, and differs from the usual commercial preparation which consists of 8-arginine and 8-lysine vasopressin; the former being a beef derivative and the latter hog. For acquired resistance to vasopressin a pure synthetic hog 8-lysine vasopressin has been introduced,[7] and other synthetic preparations, such as phenylalanine-lysine-vasopressin, have had investigational uses; one of these has been the stimulation of ACTH release.[8]

ADH is formed in the cells of the supraoptic and paraventricular nuclei as well as cells in the central and posterior portions of the hypothalamus, including the mammillary body and lateral tuberal nuclei. Fibers from all these nuclei descend to the posterior pituitary as the hypothalamohypophyseal tract, and transport neurosecretory material which is the carrier of both vasopressin and oxytocin. Within the posterior pituitary, where it is stored, ADH apparently exists in two pools; one is readily releasable and accounts for 10–20% of the total ADH of the gland, the remainder is available for release only at a greatly reduced rate.[9]

As for the regulation of ADH secretion, both an increase in plasma osmolality and a decrease in plasma volume can increase hormonal output and cause water retention. Hypertonic sodium chloride injected into the internal carotid artery in amounts raising the plasma osmolality by only 1 to 2% is sufficient to cause antidiuresis. The stimulus for increased ADH secretion in this instance is apparently dehydration of the osmoreceptor cells which, according to some evidence, are not identical to the neurosecretory cells of the hypothalamic nuclei.

As has recently been demonstrated, the most potent controller of ADH release is the circulating blood volume.[10] When plasma volume is reduced, even in the face of plasma hypo-osmolality, antidiuresis is induced. The volume receptors may be located in a number of sites such as the aorta, carotid artery, and the left atrium.

In addition to the above factors, it has been shown that stress and painful stimuli can cause an increased output of ADH. An enhanced secretion of this hormone can also be effected by ether, morphine, histamine, acetylcholine and nicotine.

In normal man more than 150 liters of water, 20,000 mEq of sodium, and 14,000 mEq of chloride are filtered through the glomeruli every twenty-four hours. About 99% of these substances are reabsorbed with only 1% appearing in the urine. The glomerular filtrate contains all the solutes of blood, except the lipids and proteins, in approximately the same concentration as the plasma. As the filtrate passes through the proximal convoluted tubules, roughly 80% of both water and electrolytes are reabsorbed with the tubular urine remaining isotonic in relation to plasma. Reabsorption of sodium and chloride greatly in excess of water then occurs in the loop of Henle, resulting in a urine hypotonic to plasma entering the distal convoluted tubules. Simultaneously, a high osmotic concentration develops in the interstitial tissue surrounding the tubules. In the distal convoluted tubules additional sodium and chloride are reabsorbed by a process of cation exchange in which hydrogen and potassium ions are secreted into the tubular lumen and an equivalent amount of sodium absorbed into the plasma. This sodium reabsorption is under the control of aldosterone.

The urine that leaves the loop of Henle is hypotonic. Without ADH the distal convoluted tubules and collecting ducts are relatively impermeable to water, so that large volumes of hypotonic urine are excreted. Under the influence of the hormone, however, an enhanced permeability of the tubules allows water to move from the hypotonic urine to the hypertonic interstitial fluid. This results in a reduction in volume and an increased concentration of the urine.

ADH has been shown to increase the permeability of cell walls and membranes by enlarging pore size. Apparently, this is accomplished by stimulating the production of cyclic 3′,5′-adenosine monophosphate (AMP) from adenosine triphosphate (ATP). Cyclic 3′,5′-AMP then increases the permeability of the membranes to water.[11] The actual mechanism involved in ADH-induced changes in membrane permeability has been envisioned as an action on two parts of the same membrane. For example, the urinary surface of mucosal cells has been hypothesized to consist of an outer dense barrier and an inner porous barrier. All substances, including water, are normally retarded at the dense barrier. ADH has been thought to act by enhancing the permeability of the dense barrier to urea and sodium, and the permeability of the porous barrier to water.[12]

Other actions of ADH have been a reduction of renal blood flow to the medulla, an increase in the permeability of the vascular bed, and modification of the glomerular filtration rate. In addition, extrarenal actions of ADH have been demonstrated. These include effects on sweat glands, salivary glands, and stomach, intestinal, pancreatic, and bile secretion. ADH has been shown to decrease salivary and gastric secretion, to decrease sodium and water reabsorption by the intestinal mucosa to decrease sweat secretion, and reduce the secretion of bile.[13] In other words, ADH seems to be a general fluid regulator, involved wherever water economy is at stake and in all organs concerned with the turnover of body fluids. Inactivation of ADH is achieved partly by the kidney and partly by the liver, but much of the process of its degradation is still unknown.

To return to the clinical situation, it was Forssman[14] who first suggested that the entity nephrogenic DI could exist. When the genetics of such cases were subsequently studied they were thought to be compatible with a sex-linked recessive mode of inheritance.[15] However, one investigator thought the inheritance might actually be sex-linked dominant.[16] It is interesting that in the former genetic pattern a partial responsiveness to ADH was found in female siblings and relatives of patients with the fully expressed disorder.[17]

Nephrogenic DI has, since its original description, been viewed as a refractoriness of the distal renal tubule cell membrane to the action of ADH. However, with the recent finding of enormously elevated levels of the parathormone antagonist, thyrocalcitonin, in a case of pseudohypoparathyroidism,[18] one wonders if, in cases of nephrogenic DI, there is really a circulating ADH-antagonist rather than a faulty tubular response to ADH itself. Recently, prostaglandin E_1 was shown to reverse ADH-induced antidiuresis.[19]

In testing for the presence and type of DI in any given patient several procedures can be used. The simplest one is to withhold water beginning in the morning. The volume and osmolality of the urine is then measured at specified intervals throughout the day. In patients with DI there is the continued excretion of large volumes of urine having low osmolality, body weight is lost, and plasma osmolality, usually higher than normal to start with, rises still further. If the underlying condition is psychogenic polydipsia, the urine volume decreases and the osmolality rises while the body weight decreases and plasma osmolality, lower than normal at the outset, rises into the normal range. However, it must be realized that withholding all fluid is an extremely distressing procedure in any patient with polydipsia and actually can be dangerous in small children. For these reasons it is not recommended. It should be mentioned that some patients, especially those with psychogenic polydipsia, will resort to almost anything to obtain fluid during a dehydration procedure, including the drinking of their own urine. That patients should be taken off all medication during such diagnostic work-up was emphasized in a recent study showing that phenothiazine derivatives, chlorprothixene, tetrabenazine, dibenzazepine anti-depressants, and monoamine oxidase inhibitors all block the secretion of ADH which occurs in response to dehydration.[20]

Another diagnostic method, employed in adult cases, is the use of nicotine. Lewis and Chalmers[21] suggested that the supraopticohypophyseal system may be presumed to be largely destroyed if the inhaled smoke of one to three cigarettes does not result in satisfactory antidiuresis. A more refined form of the test involves the i.v. administration of 1 mg of nicotine base over a period of three to five minutes; a prompt antidiuresis is seen in normal patients who have been water loaded as for the tests utilizing hypertonic saline infusions.

The infusion of hypertonic saline has been widely employed to test the integrity of the hypothalamohypophyseal-renal system in DI. For the desired effect the renal tubules must be responsive to ADH. There are actually several procedures which can be used. In addition to the Hickey-Hare[22] and Carter-Robbins[23] tests, there have been several recent modifications which have the intended purpose of improved accuracy and ease of testing.[24,25] If in these procedures the urine volume decreases and the osmolality increases, a functioning supraopticohypophyseal system and responsive renal tubules are present. This will be observed in normal patients and in those with psychogenic polydipsia. If the urine osmolality does not rise and the volume does not decrease, true DI rather than psychogenic polydipsia is present. If a state of DI is indicated, the vasopressin test is performed to decide whether or not the condition is nephrogenic. In this test the 100 milliunits (0.1 unit) of aqueous material that is used should produce a maximal antidiuresis in twenty to thirty minutes. Failure to achieve a significant antidiuresis indicates that the DI is of the nephrogenic form, presuming the absence of the various forms of renal disease known to be associated with polyuria. DI secondary to an underlying condition such as Hand-Schuller-Christian disease usually offers no serious diagnostic difficulties. Before leaving the subject of hypertonic saline infusions it should be mentioned that cortisol has been shown to raise the osmotic threshold necessary for release of ADH.[26]

Several disturbing clinical exceptions make the diagnostic format outlined above subject to flaws. There has been one report of ADH-resistant DI associated with pathologic changes in the supraoptic and paraventricular nuclei.[27] In addition, and more significantly, De Wardener and Herxheimer[28] demonstrated that excessive consumption of water by normal volunteers over a three to eleven day period leads to a state of vasopressin-resistant hyposthenuric polyuria. It has been suggested that the mechanism of this resistance is a washout of renal medullary hypertonicity. Thus, a patient may still have psychogenic polydipsia and not respond as expected to the various tests.

In recent review of DI[29] this author advocated the use of an i.v. ADH test which would separate cases of idiopathic DI from nephrogenic DI, in addition to uncovering those instances of partial ADH deficiency and partial ADH unresponsiveness (FIGURE 1). In this procedure all fluid is withheld, and the urine osmolality is determined at twenty minute intervals. As soon as the urine osmolality gives evidence of reaching a plateau (this can usually be determined over the span of three specimens), 100 milliunits of aqueous vasopressin are injected intravenously. The procedure is terminated when maximum effect has

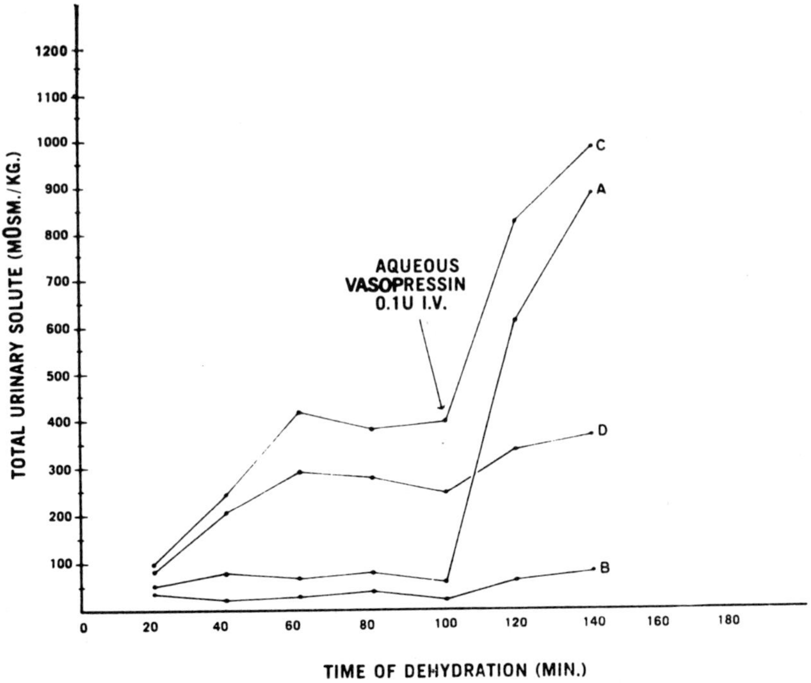

FIGURE 1. Representative examples of (A) supraopticohypophyseal diabetes insipidus, (B) nephrogenic diabetes insipidus, (C) partial deficiency of ADH, and (D) partial unresponsiveness to ADH. (Reproduced from the N. Y. State Journal of Medicine Nov. 1966.)

been achieved from the vasopressin. In a normal patient the urine osmolality will show an essentially steady increase as long as there is dehydration. The same applies, with the previous proviso, to cases of psychogenic polydipsia. In patients with DI, vasopressin will produce a dramatic rise in urine osmolality, ideally in the neighborhood of 900 mOsm/kg. Patients with nephrogenic DI will exhibit a low plateau of osmolality showing no further increase with vasopressin.

The treatment of choice in cases of idiopathic DI consists of ADH. In addition, three other drugs have been found to have a beneficial effect in the treatment of this condition. One is chlorthiazide, to be discussed later, and another is chlorpropamide.[30] The latter drug was first tested in three patients with idiopathic DI and two patients with nephrogenic DI. While there was no salutory effect in the nephrogenic cases, the three patients with idiopathic DI showed an impressive fall in free water clearance. The authors concluded that, regarding free water clearance, chlorpropamide has an effect similar to that of ADH, in that both cause a decrease of free water clearance in idiopathic DI and are without effect in nephrogenic DI. While the exact mechanism of chlorpropamide's effect in DI is still speculative it should be mentioned that the drug also seems to have an antidiuretic effect in cases of diabetes mellitus, even when it does not affect the blood sugar. Furthermore, while the drug was being studied in the three patients with idiopathic DI it was noted that no clinical manifestations of hypoglycemia were produced, the lowest recorded blood sugar being 64 mg%.

The third drug used in cases of idiopathic DI has been furosemide, given intravenously.[31] This drug has been shown to affect sodium transport so that the potential difference across the cell membrane decreases by 50–80%, ADH having the opposite effect;[32] its mechanism of action is apparently quite similar to that of chlorthiazide.

While ADH appears to be of little use in cases of nephrogenic DI, it should be noted that there is some evidence, from the Brattleboro strain of rats mentioned earlier, that prolonged administration of ADH may overcome primary ADH resistance.[33]

The agent used most frequently in nephrogenic DI is chlorothiazide. Its use in this condition, as in idiopathic DI, was originally described by Kennedy and Crawford.[34] These investigators found that the drug enabled a doubling of urine osmolality and a halving of urine volume. The mechanism of the drug's action, however, is still not completely resolved. It had been thought that its effect was mediated via a reduction in plasma volume and glomerular filtration rate.[35] The effects on urine osmolality and volume seen with chlorthiazide seem to be a consequence of a deficit of sodium, induced by the diuretic rather than being caused by a primary influence on the permeability of the distal tubule to water.[36] It has been presumed that the primary deficit of sodium induced by chlorthiazide somehow results in the reabsorption of a greater amount of filtered sodium in the proximal tubule. Thus, less fluid is delivered to the distal tubule, imposing a limitation on the volume of water available for excretion. Recent work has offered further evidence along these lines, tending to support such hypotheses.[37]

While there have been advocates of the use of a low-solute diet alone in the treatment of nephrogenic DI, results have been mostly disappointing. Such a diet is best used in conjunction with chlorothiazide.

A final word should be said about the use of chlorthiazide in cases with idiopathic DI. Since these patients are usually well controlled by injections of vasopressin tannate in oil, the main advantage in introducing chlorthiazide is its potential for lessening the number of injections. Actually, there is no point in administering chlorthiazide with vasopressin, thereby using two drugs where one will suffice. Although both medications would then be used in lower doses than when either is used alone, the only desirable regimen is one in which the two drugs can be alternated. In this manner the patient is subjected to half as many injections. Since chlorothiazide will not reduce the renal water requirement any more in idiopathic DI than in nephrogenic DI, the author has not been surprised to experience little success when such an alternating therapeutic regimen has been attempted.

References

1. BLOTNER, H. 1942. The inheritance of diabetes insipidus. Am. J. Med. Sci. **204**: 261.
2. MARTIN, F. I. 1959. Familial diabetes insipidus. Quart. J. Med. **28**: 573.
3. FORSSMAN, H. 1945. On hereditary diabetes insipidus: with special regard to a sex-linked form. Acta Med. Scand. Supp. **159**: 1.
4. BRAVERMAN, L. E., J. P. MANCINI & D. M. MCGOLDRICK. 1965. Hereditary idiopathic diabetes insipidus. A case report with autopsy findings. Ann. Int. Med. **63**: 503.
5. VALTIN, H. 1967. Hereditary hypothalamic diabetes insipidus in rats (Brattleboro strain). Am. J. Med. **42**: 814.
6. ROTH, J., S. M. GLICK, L. A. KLEIN & M. J. PETERSEN. 1966. Specific antibody to vasopressin in man. J. Clin. Endocrinol. & Metab. **26**: 671.
7. BARLTROP, D. 1963. Diabetes insipidus treated with synthetic lysine vasopressin. Lancet **2**: 276.
8. STROTT, C. A., K. NAKAGAWA, H. NANKIN & C. A. NUGENT. 1967. A phenylalanine-lysine-vasopressin test of ACTH release. J. Clin. Endocrinol. & Metab. **27**: 448.
9. SACHS, H. 1967. Biosynthesis and release of vasopressin. Am. J. Med. **42**: 687.
10. SHARE, L. 1967. Vasopressin, its bioassay and the physiological control of its release. Am. J. Med. **42**: 701.
11. ORLOFF, J. & J. S. HANDLER. 1964. The cellular mode of action of antidiuretic hormone. Am. J. Med. **36**: 686.
12. LEAF, A. 1967. Membrane effects of ADH. Am. J. Med. **42**: 746.
13. WAKIM, K. G. 1967. Reassessment of the source, mode and locus of action of antidiuretic hormone. Am. J. Med. **42**: 394.
14. FORSSMAN, H. 1942. Om arftlighetsgangen vid diabetes insipidus. Nord. Med. **16**: 3211.
15. WILLIAMS, R. H. & C. HENRY. 1947. Nephrogenic diabetes insipidus: transmitted by females and appearing during infancy in males. Ann. Int. Med. **27**: 84.
16. SCHOEN, E. J. 1960. Renal diabetes insipidus. Pediatrics **26**: 808.
17. CARTER, C. & M. SIMPKISS. 1956. The "carrier" state in nephrogenic diabetes insipidus. Lancet **2**: 1069.
18. ALIAPOULIOS, M. A., E. F. VOELKEL & P. L. MUNSON. 1966. Assay of human thyroid glands for thyrocalcitonin activity. J. Clin. Endocrinol. & Meta. **26**: 897.
19. JOHNSTON, H., J. HERZOG & D. LAULER. 1967. Reversal of pitressin-induced antidiuresis by prostaglandin E_1. Clin. Res. **15**: 360.
20. BORIS, A. & R. H. STEVENSON. 1967. The effects of some psychotropic drugs on dehydration induced antidiuretic hormone activity in the rat. Archs. int. Pharmacodyn. Ther. **166**: 486.
21. LEWIS, A. A. G. & T. M. CHALMERS. 1951. A nicotine test for the investigation of diabetes insipidus. Clin. Sci. **10**: 137.
22. HICKEY, R. C. & K. HARE. 1944. The renal excretion of chloride and water in diabetes insipidus. J. Clin. Invest. **23**: 768.
23. CARTER, A. C. & J. ROBBINS. 1947. The use of hypertonic saline infusions in the differential diagnosis of diabetes insipidus and psychogenic polydipsia. J. Clin. Endocrinol. & Metab. **7**: 753.
24. PRICE, J. D. E. & R. W. LAUENER. 1966. Serum and urine osmolalities in the differential diagnosis of polyuric states. J. Clin. Endocrinol. & Metab. **26**: 143.
25. MOSES, A. M. & D. H. P. STREETEN. 1967. Differentiation of polyuric states by measurement of responses to changes in plasma osmolality induced by hypertonic saline infusions. Am. J. Med. **42**: 368.
26. AUBRY, R. H., H. R. NANKIN, A. M. MOSES & D. H. P. STREETEN. 1965. Measurement of the osmotic threshold for vasopressin release in human subjects, and its modification by cortisol. J. Clin. Endocrinol. & Metab. **25**: 1481.
27. CAMPBELL, W. G., JR. 1961. Vasopressin-resistant diabetes insipidus associated with cytological changes in the supraoptic and paraventicular nuclei. Lancet **2**: 522.

28. De Wardener, H. E. & A. Herxheimer. 1957. The effect of high water intake on the kidney's ability to concentrate the urine in man. J. Physiol. **139:** 42.
29. Relkin, R. 1966. Diabetes insipidus. N. Y. State J. Med. **66:** 2789.
30. Arduino, F., F. P. J. Ferraz & J. Rodrigues. 1966. Antidiuretic action of chlorpropamide in idiopathic diabetes insipidus. J. Clin. Endocrinol. & Metab. **26:** 1325.
31. Torretti, J. & I. Zanzi. 1967. Intravenous furosemide in diabetes insipidus. Metabolism **16:** 529.
32. Molina, G., J. O. Gonzales & J. G. Orozco. 1967. Einfluss des antidiuretischen Hormons und des Furosemid auf den Natriumtransport. Arzneimittel-forsch. **17:** 382.
33. Harrington, A. R. & H. Valtin. 1965. Vasopressin effect on urinary concentration in rats with hereditary hypothalamic diabetes insipidus (Brattleboro strain). Proc. Soc. Exper. Biol. & Med. **118:** 448.
34. Kennedy, G. C. & J. D. Crawford. 1959. Treatment of diabetes insipidus with hydrochlorothiazide. Lancet **1:** 866.
35. Havard, C. W. & P. H. Wood. 1960. Antidiuretic properties of hydrochlorothiazide in diabetes insipidus. Brit. Med. J. **1:** 1306.
36. Earley, L. E. & J. Orloff. 1962. The mechanism of antidiuresis associated with the administration of hydrochlorothiazide to patients with vasopressin-resistant diabetes insipidus. J. Clin. Invest. **41:** 1988.
37. Skadhauge, E. 1966. Studies of the antidiuresis induced by natrichloruretic drugs in rats with diabetes insipidus. Quart. J. Exper. Physiol. **51:** 297.

PART III. GENETIC VARIATIONS THAT MODIFY DRUG RESPONSE

VARIATIONS IN DETOXICATION ENZYMES DURING MAMMALIAN DEVELOPMENT*

Sumner J. Yaffe, Joseph Krasner and Charlotte S. Catz

Department of Pediatrics, School of Medicine
State University of N. Y. at Buffalo

It has been repeatedly demonstrated that the developing fetus and newborn infant are more sensitive than the adult to the effects of many pharmacologic agents.[1,2] Differences in absorption, distribution, and excretion may be present in the newborn organism, but the principal factor in this response differential appears to be variation in the rates of detoxication. Drug metabolic processes have been studied in vitro in several animal species and, in most instances, activities are lower in the newborn organism compared with the adult.[3,4] Variations in drug metabolism appear to be genetically determined and the enzymic activity observed at any given age is dependent upon the species and strain of organism as well as the substrate employed in the reaction. Our primary objective in our initial studies was to determine how soon after birth one could detect and differentiate the contribution to drug metabolism made by genetic endowment.

To study drug response, hexobarbital was selected because its pharmacologic effect, sleeping time (loss of righting reflex), is easily measurable, its metabolism has been carefully studied, and the correlation between pharmacologic effect and biotransformation of the drug is fairly well established. In the following studies[5] the hypnotic effect of hexobarbital was measured as the sleeping time or time interval in minutes from injection of the drug until restoration of the righting reflex. The drug was administered i.p. (0.7% (w/v) aqueous solution) in a dosage of 50 or 100 mg/kg except in the newborn, for whom the s.c. route was used. To maintain body temperature, the newborn mice were kept in a ventilated, warm room at 35°C. Hypnotic investigations of all other ages were carried out at room temperature (24–26°C). Animals were used only once for the experimental studies because of the well-documented increase in drug-metabolizing ability which is known to accompany prior administration of barbiturates. The mean values for sleeping time in adult mice following i.p. injection of 100 mg/kg of hexobarbital are shown in FIGURE 1.

Twelve animals of each sex and strain were used in the assay procedure. The actual values (with standard errors of the mean) in the male animals are as follows: C_{57}BL, 18.70±0.96 minutes; Balb/C, 33.64±1.28 minutes; 129J, 61.67 ± 5.70 minutes. The differences between the strains are statistically significant at the $P < .01$ level. Within any given strain there was remarkably little variation in hypnotic response in animals of the same sex and age, but in all strains tested there was a distinct male sex preponderance with the male sleeping more than twice as long as his female counterpart. This sex difference was of considerable interest since it suggested a hormonal mediation of drug response. In the C_{57} BL strain where detailed inquiry was made, sleeping times in the female were correlated with the estrus cycle determined by vaginal smear. The shortest sleeping times (4.93 ± 1.9 minutes) in this strain occurred during the phase of estrus and proestrus, when estrogenic effect is known to be greatest. Sleeping

* These investigations were supported in part by a research grant from the U.S. Public Health Service (HD–01219).

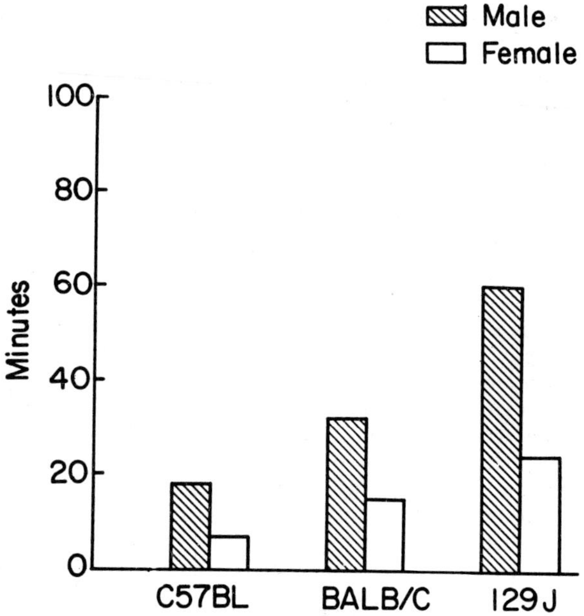

FIGURE 1. Strain variation in sleeping time. The height of each bar represents the mean value for sleeping time in minutes following i.p. injection of 100 mg/kg of hexobarbital. Twelve adult animals of each sex and strain were used in the assay procedure.

times (9.87 $\pm$ 1.08 minutes) during diestrus and metestrus were significantly longer ($P < .05$). However, attempts to modify the duration of hypnosis by in vivo administration of several female sex hormones were unsuccessful.

Mean sleeping time following administration of 50 mg/kg hexobarbital in male mice of different ages is depicted graphically in FIGURE 2. The dose of 100 mg/kg used in the adult mice was uniformly lethal in the newborn animals and a smaller dose had to be given in order to investigate age-dependent variations in hypnotic response. The results shown in FIGURE 2 indicate that there were significant differences between strains in hypnotic effect present on the day of birth and that these differences persisted into adult life. The gradual decrease in sleeping time with increasing age correlates with hexobarbital-metabolizing ability as determined in vitro in liver homogenates. The striking decrease in sleeping time at age three weeks to below adult values for this dose of hexobarbital (100 mg/kg) assumes even greater significance when viewed in the context of previous and subsequent postnatal development (FIGURE 3). At age three weeks, half of the animals tested did not lose their righting reflex, and the mean value used in the figure is based upon sleeping times determined in those animals in whom the hypnotic effect was evident.

The changing quantitative patterns of drug action during development are paralleled by appropriate variations in the level of activity of the reduced triphosphopyridine nucleotide-dependent hepatic oxidizing enzyme. As a result, plasma concentration of hexobarbital determined at the time of awakening are similar (TABLE 1), indicative of no change of sensitivity to the injected hypnotic agent with increasing age. (No measurements were made of plasma concentration in newborn mice because of inadequate sample size.) This marked reduction in

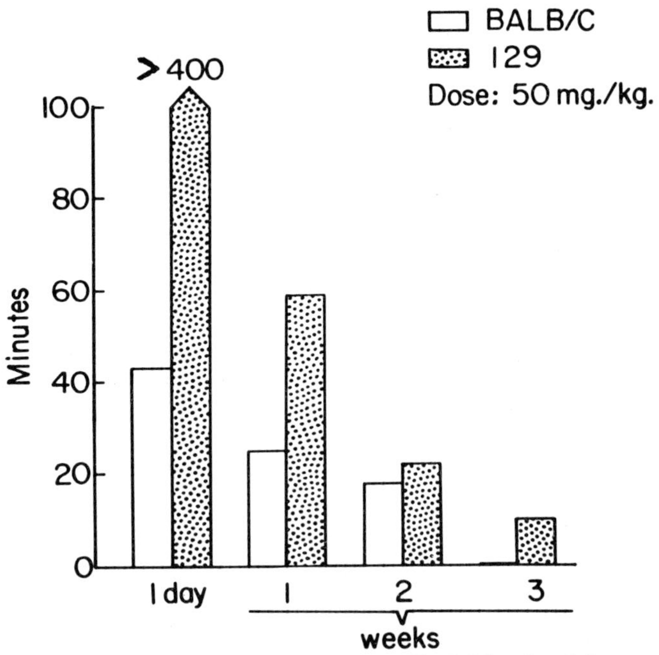

FIGURE 2. Strain and age variation in sleeping time. The height of each bar represents the mean value for sleeping time (in minutes) following i.p. administration of 50 mg/kg of hexobarbital. Twelve (or more) male mice of each age and strain were used for the determination.

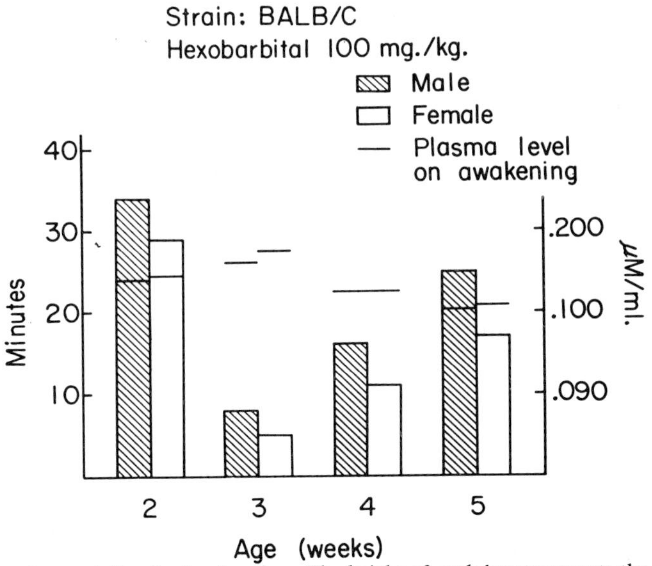

FIGURE 3. Age variation in sleeping time. The height of each bar represents the mean value for sleeping time (in minutes) following i.p. administration of 100 mg/kg of hexobarbital. – indicates the plasma concentration of hexobarbital determined at the time of awakening. Twelve mice of the Balb/C strain of varying ages were used for each determination.

TABLE 1
AGE VARIATION IN SLEEPING TIME IN BALB/C MICE*

Age weeks	Sleeping Time minutes		Plasma Concentration µmole/ml	
2	36 ± 1.8†	(14)‡	0.140 ± 0.012	(9)
3	9 ± 1.2	(18)	0.153 ± 0.080	(15)
4	16 ± 2.6	(9)	0.126 ± 0.02	(10)

* Following a single 100 mg/kg intraperitoneal injection of hexobarbital.
† Standard error of the mean.
‡ Figures in parentheses refer to number of animals.

sleeping time at age three weeks was a surprising finding. This age in the mouse coincides with weaning and increased physical activity. It is also correlated with a sudden and significant increase in the rate of hexobarbital degradation by liver homogenate as measured in vitro. No clear explanation for this finding is available at the present time. Teleologically, this phenomenon would appear sound, since, at weaning, greater possibilities of exposure to foreign compounds occur and the "detoxifying mechanism" becomes of prime importance. One can only speculate about the analogy of this finding to the human organism. There are, unfortunately, no data available concerning similar periods during the development of man. Most clinical investigators have concentrated their efforts on the newborn period and have demonstrated qualitative and/or quantitative variations in drug-metabolizing ability at this age. It seems reasonable to suppose that there will be other periods during postnatal human development in which alterations in drug metabolic activity will be found. Puberty, with its associated adolescent growth spurt and marked increase in the secretion of several hormones, is most likely to be associated with changes in the ability of the organism to metabolize drug substrates. Assay of enzymic activity during postnatal development is a necessary prerequisite to rational therapeutics in infants and children.

The developmental approach also can be utilized to gain insight into the nature and specificity of the metabolic process. The number of enzyme systems capable of glucuronide formation in mammalian liver remains uncertain. A definitive study of the microsomal enzyme, UDP-glucuronyltransferase, which is known to participate in this reaction is difficult, because the enzyme is insoluble and solubilization procedures in general tend to inactivate the enzyme. Early work[6,7] supported the concept of a single enzyme, but more recently, a number of authors[8–10] have reported results indicating that there are several enzymes for 0-glucuronide formation, each with a unique substrate specificity. In these later experiments, significant variations were found in the conjugating abilities of liver preparations from different species of animals, depending upon which substrate and what assay conditions were used. All these experiments were done with particulate preparations. The necessity of working with an insoluble enzyme source and the frequent choice of an unnatural substrate has obvious and recognized drawbacks, particularly when conclusions are reached with respect to the human organism. Since evidence for the formation of 0-glucuronide with foreign substrates has accumulated, it seemed worthwhile to investigate the conjugating enzyme by using bilirubin which is a more refractory but biologically important substrate. Male New Zealand rabbits were used throughout the study. When newborn or young rabbits were employed, the animals were supplied directly from the breeder on the day of the experiment. Older animals were maintained on a diet of Purina Chow and water ad libitum. Adults were killed by an i.v. injection of air into an ear vein, and young rabbits were decapitated. After removal of the gallbladders, the livers were rinsed immediately with cold 0.1 M KCl and homogenized with three volumes of the KCl for two minutes in the cold. Homogenates were prepared using a glass homogenizer with a Teflon pestle. All subsequent procedures were carried out in the cold. Assays were performed using either the homogenate or the microsomal suspension obtained after centrifugation at 105,000 × g for two hours. The assay procedures have been described previously.[11]

FIGURE 4 shows graphically the conjugating activities, as percentages of the adult male activity (based on conjugation per mg of protein) for p-nitrophenol and bilirubin, with liver homogenates as the source of enzyme. Each point is the average of at least four separate experiments. The enzyme activity at any given age was reproducible to within ± 8%. It is evident that the development of glucuronide conjugating activity with these two substrates does not follow the same course. P-nitrophenol conjugation is much higher at birth and reaches the adult levels of activity faster than does bilirubin conjugation. Similar results for the formation of p-nitrophenyl and o-aminophenyl glucuronides in the perinatal mouse have been noted by Dutton.[10] O-aminophenol conjugating ability, as shown here for bilirubin, developed more slowly than that for p-nitrophenol. Lack of

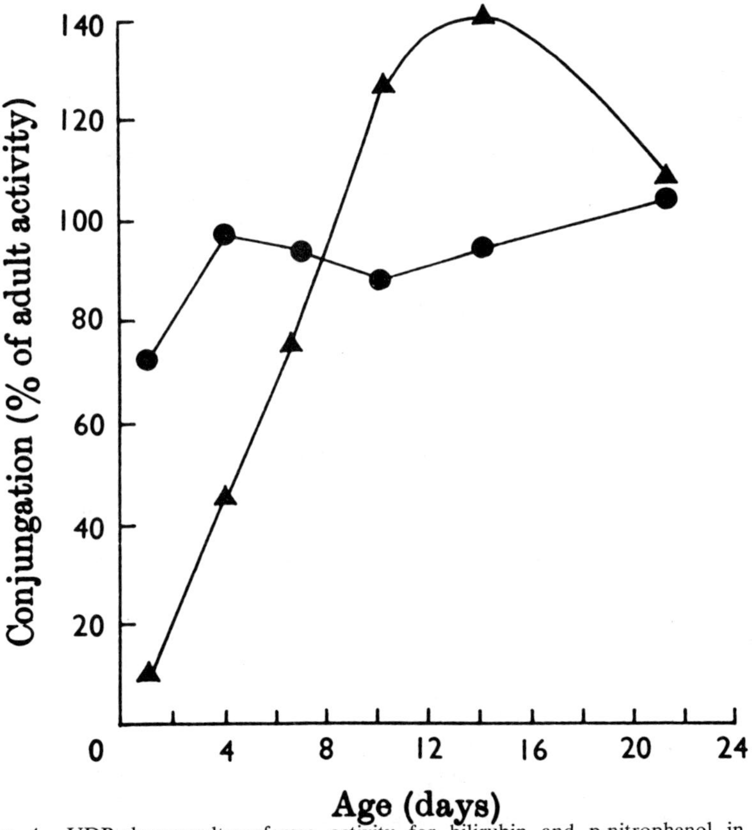

FIGURE 4. UDP-glucuronyltransferase activity for bilirubin and p-nitrophenol in liver homogenates of rabbits of different ages. Assay mixtures were incubated at 37°C for 20 min. ▲, Bilirubin; ●, p-nitrophenol. (Reproduced through the courtesy of Biochemical Journal.)

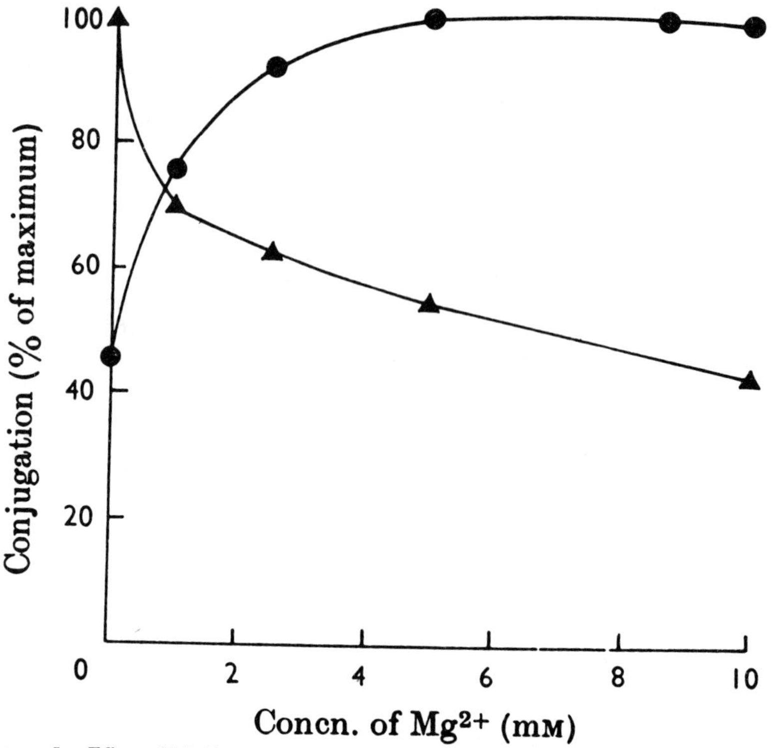

FIGURE 5. Effect of Mg^{2+} concentration of glucuronide formation of bilirubin and, p-nitrophenol by rabbit-liver microsomes after 20 min. incubation at 37° C. ●, Bilirubin; ▲, p-nitrophenol. (Reproduced through courtesy of Biochemical Journal.)

parallelism between rates of synthesis of bilirubin and o-aminophenyl glucuronides in both tissue slices and suspensions of livers from a number of animals were reported also by Lathe and Walker.[12] Another aspect of the situation has been investigated by van Leusden[9] who studied p-nitrophenol and bilirubin conjugation in livers of adult homozygous Gunn rats. These animals, which are jaundiced, presumably due to low activity of the enzyme necessary for bilirubin glucuronide formation, nevertheless possess the ability to conjugate p-nitrophenol. Our results and the results cited by others strongly suggest the presence of not one nonspecific enzyme, but of a family of enzymes, each with its own substrate specificity.

Additional evidence obtained from co-factor requirements supports this contention. The concentration of magnesium (8.6 mM) used in the bilirubin assays, which was optimum for conjugation of this substrate, inhibited p-nitrophenol conjugation. FIGURE 5 shows the effects of magnesium on the conjugation of both substrates. Magnesium at 10 mM decreased p-nitrophenol conjugation by 43%, whereas the elimination of magnesium from the reaction mixture with bilirubin as the substrate resulted in a 55% decrease in activity. Similar results were obtained with either tris, KCl, or phosphate buffer. The difference in response to magnesium for the several substrates is probably not only one of permeability (which can be a factor when particulate enzyme preparations are used) but also could be a manifestation of the presence of several enzymes rather than one. Alternatively, the ion may influence active-center interactions for different substrates on the same enzyme.

Kinetic data lend further credence to the existence of more than one enzyme system. P-nitrophenol was a potent inhibitor of bilirubin glucuronidation, giving nearly 25% inhibition at 5 mM, but the effect was noncompetitive (FIGURE 6). If the same enzyme conjugated both substrates, one would expect a competitive type of inhibition to occur. On the other hand, in the same system bilirubin, even at a 10-fold excess, was unable to decrease p-nitrophenol conjugation. Attempts to solubilize the enzyme responsible for bilirubin glucuronide conjugation were unsuccessful using a variety of techniques (snake venom, deoxycholate, ribonuclease plus digitonin, lecithinase C, butanol, and ultrasonic oscillation). With p-nitrophenol as a substrate, not only was some solubilization of the conjugating enzyme obtained (21%) using snake venom, but, in addition, assays on the reaction mixture after treatment with snake venom, but before high-speed centrifugation, showed that enzyme activity was enhanced. This enhancement (3-fold) of p-nitrophenol conjugation occurred when there was an 80% loss of bilirubin glucuronidation. Thus, assay of activities with two substrates during the process of purification and solubilization also supports the concept of two enzymes rather than one.

Activity of the enzyme, phenolsulfotransferase, in mouse liver suspensions shows an unusual variation with postnatal age. The phenolsulfotransferase assay system is a modification of the method used by Percy and Yaffe.[31] The reaction mixture contains p-nitrophenolsulfate (p-NPS) as substrate, Tris buffer pH 7.8, EDTA, reduced glutathione, co-factor 3′–5′ diphosphoadenosine (PAP) which

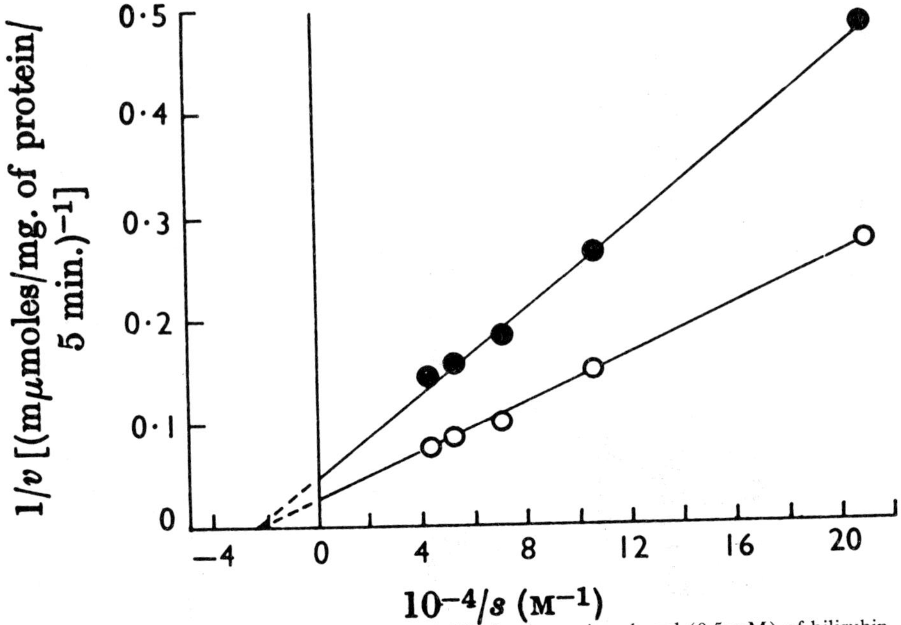

FIGURE 6. Lineweaver-Burk plot showing inhibition by p-nitrophenol (0.5 mM) of bilirubin glucuronide formation after 5 min. incubation at 37° C. ○, no inhibitor; ●, p-nitrophenol added. (Reproduced through the courtesy of Biochemical Journal.)

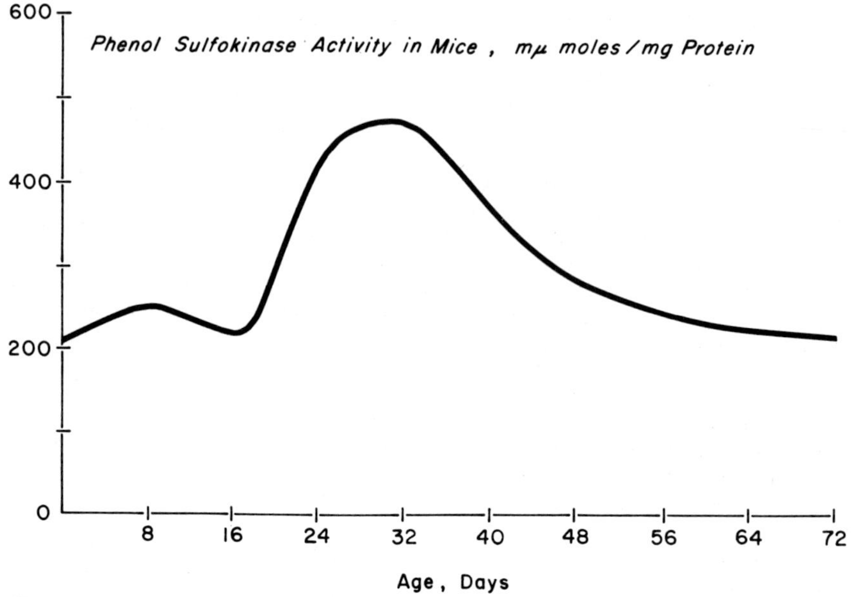

FIGURE 7. Phenolsulfotransferase activity during postnatal development in the mice. High speed supernatant from liver homogenate was used as the enzyme source with p-nitrophenyl sulfate as substrate.

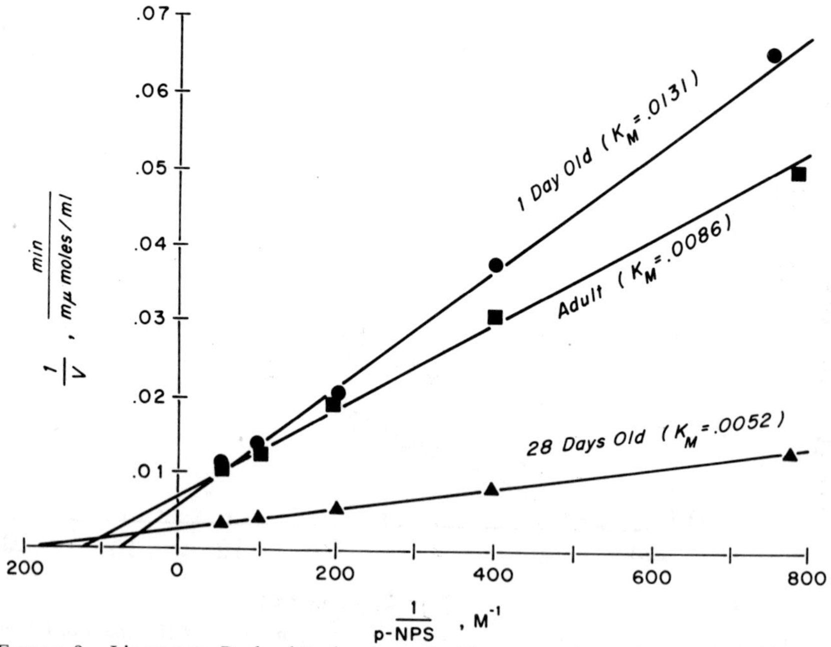

FIGURE 8. Lineweaver-Burk plot showing velocities at varying substrate (p-NPS) concentrations in enzyme preparations from 1 day, 28 day, and adult mice.

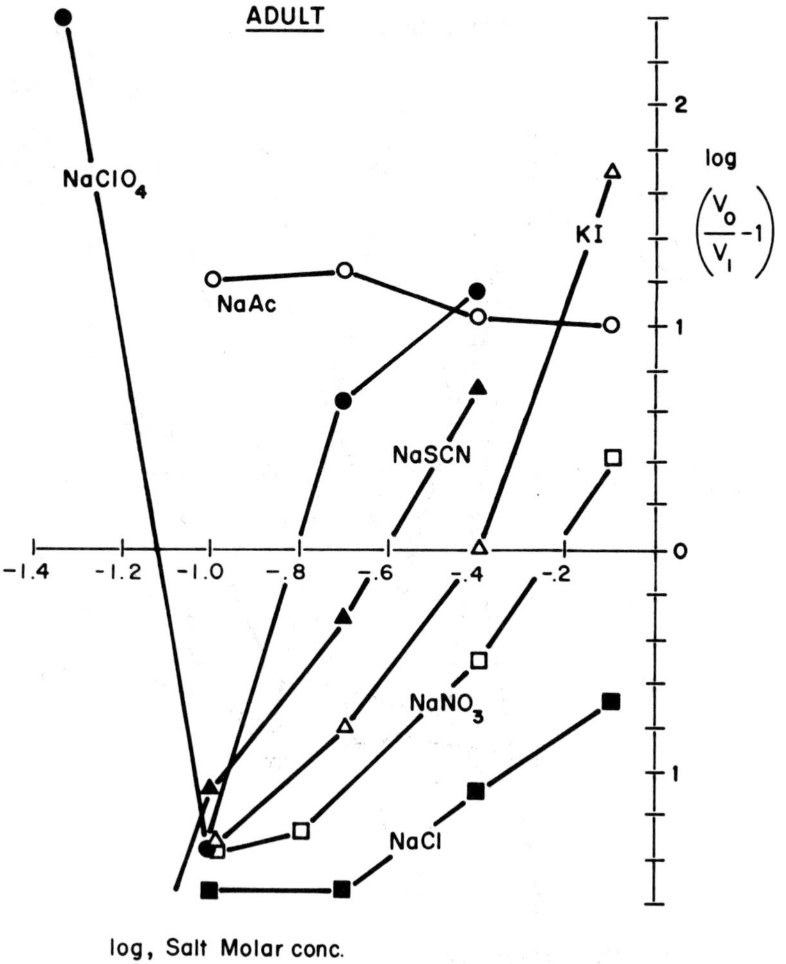

FIGURE 9. The effect of neutral salts on phenolsulfotransferase activity in high-speed supernatant obtained from adult mouse liver. p-NPS was the substrate (0.02 M).

is contained in a crude preparation of adenosinediphosphate (ADP), m-aminophenol (m-AP) as a sulfate acceptor and a particle-free high-speed supernatant as the enzyme source. The supernatant is prepared after fractional ultracentrifugation at 104,000 × g of mouse liver homogenized in 0.1 M KCl. The reaction is carried out at 37°C with appropriate controls. Enzyme activity is measured by the amount of free p-NP released as follows:

$$\text{p-NPS} + \text{PAP} \rightleftharpoons \text{p-NP} + \text{PAPS} \quad (1)$$

$$\text{PAPS} + \text{m} - \text{AP} \rightleftharpoons \text{PAP} + \text{m} - \text{APS} \quad (2)$$

The liberation of p-nitrophenol was measured at its absorption maximum of 400 mμ in a Cary model 15 recording spectrophotometer. No color change is produced when either co-factor or acceptor is omitted from the assay mixture.

Using m-aminophenol as sulfate acceptor, newborn and adult levels of activity are similar but a three-fold increase occurs at 28 days of age (FIGURE 7). Because

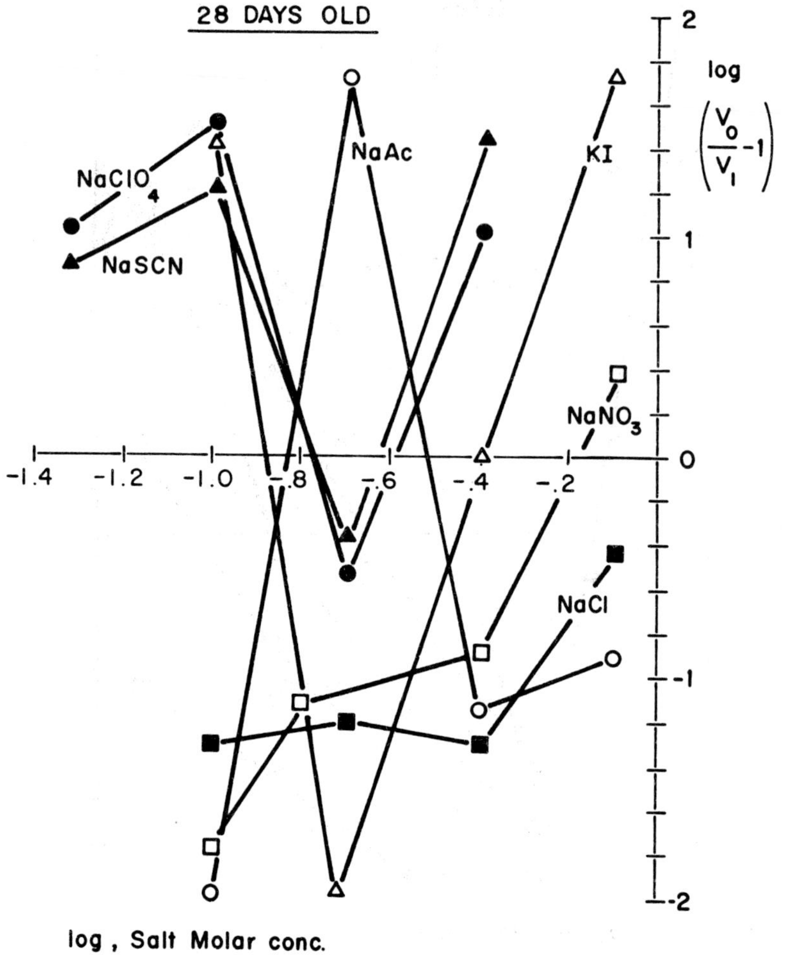

FIGURE 10. The effect of neutral salts on phenolsulfotransferase activity in high-speed supernatant obtained from 28-day-old mouse liver. p-NPS was the substrate (0.02 M).

the sulfotransferase conjugating enzyme exhibited these unusual characteristics during postnatal development it was decided to compare the properties of the enzyme at these three different ages. Chromatographic separation on a Sephadex G-200 column showed similar patterns for the 1-day, 28-day, and adult supernatant preparations, insofar as enzyme activity and protein are concerned. Also, electrophoretic mobilities using acetate or starch-gel were similar for the three preparations. Apparent enzyme-substrate affinity as determined by Michaelis-Menten constants derived from Lineweaver-Burk plots, are markedly different in preparations from newborn (0.0131), 28-day-old (0.0052), and adult (0.0086) mice (FIGURE 8).

Additions of high concentrations of neutral salts such as sodium chloride (NaCl), sodium acetate (NaAc), sodium nitrate ($NaNO_3$), sodium thiocynate (NaSCN), sodium perchlorate ($NaClO_4$), and potassium iodide (KI) markedly

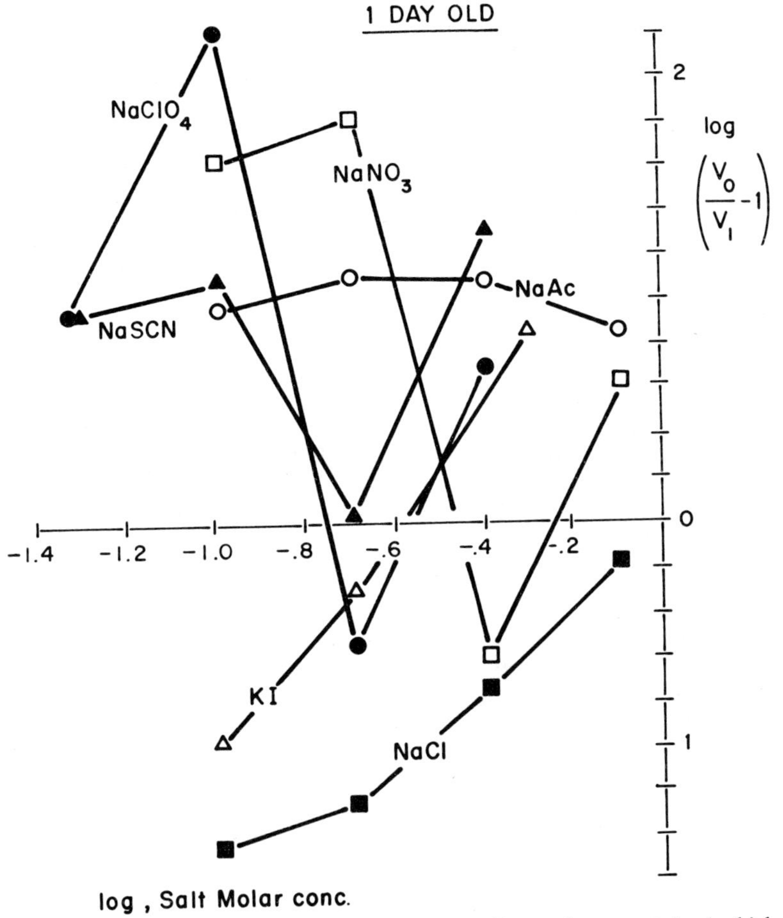

FIGURE 11. The effect of neutral salts on phenolsulfotransferase activity in high-speed supernatant obtained from 1-day-old mouse liver. p-NPS was the substrate (0.02 M).

inhibited enzyme activity. Analysis of the kinetics of the inhibition produced by each of the salts showed this to be noncompetitive.

The salts were added in gradually increasing concentrations to the assay mixture using p-nitrophenylsulfate (0.02 M) as substrate, and the results with each concentration of salt compared to the activity obtained without salt were added. Results were plotted using the equation derived by Johnson, Eyring, and Williams.[14] Here the log of the salt concentration in moles is plotted against log $\left(\frac{Vo}{Vi}-1\right)$ where the Vo is the initial velocity without salt and Vi is the velocity in the presence of salt. The advantages of this method for expressing results are that one can derive readily, by visual inspection, the concentration of salt producing 50% inhibition and the relative amount of salt bound to protein can be ascertained from the slope of the lines. In the adult preparation, all the salts produced inhibition with increasing salt concentrations except sodium acetate which showed relatively little effect (FIGURE 9). Inhibition with NaSCN, KI, and $NaNO_3$ is noted at salt concentrations of 0.1 M. With NaCl no effect is noted until 0.2 M salt concentration is present. The degree of inhibition increases with increasing salt concentration. On the other hand, $NaClO_4$ activated or enhanced the activity of the enzyme at .05 M and inhibition did not occur until 0.1 M and then gradually increased with increasing concentrations of the salt. The intercept of the curves with the abscissa represents that salt concentration producing 50% inhibition.

In the 28-day-old preparation using the same coordinates, differences in salt effects were noted (FIGURE 10). Sodium acetate showed slight inhibition at 0.1 M, with slight stimulation of activity at 0.2 M, and then increasing amounts of inhibition with increasing salt concentrations (0.4 and 0.8 M). This is in contrast to the absence of effect in the adult preparation. NaCl did not produce noticeable inhibition until a concentration of 0.4 M was present. KI, $NaClO_4$ and NaSCN enhanced the activity at low concentrations before inhibiting.

In the preparation derived from the newborn animal markedly different patterns of inhibition were noted from those seen at 28 days and in the adult (FIGURE 11). NaAc effects were similar to those found in the adult. $NaNO_3$, on the other hand, enhanced activity at 0.1 and 0.2 M as did NaSCN and $NaClO_4$ at .05 and 0.1 M. KI and NaCl behaved as they did in the adult preparation but differently from that seen in the 28-day-old preparation. Even though there may be similarities with these two salts and with some of the others in the shape of the curves, the different slopes would indicate different amounts of salt being bound to the enzyme protein.

Neutral salts in sufficiently high concentrations have been shown to alter the conformation of proteins.[15–17] This salt effect, by altering the structure of the protein, results in a loss of enzyme activity which is noncompetitive when expressed on a kinetic basis. The markedly different patterns of salt effects and inhibitions noted in the preparations obtained from mice of three different ages would suggest that three enzyme protein configurations exist at these stages of postnatal development. If the same protein structure were present, one would expect that the salt effects would be similar at each age.

Summary

Three different approaches to the study of the characteristics of detoxifying enzymes have been presented. Developmental and maturational changes in the host have been utilized not only to characterize processes of drug metabolism in the developing organism, but also as a tool to sharpen our inquiry into the basic nature of these processes. Variations in sleeping time following hexobarbital administration were noted between different strains of mice, and these effects were apparent throughout postnatal development beginning at one day of age. The application of several substrates to the study of glucuronidation suggests, from differences in developmental patterns and co-factor requirements, that different enzyme proteins are present for each aglycone acceptor. Finally, the structural alterations produced by neutral salts using a single substrate suggest that the protein responsible for the enzymatic transfer of sulfate undergoes a change in configuration at the three stages of postnatal development studied.

References

1. KRETCHMER, N. 1959. Practical therapeutic implications of immaturity. Pediatrics **23:** 638–640.
2. NYHAN, W. L. 1961. Toxicity of drugs in the neonatal period. J. Pediat. **59:** 1–20.
3. FOUTS, J. R. & R. H. ADAMSON. 1959. Drug metabolism in the newborn rabbit. Science **129:** 897–898.

4. JONDORF, W. R., R. P. MAICKEL & B. B. BRODIE. 1959. Inability of newborn mice and guinea pigs to metabolize drugs. Biochem. Pharmacol. **1**: 352–354.
5. CATZ, C. S. & S. J. YAFFE. 1967. Strain and age variations in hexobarbital response. J. Pharmacol. Exp. Thera. **115**: 152–156.
6. AXELROD, J., R. SCHMID & L. HAMMAKER. 1957. A biochemical lesion in congenital, non-obstructive, non-haemolytic jaundice. Nature **180**: 1426–1427.
7. BROWN, A. K. & W. W. ZUELZER. 1958. Studies on the neonatal development of the glucuronide conjugating system. J. Clin. Invest. **37**: 332–340.
8. CHOJECKI, A. & F. KERN, JR. The effect of dietary cirrhosis and carbon tetrachloride poisoning on glucuronyl transferase activity of rat liver. Gastroenterology **40**: 521–531.
9. VAN LEUSDEN H. A. I. M., J. A. J. M. BAKKEREN, F. ZILLIKEN & L. A. M. STOLTE. 1962. p-Nitrophenylglucuronide formation by homozygous adult Gunn rats. Biochem. Biophys. Res. Comm. **7**: 67–69.
10. DUTTON, G. J. 1966. Variations in glucuronide formation by perinatal liver. Biochem. Pharmacol. **15**: 947–951.
11. TOMLINSON, G. A. & S. J. YAFFE. 1966. The formation bilirubin and p-nitrophenyl glucuronides by rabbit liver. Biochem. J. **99**: 507–512.
12. LATHE, G. H. & M. WALKER. 1958. The synthesis of bilirubin glucuronide in animal and human liver. Biochem. J. **70**: 705–712.
13. PERCY, A. K. & S. J. YAFFE. 1964. Sulfate metabolism during mammalian development. Pediatrics **33**: 965–968.
14. JOHNSON, F. H., H. EYRING & R. W. WILLIAMS. 1942. The nature of enzyme inhibitions in bacterial luminescence: sulfanilamide, urethane, temperature and pressure. J. Cell Comp. Physiol. **20**: 247–268.
15. VON HIPPEL, P. H. & K. Y. WONG. 1964. Neutral salts: the generality of their effects on the stability of macromolecular conformations. Science **145**: 577–580.
16. WARREN, J. C.. L. STWORING & M. F. MORALES. 1966. The effect of structure-disrupting ions on the activity of myosin and other enzymes. J. Biol. Chem. **241**: 309–316.
17. WARREN, J. C. & D. M. PETERSON. 1966. Structure-destroying ions: Detection of qualitative change in an enzyme. Science **152**: 1245–1246.

GENETIC AND ENVIRONMENTAL FACTORS AFFECTING HEXOBARBITAL METABOLISM IN MICE

Elliot S. Vesell

Section on Pharmacogenetics, Laboratory of Chemical Pharmacology
National Heart Institute, National Institutes of Health
Bethesda, Md.

Introduction

Knowledge of the genetic and environmental factors that influence man's pharmacologic responsiveness is scant. Recently, genetic conditions have been recognized in which drugs may cause toxicity in individuals lacking certain enzymes. But with the exception of polyneuritis in slow inactivators of isoniazid and of hemolytic anemia following ingestion of various drugs by individuals with glucose-6-phosphate dehydrogenase deficiency, most of the toxic reactions resulting from inborn errors of metabolism are rare. None have been described affecting the drug-metabolizing enzymes located in liver microsomes.

How other, more 'normal' genetic differences and various environmental factors affect man's response to drugs requires more investigation. Two broad genetic categories of response to drugs are readily distinguishable. The first, and probably the most frequent type, results from the operation of multiple genes. This category is therefore termed polygenic, and produces a unimodal, continuous or Gaussian distribution curve. The second category results from the operation of a mutant gene or genes at a single locus, and produces a bi- or trimodal distribution curve that is clearly discontinuous. The latter is more readily investigated because of the separation of individuals into genotypes by their position on the distribution curve and because of the ease of analyzing the segregation of a single factor in a pedigree.

Experiments in animals have numerous advantages; drugs can be given with impunity in dosages and with frequencies that could not be attempted in man. In contrast to the human situation, matings can be controlled; large and frequently produced litters are generally available and can be studied at any point in development to search for genetic effects, without the frequently encountered human refusal of examination. Finally, numerous environmental conditions affecting the response to drugs can be rigidly controlled in animals with much greater ease than in man.

The present study was designed to determine some of the genetic and environmental factors affecting the response of animals to barbiturates. Although earlier investigations of the subject[1-11] clearly established the importance of certain genetic and environmental factors in animal responsiveness, the present experiments describe previously unrecognized factors as well as new aspects and interpretations of former studies and thus may be useful in guiding the selection of appropriate conditions of drug study. The existence of genetic and environmental factors altering the metabolism of barbiturates in animals raises the question of whether similar factors operate in man.

Materials and Methods

Several strains of mature male and female mice were employed in this study [A/HeN, AL/N, AKR/N, BALB/cAnN, BRSUNT/N, C3H/HeN, C57BL/6N, DBA/2N, NBL/N, STR/N, CAF_1, CdF_1, NIH, CFW and G.P. (General

TABLE 1

MEAN SLEEPING TIME IN MINUTES AND MEAN BRAIN HEXOBARBITAL LEVELS (γ /GRAM) IN FIVE GROUPS OF STIMULATED AND UNSTIMULATED GP MALE MICE WITH STANDARD ERROR OF MEAN*

Group	No Stimulation		1 Stimulus/min		1 Stimulus/5 min	
	Sleeping Time	Brain Hexobarbital (γ/gm)	Sleeping Time	Brain Hexobarbital	Sleeping Time	Brain Hexobarbital
1	71 ± 3	30 ± 3	44 ± 3	46 ± 2	60 ± 3	38 ± 2
2	62 ± 3	24 ± 1	40 ± 2	36 ± 2	53 ± 3	29 ± 1
3	38 ± 3	26 ± 2	34 ± 4	42 ± 2	31 ± 3	34 ± 1
4	41 ± 2	27 ± 1	34 ± 3	43 ± 1	38 ± 2	35 ± 1
5	44 ± 4	28 ± 2	34 ± 2	44 ± 2	38 ± 2	37 ± 2

* Twelve animals were used in each group and condition. In combining the results of all five groups, differences between unstimulated and stimulated animals (1 stimulus/minute) in sleeping time and brain hexobarbital level on awakening are significant ($P < 0.05$).

Purpose) White Swiss]. Reciprocal crosses between AL/N and DBA/2N mice were made. Male Sprague-Dawley rats (200 g) were used in some experiments. Weights of mice were 20 to 30 g except where developmental studies were performed, in which case they were less.

Sleeping times were measured by stopwatch from i.p. injection of sodium hexobarbital (125 mg/kg in mice and 200 mg/kg in rats) to restoration of the righting response, defined as the capacity of the animal to place both forefeet simultaneously on the ground twice within 15 seconds. Animals were stimulated at two-minute intervals by pressure on their tails from a forceps. This practice had been used routinely in previous studies because it was felt that unstimulated sleeping animals would fail to right themselves when they were capable of doing so. To test this hypothesis we compared the sleeping times of male NIH mice that received either no stimulation, one per minute, and one per five minutes. The mean sleeping times with standard error are given in TABLE 1. The results in each of five separate experiments show that unstimulated animals slept longer than ones stimulated every five minutes and that more frequent stimulation caused further shortening of sleeping time. However, TABLE 1 also shows that the magnitude of the difference between unstimulated and stimulated animals changes from one experiment to the other, as does the sleeping time of unstimulated animals.

When the righting response was restored, the animals were sacrificed and the brains and livers removed. The hexobarbital content of the brain was determined by extraction of the drug from brain homogenized with phosphate buffer pH 8.0, 0.5 M, into spectrally pure heptane containing 1.5% isomyl alcohol according to the method of Cooper and Brodie.[12] The heptane was then washed with citric acid buffer pH 5.5 to remove metabolites of hexobarbital. The hexobarbital in the heptane was then extracted into phosphate buffer (pH 11.0, 0.8 M). Differences between readings at wavelengths 245 and 260 mμ in a Beckman DU Spectrophotometer were related to readings at these wavelengths of a standard solution of hexobarbital. When the brain is homogenized in phosphate buffer pH 8 and the above procedure is followed, the blanks are close to zero. Recovery of a known quantity of hexobarbital added to the brain homogenate from a control mouse is approximately 90%.

The hexobarbital metabolizing activity of the 9000 × g supernatant prepared from a 20% homogenate of liver was assayed as previously described.[12] The 9000 × g supernatant (2 ml) was incubated for 15 minutes at 37°C with sodium hexobarbital (1 μmole) in phosphate buffer (pH 7.5, 0.2 M, 3 ml) to give a

TABLE 2

SLEEPING TIME, HEXOBARBITAL OXIDASE ACTIVITY AND BRAIN HEXOBARBITAL LEVEL ON AWAKENING IN VARIOUS STRAINS OF MALE MICE*

Strain		Sleeping Time ± S. D. Min	Hexobarbital Oxidase µmole/gram liver/15 min	Brain Hexobarbital Level (γ/gm)
AL/N	(24)†	86 ± 16	0.20 ± 0.01	45 ± 6
BALB/C	(24)	46 ± 6	0.34 ± 0.02	46 ± 4
C3H/HeN	(24)	41 ± 7	0.34 ± 0.02	53 ± 5
C57BL/6N	(24)	73 ± 13	0.23 ± 0.01	52 ± 5
DBA/2N	(24)	85 ± 17	0.21 ± 0.01	48 ± 4
STR/N	(24)	47 ± 6	0.36 ± 0.01	49 ± 4
CAF_1	(24)	72 ± 10	0.24 ± 0.02	46 ± 4
CdF_1	(24)	58 ± 9	0.28 ± 0.02	54 ± 5
NIH	(24)	37 ± 5	0.32 ± 0.03	48 ± 4
CFW/N	(24)	40 ± 7	0.37 ± 0.02	46 ± 3
GP	(24)	42 ± 8	0.37 ± 0.03	52 ± 5

* Differences in sleeping time and liver hexobarbital oxidase activity between AL/N, DBA/2N, C57BL/6N, CAF_1 and CdF_1 mice and other strains are significant ($P < 0.05$).

† The numbers in parenthesis indicate the number of animals used.

final volume of 5.0 ml. The amount of hexobarbital remaining after a 15 minute incubation was determined by the procedure described above. Similar studies were performed on the microsomal fraction prepared by spinning the 9000 × g supernatant for 60 minutes at 105,000 × g. Aniline hydroxylase and morphine N-demethylase were assayed by the methods used by Kato and Gillette.[13]

In all experiments except those in which red cedar bedding was specified, hardwood bedding, composed of a combination of beech, birch and maple, was used. The mice were offered water and standard Purina Chow *ad libitum*. The mice received hexobarbital between 9 and 11 a.m. except the group in which diurnal variations were studied.

Results

TABLE 2 shows the sleeping times with standard deviations, the hexobarbital oxidase activity of the 9000 × g supernatant of liver homogenate, and the brain hexobarbital level on restoration of the righting reflex in various strains of mice. All strains gave similar results except for the AL/N, DBA/2N and C57BL/6N strains, which slept longer than the others, had greater standard deviations and lower hexobarbital oxidase activity. CAF_1 and CdF_1 mice, hybrids between female BALB/C and male AL/N and male DBA/2N respectively, had sleeping times and hexobarbital oxidase activities intermediate between that of their parents. Reciprocal crosses between AL/N and DBA/2N mice retained the long sleeping time and low hexobarbital oxidase activity of their parents. No mouse among the 3,000 examined had undetectable or very low hexobarbital oxidase activity.

The longer sleeping animals exhibited greater standard deviations. To explore this relationship further we divided animals from a single strain (AL/N) into three groups. The first was made to sleep a short time by keeping them for three days on red cedar bedding, the second group was kept on hardwood bedding and slept an intermediate time, and the third group was treated with SKF 525A (50 mg/kg i.p.) one-half hour before hexobarbital administration and slept an extremely long time. The sleeping times in minutes and the standard deviations in these three groups were 23 ± 2, 84 ± 8, and 852 ± 91 respectively. The standard deviations increased in direct proportions to the sleeping times (FIGURE 1).

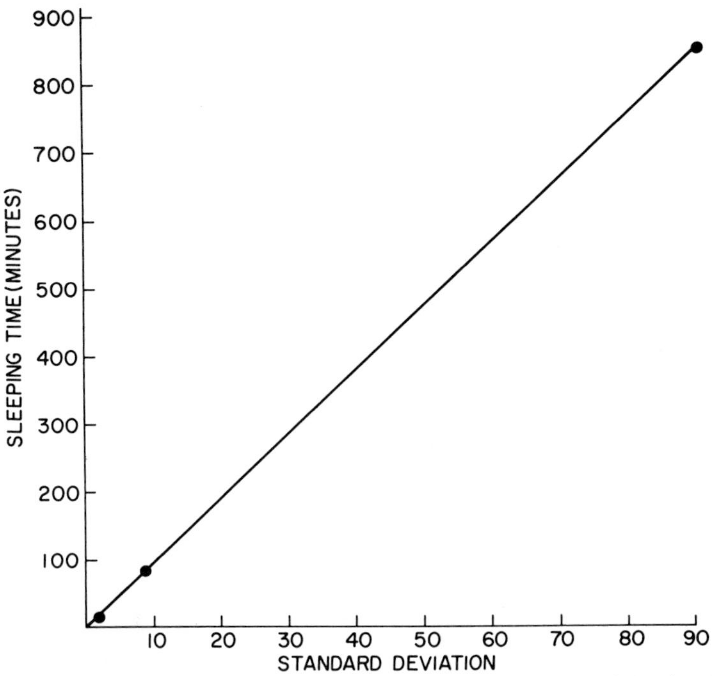

FIGURE 1. Relationship between sleeping time and standard deviation of sleeping time.

TABLE 3
SLEEPING TIME WITH STANDARD DEVIATION OF CdF_1 AND AL/N MALE MICE ANALYZED BY LITTER*

Litter No.	Sleeping time ± S. D. Min
CdF_1	
1 (6)†	25.6 ± 4.2
2 (4)	42.0 ± 0.8
3 (2)	34.0 ± 0.0
4 (3)	47.7 ± 5.8
5 (4)	34.7 ± 7.7
6 (2)	50.9 ± 0.4
7 (4)	28.9 ± 7.0
8 (3)	42.0 ± 1.4
All 28 mice	36.2 ± 9.0
AL/N	
1 (6)	79 ± 1.0
2 (4)	68 ± 0.9
3 (3)	58 ± 7.0
4 (5)	90 ± 8.0
All 18 mice	77 ± 13.0

* The intra litter variance is significantly lower than the inter litter variance for CdF_1, and AL/N ($P < 0.01$). All mice weighed between 22 and 27 grams.
† The numbers in parenthesis indicate the number of animals used.

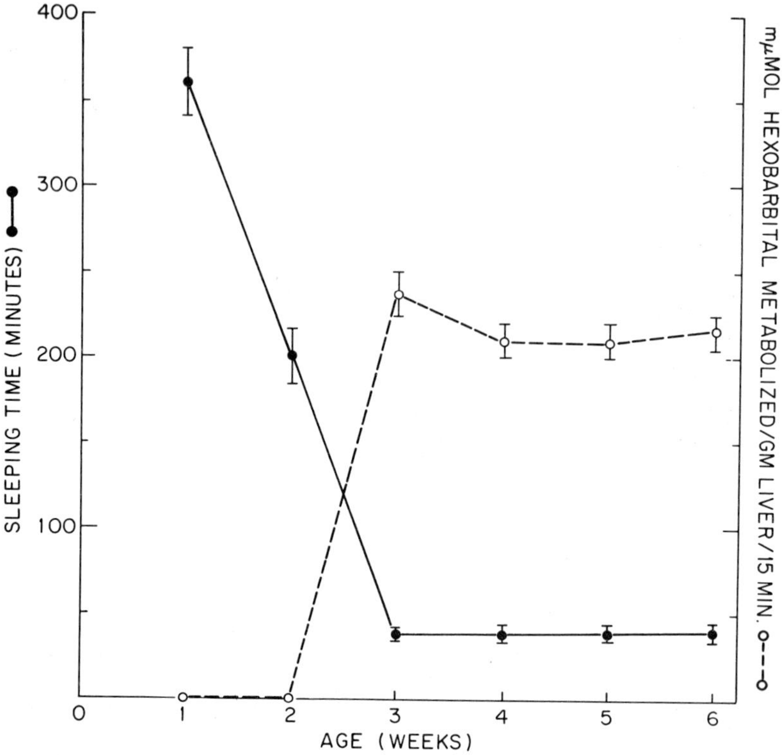

FIGURE 2. Development of hexobarbital oxidase activity of 9000 × g supernatant of liver homogenate and decrease of sleeping time with age. Each point represents the mean of 12 male NIH mice with standard deviations. Each mouse received sodium hexobarbital (125 mg/kg) i.p.

The standard deviations of the sleeping time could be substantially reduced within a strain if the mice were treated by litter rather than in groups of 24 composed of several litters. TABLE 3 shows that the standard deviations of the intra litter sleeping times are substantially lower than those for inter litter sleeping times.

A sex difference in hexobarbital sleeping time has been established.[9] Male mice sleep longer than females.[9] The present study reveals that this sex difference is maximal in inbred strains and diminishes as the strains are outbred (TABLE 4).

It has been demonstrated that at birth many animals lack microsomal drug-metabolizing enzymes that appear later in life.[11] FIGURE 2 shows that during the development with age of increasing hexobarbital oxidase activity in the 9000 × g supernatant of liver homogenate there is a corresponding decrease in sleeping time.

A wide variety of environmental influences modified the response of mice to hexobarbital. Induction of various drug-metabolizing enzymes in the liver microsomes were produced by softwood beddings (red cedar, white pine or ponderosa pine) (TABLE 5). Induction of these three enzymes also occurred in the liver microsomes of Sprague-Dawley rats after three days on red cedar bedding. When mice were taken from their usual hardwood bedding and placed on red cedar for six days, there was a rapid decrease in sleeping time and increase in hexobarbital metabolizing activity of the 9000 × g supernatant of liver homogenate (FIGURE 3). No change occurred in the brain level of hexobarbital on awakening; on these six days the brain levels were 48, 50, 49, 50, 47 and 51 γ/gram. Changes in sleeping time and enzyme activity were reversed by putting mice back on hardwood bedding (FIGURE 3).

In an attempt to eliminate the substance(s) responsible for the induction of these drug-metabolizing enzymes, the red cedar shavings were extracted in hexane for two hours at 25°C and for 30 minutes at 61°C. This treatment removed much of the inducing material, as indicated by the fact that mice kept on the dried, hexane-extracted, red cedar bedding for seven days exhibited only 25% decrease in their hexobarbital sleeping times as compared to an 80% decrease in mice kept on untreated red cedar bedding. Both red cedar heart wood and sap wood contain the inducing substance(s). Synthetic beddings did not cause enzyme induction. The rapidity of induction suggested that terpenes might be involved rather than DDT or the chlordane-type insecticides which are known inducers of drug-metabolizing enzymes but which take longer to act and to which neither softwood nor hardwood beddings were exposed. It is not clear whether induction in mice and rats on softwood bedding follows ingestion or inhalation of these compounds.

The temperature of the ambient atmosphere also influences the sleeping times after hexobarbital administration. NIH mice slept 50% longer and had correspondingly lower hexobarbital oxidase activity of the 9000 × g supernatant of liver homogenate in an environment maintained at 20°C than in one kept at 25°C or 30°C. The effect of prolonging sleeping time by lowering the temperature of the environment from 25°C to 20°C was consistently demonstrated with other strains. Mice given hexobarbital are unable to survive at environments of 15°C or

TABLE 4

SEX DIFFERENCES IN DURATION OF ACTION OF HEXOBARBITAL IN VARIOUS STRAINS OF MICE*

	Sleeping Time (min) ± S. D. Male	Female
General Purpose (12)	34 ± 5	31 ± 5
CFW (12)	29 ± 5	31 ± 5
AL/N (12)	99 ± 6	58 ± 4
NBL/N (12)	73 ± 5	35 ± 2

* The numbers in parenthesis are the numbers of animals used. Sex differences between GP's and between CFW's are not significant. Sex differences between AL/N's and between NBL/N's are significant ($P < 0.01$).

TABLE 5

SLEEPING TIME AND ACTIVITIES OF HEPATIC MICROSOMAL HEXOBARBITAL OXIDASE, ANILINE HYDROXYLASE AND ETHYLMORPHINE N-DEMETHYLASE OF NIH MALE MICE KEPT THREE DAYS ON HARDWOOD OR RED CEDAR BEDDING (MEAN ± S. D.)*

	Sleeping Time (minutes)	Hexobarbital Oxidase	Aniline Hydroxylase	Ethylmorphine N-demethylase
Hardwood (12)	44 ± 6.2	0.35 ± 0.04	0.44 ± 0.09	3.1 ± 0.1
Red Cedar (12)	17 ± 4.1	0.85 ± 0.09	0.83 ± 0.07	6.0 ± 0.9

* All activities are expressed in μmole of substrate metabolized per gram of liver for 10 minutes except for hexobarbital, which is 15 minutes. The number of animals is given in parenthesis. All differences are significant ($P < 0.01$).

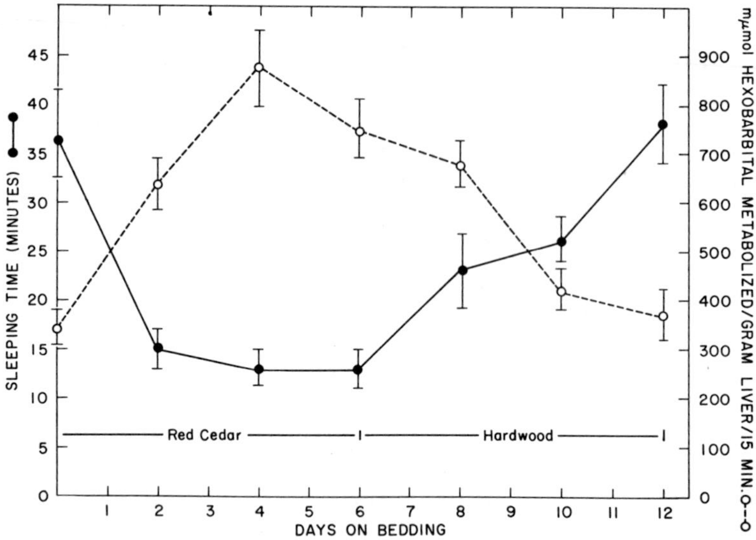

FIGURE 3. Each point represents sleeping time (with standard deviations) of 10 NIH male mice and hexobarbital oxidase activity of 9000 × g supernatant. Mice were on red cedar bedding for six days and then on a combination of beech, birch and maple bedding for six subsequent days.

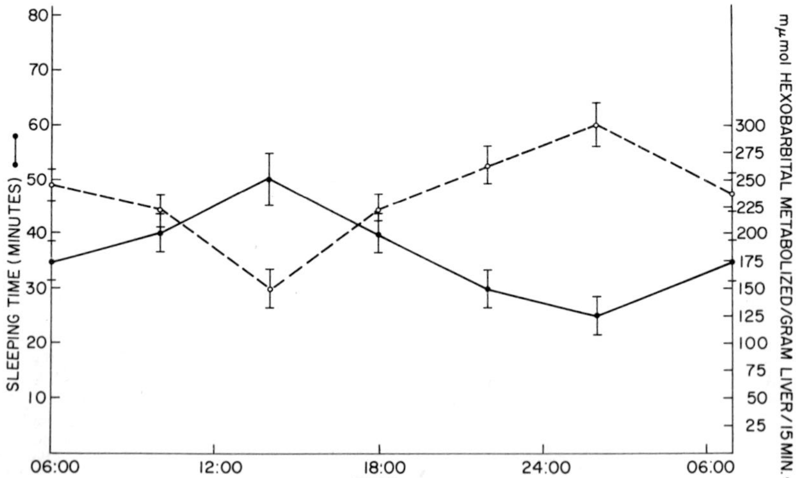

FIGURE 4. Diurnal variations in sleeping time and hexobarbital oxidase activity of 9000 × g supernatant of liver homogenate over a 24-hour period beginning at 6 a.m. Each point represents 12 male NIH mice with standard deviations. Mice were kept in light from 7 a.m. to 7 p.m. and without light from 7 p.m. to 7 a.m.

37°C. This may be due to the effect of hexobarbital on the temperature-regulating centers in the central nervous system.

Crowding also alters sleeping times. Mice grouped in cages which provide each mouse with 4 square inches of space exhibit approximately 30% shorter sleeping times than mice given 12 square inches.

Finally, diurnal variations in sleeping time reported by Davis[10] have been confirmed and extended to include a study of hexobarbital metabolism and receptor sensitivity. Sleeping time is longer and hexobarbital oxidase activity lower during the light than the dark period (FIGURE 4). The brain hexobarbital level on awakening was unchanged during a 24-hour period. For this study NIH mice were placed in a room illuminated by bright artificial light and sunlight from 7 a.m. to 7 p.m. The room was darkened from 7 p.m. to 7 a.m. The mice were kept on this schedule for several days before hexobarbital was administered.

Discussion

Genetic and environmental factors affecting the response of mice to hexobarbital include age, sex, litter, strain, bedding, painful stimuli, ambient temperature, grouping, and hour of drug administration. Additional factors altering pharmacologic responsiveness not studied in the present experiments are dilution of oral doses of pentobarbital which increases toxicity,[6] starvation which depresses hepatic metabolism of hexobarbital,[7] and the presence in cages of sheet metal floors which cause higher mortality than mesh floors.[8] Other factors such as loss of body weight, adrenalectomy of male rats, and composition of inspired air are discussed by Gillette.[2] In female mice the sleeping times vary with the menstrual cycle, the shortest sleeping times occurring when the estrogenic effect is greatest.[14]

The existence of still other, as yet undefined, factors is suggested by the data in TABLE 1. Although it was thought that each of the five groups of the same age, sex and strain was treated similarly, the decrease of sleeping time in the last three groups of unstimulated animals implies some alteration in conditions and an unknown factor. These day to day differences in the mean sleeping time of animals of the same age, sex and genetic background occurred in all strains. Furthermore, on occasion the sleeping time of a few animals was markedly different from that of the majority in the group. Such animals were kept and several weeks later given a second dose of hexobarbital. Following the second dose the sleeping time was nearer the mean and the liver hexobarbital oxidase activity was proportional to the sleeping time. Thus, unusually high or low sleeping times should be repeated after a long interval. Aberrant sleeping times in individual animals may be related to technical errors during drug administration, including the amount given and site of injection, or to ill-defined environmental factors such as the relative health of the animals. In any event, these possibilities should be explored if the sleeping times of individuals appear unrelated to their hexobarbital oxidase activities. When large numbers of animals were employed, the mean sleeping times are proportional to the mean enzyme activities: longer sleeping mice have lower microsomal hexobarbital oxidase activities than shorter sleeping animals (TABLE 2).

Numerous technical considerations involved in the preparation of liver microsomes and the assay of drug-metabolizing enzymes might be discussed were the present study not limited to genetic and physiologic conditions. It has been emphasized that alterations in the complex system employed to determine the activities of drug-metabolizing enzymes may dramatically affect the results.[15]

Recognition of the fact that pharmacologic responsiveness may be altered by numerous genetic and environmental factors will help increase the reproducibility of results within a given laboratory and decrease the widespread differences in the literature. However, the operation of so many factors influencing drug metabolism suggests the futility of standardizing all the pertinent conditions but the need to specify details concerning them in publication of experimental results.

Introduction at regular intervals of a painful stimulus significantly shortens sleeping time. As shown in TABLE 1 such a stimulus shortens sleeping time by raising the threshold for brain hexobarbital at which the righting reflex occurs. Liver hexobarbital oxidase activity was similar in the five groups, indicating that painful stimulation did not alter the rate of hexobarbital metabolism. Barbiturates possess no analgesic action, and even antagonize the analgesic effect of other anesthetics.[16] Thus pain decreases the duration of anesthesia induced by barbiturates.

Genetic factors affect the metabolism of hexobarbital in mice. In the present study three inbred strains, AL/N, DBA/2N and C57BL, slept longer than others and had lower hexobarbital oxidase activity in liver microsomes (TABLE 2). Two hybrids, CAF_1 and CdF_1, the products of mating BALB/C females with AL/N and DBA/2N males respectively, had sleeping times and liver microsomal hexobarbital oxidase activities intermediate between that of their parents, a result suggesting polygenic control. Reciprocal crosses between AL/N and DBA/2N mice gave animals that retained the long sleeping time and low hexobarbital oxidase activity of their parents. Of the 3,000 mice studied, none displayed undetectable or very low hexobarbital oxidase activity. Differences in hepatic microsomal hexobarbital oxidase activity rather than decreased sensitivity of drug receptor sites caused the heritable increase in sleeping time. If there had been altered sensitivity of drug receptors in the central nervous system of the longer sleeping mice, levels of brain hexobarbital on awakening would have been different in them, but the brain levels of hexobarbital on awakening were the same in all strains examined (TABLE 2).

Previous studies demonstrated differences among strains of mice in sleeping time after hexobarbital administration.[3,4] Neither hexobarbital-metabolizing activity in liver microsomes nor brain levels of hexobarbital on awakening were measured so that the nature of the genetic differences could not be determined. Standard deviations of sleeping times were employed to decide whether inbred or outbred animals responded more uniformly to the environmental alteration of unconsciousness induced by hexobarbital. Opposite conclusions were drawn on this issue.[3,4] The present experiments suggest that the standard deviation of the sleeping time may be a dangerous guideline because it varies directly with the sleeping time (FIGURE 1). Neither the AL/N, DBA/2N or C57BL/6N mice investigated 12 years ago, presumably the ancestors of those used in this study, were distinguished in 1955 by longer sleeping times.[3] On the other hand, in 1967 the outbred strains (CFW and GP) do not exhibit the greater standard deviations that they did in 1955. The sleeping times presented in TABLE 2 reveal greater standard deviations than would have been obtained if litter mates had been used (TABLE 3), but to gather large enough numbers litters had to be mixed. Reexamination of data of McLaren and Michie[4] failed to support the claim that heterozygosity increases uniformity of response to pentobarbital and the conclusion that outbred rather than inbred animals should be employed for experimental purposes to lessen variability. The authors plotted their data on a log scale but when transposed to an arithmetic scale the data show no differences in variability of sleeping time among inbred, hybrid or outbred animals. The data of the present study also reveal no differences among inbred and outbred strains in response to hexobarbital except for the AL/N, DBA/2N and C57BL/6N strains. The greater standard deviations in these strains may be attributable to longer sleeping times (FIGURE 1), rather than to any of the theoretical disadvantages of homozygosity discussed by McLaren and Michie.[4] Other inbred strains in the present study exhibited no differences in standard deviation from outbred strains (TABLE 2).

The demonstration that variability within some litters is much lower than inter litter variability (TABLE 3) suggests that certain loci may remain heterozygous in spite of extensive inbreeding, and that increased genetic similarity occurs in litter mates of certain litters whether these be in heterozygous (the F_1 generation produced by crossing two inbred strains) or maximally homozygous (inbred) mice (TABLE 3). There is, however, great variability among litters in standard deviations and the decreased variability of litter mates may be due to environmental factors.

Sex differences in the response of Swiss-Webster mice to pentobarbital have been reported.[9] TABLE 4 reveals that this sex difference is maximal in certain inbred strains, whereas several outbred strains fail to exhibit it. The reasons for diminution of this sex difference with outbreeding are not known.

It is known that a variety of animals including mice have low activity of several drug-metabolizing enzymes at birth, but that activity increases rapidly with age.[11] The course of this development in mice is illustrated in FIGURE 2. For two weeks after birth, mice show negligible hexobarbital oxidase activity and exceedingly long sleeping times. Development of adult enzyme activities occurs during the next few weeks, with corresponding decreases in sleeping time. The appearance of drug-metabolizing enzymes coincides with the period at which such a function would be required; in utero and during the first several weeks of life the mouse has no need for the metabolism of alkaloid materials in food since this would be accomplished by the mother. Only after weaning occurs at approximately three weeks of age would the animal become dependent on its own enzymes to metabolize exogenous lipid soluble compounds. The rapid increase of hexobarbital oxidase activity shortly after weaning confirms observations of Catz and Yaffe.[14]

Of the various environmental factors affecting pharmacologic responsiveness studied in this investigation, discovery of the induction in mice and rats of three drug-metabolizing enzymes by various softwood beddings was most dramatic. Abrupt alterations of sleeping time of mice on red cedar has previously been reported.[5] The present study reveals that for each of three distinct enzymes there was an approximate doubling of activity after mice taken from hardwood bedding were put on red cedar bedding for three days. The widespread dissemination of various organic compounds in the environment raises questions concerning the contribution such substances make to total drug-metabolizing activity, and the activity an organism would possess in an environment free of such contamination. Differences in the results of studies on drug-metabolizing enzymes may arise from the presence or absence of inducers. Such inducers may make it extremely difficult to construct a scheme for the phylogenetic evolution of drug-metabolizing enzymes, since these enzymes are measured in various species exposed to varying amounts of inducing substances. Further complication results from the possibility that the geographical distribution of inducing substances and of various species changed during evolution.

The last three environmental factors to be considered are ambient temperature, grouping and diurnal variation. By elevating the ambient temperature from 20°C to 25°C the sleeping times are approximately halved and the hexobarbital oxidase activity doubled. The sleeping times are also depressed by increasing the number of mice in a given area. Since crowding increases body temperature the effect of grouping on hexobarbital metabolism may be temperature-dependent. Similarly, temperature may be implicated in the diurnal variations of sleeping time and hexobarbital oxidase activity shown in FIGURE 4. Mice are nocturnal; their activity at night and early morning raises their body temperature above that existing during sleep. These results confirm the circadian periodicity in the sleeping time of mice following pentobarbital administration reported by Davis, who also demonstrated that raising the ambient temperature leveled the diurnal pattern.[10] The present studies reveal that these changes in sleeping time are produced by diurnal variations in liver hexobarbital oxidase activity, rather than by alterations in the sensitivity of the receptor site. The mechanism by which temperature affects hexobarbital oxidase activity is not clear. Mediation through altering the release of adrenocortical hormones has been suggested,[10,2] and diurnal periodicity in the secretion of such hormones has been established.[17]

Summary and Conclusions

1) The pharmacologic responsiveness of mice to hexobarbital is altered by both genetic and environmental factors including age, sex, litter, strain, bedding, painful stimuli, ambient temperature, grouping and hour of drug administration. These factors have been analyzed by their effect on the sleeping time, the hexobarbital oxidase activity of liver microsomes and the brain hexobarbital level on awakening. Such an approach permitted determination of whether a particular effect on sleeping time was due to altered metabolism or sensitivity of drug receptor sites.

2) Of the strains studied, most of the inbred and outbred mice did not differ in sleeping time, hexobarbital oxidase activity and brain hexobarbital levels on awakening. AL/N, DBA/2N and C57BL/6N mice had longer sleeping time due to lower hexobarbital metabolism, as indicated by the decreased liver microsomal enzyme activity, but normal brain hexobarbital level on awakening. Crosses between male AL/N and female BALB/C mice and between male DBA/2N and female BALB/C mice produced animals with sleeping time and hexobarbital oxidase activity intermediate between that of their parents, a result suggesting polygenic inheritance of the enzyme level.

3) Standard deviations of sleeping times were similar in all strains except for the greater values in AL/N, DBA/2N, C57BL/6N, CAF_1 and CdF_1 mice. Standard deviations rose in direct proportion to increases of the sleeping time. Therefore the standard deviation of sleeping time appears to be an unreliable indication of whether inbred or outbred animals respond more uniformly to an environmental alteration. Standard deviations could be appreciably reduced by treating litters individually, rather than mixing them. Litter mates appeared more uniform than non-litter mates in response to hexobarbital. This greater similarity of litter mates may have been due to closer similarity of the environment or of their genetic material or to both.

4) Sleeping times decreased and hexobarbital oxidase activity increased markedly after two weeks of age to reach adult levels at three weeks, the time when mice are weaned and become dependent on their own enzymes to detoxify and excrete exogenous compounds. The sex difference in hexobarbital metabolism was maximum in inbred mice and disappeared in the outbred strains.

5) Of the environmental factors affecting hexobarbital metabolism, painful stimulation decreased sleeping time by raising the threshold of the central nervous system as shown by higher brain levels of hexobarbital at which stimulated mice awoke.

6) On the other hand, keeping mice on softwood bedding lowered sleeping time by elevating hexobarbital oxidase activity without change in the brain level of hexobarbital on awakening. Induction by softwood bedding of aniline hydroxylase and morphine N-demethylase in hepatic microsomes of rats and mice was also demonstrated.

7) Temperature elevation of the ambient environment from 20°C to 25°C decreased sleeping time and increased hexobarbital oxidase activity. Crowding of mice also decreased sleeping time.

8) The effects of grouping and diurnal variations on hexobarbital metabolism may be related to changing concentrations of adrenocorticalsteroids or to increased temperature, since both crowding and greater activity during waking hours raise body temperature. The mechanism by which small increases of temperature elevate hexobarbital oxidase activity, thereby decreasing sleeping time, is unknown.

9) These genetic and environmental factors affecting the pharmacologic responsiveness of mice to hexobarbital may influence the behavior of other animals to a variety of drugs. With the emergence of drugs as a new feature of our environment and the development of sensitive techniques for the measurement of drug levels and the enzymes metabolizing drugs, genetic and environmental variables that alter pharmacologic responsiveness become critical for a variety of reasons. These include choice of appropriate species, strains and conditions for experimentation, reproducibility of results, understanding mechanisms of drug action, and maintenance of effective drug concentrations at sites of action.

Acknowledgments

Expert technical assistance of Wallace W. Holland is gratefully acknowledged. Drs. Jordan L. Holtzman, James R. Gillette and Bernard B. Brodie generously gave their help and advice. The Animal Production Section helped at all stages of the work. Sodium hexobarbital was generously provided by Sterling Winthrop.

References

1. QUINN, G. P., J. AXELROD & B. B. BRODIE. 1958. Species, strain and sex differences in metabolism of hexobarbitone, amidopyrine, antipyrine and aniline. Biochem. Pharmacol. **1:** 152.
2. GILLETTE, J. R. 1967. Individually different responses to drugs according to age, sex and functional or pathological state. *In* Ciba Foundation Symposium on Drug Responses in Man. Ed. G. E. W. Wolstenholme & R. Porter. 24–49.
3. JAY, G. E., JR. 1955. Variation in response of various mouse strains to hexobarbital (Evipal). Proc. Soc. Exptl. Biol. Med. **90:** 378.
4. MCLAREN, A. & D. MICHIE. 1956. Variability of response in experimental animals: a comparison of the reactions of inbred, F_1 hybrid and random bred mice to a narcotic drug. J. Genet. **54:** 440.
5. FERGUSON, H. C. 1966. Effect of red cedar chip bedding on hexobarbital and pentobarbital sleep time. J. Pharm. Sci. **55:** 1142.
6. FERGUSON, H. C. 1962. Dilution of dose and acute oral toxicity. Toxicol. Appl. Pharmacol. **4:** 759.
7. DIXON, R. L., R. W. SHULTICE & J. R. FOUTS. 1960. Factors affecting drug metabolism by liver microsomes. IV. Starvation. Proc. Soc. Exptl. Biol. Med. **103:** 333.
8. WINTER, C. A. & L. FLATAKER. 1962. Cage design as a factor influencing acute toxicity of respiratory depressant drugs in rats. Toxicol. Appl. Pharmacol. **4:** 650.

9. WESTFALL, B. A., B. M. BOULOS, J. L. SHIELDS & S. GARB. 1964. Sex differences in pentobarbital sensitivity in mice. Proc. Soc. Exptl. Biol. Med. **115**: 509.
10. DAVIS, W. M. 1962. Day-night periodicity in pentobarbital response of mice and the influence of socio-psychological conditions. Experientia **18**: 235.
11. JONDORF, W. R., R. P. MAICKEL & B. B. BRODIE. 1958. Inability of newborn mice and guinea pigs to metabolize drugs. Biochem. Pharmacol. **1**: 352.
12. COOPER, J. R. & B. B. BRODIE. 1955. The enzymatic metabolism of hexobarbital (Evipal). J. Pharmacol. Exptl. Therap. **114**: 409.
13. KATO, R. & J. R. GILLETTE. 1965. Effect of starvation on NADPH-dependent enzymes in liver microsomes of male and female rats. J. Pharmacol. Exptl. Therap. **150**: 279.
14. CATZ, C. & S. J. YAFFE. 1967. Strain and age variations in hexobarbital response. J. Pharmacol. Exptl. Therap. **155**: 152.
15. GRAM, T. E. & J. R. FOUTS. 1966. Time course differences in the metabolism of drugs by hepatic microsomes from rats, rabbits and mice. J. Pharmacol. Exptl. Therap. **152**: 363.
16. CLUTTON-BROCK, J. C. 1961. Pain and the barbiturates. Anaesthesia **16**: 80.
17. BARTTER, F. C., C. S. DELEA & F. HALBERG. 1962. A map of blood and urinary changes related to circadian variations in adrenal cortical function in normal subjects. Ann. N. Y. Acad. Sci. **98**: 969.

DISCUSSION OF THE PAPER

DR. VICTOR COHN (*George Washington Medical Center, Washington, D.C.*): We have been trying to study the genetic transmission of response to hexobarbital and of the metabolic basis for the termination of the drug's response. We have studied highly inbred mouse strains, one with a long sleeping time response to hexobarbital, DBA/2J; two with very short sleeping times, SWR/J and C3H/J; the F_1 hybrids between DBA/2J and each of the others; and the progeny of back crosses between these F_1 hybrids and the parent strains. With respect to both the sleeping time response and the activity of liver microsomal hexobarbital oxidase segregation patterns expected for a single gene inheritance were not found; it would appear that each of these parameters is under multigenic control.

It is also obvious from these studies that metabolism is not the only factor responsible for the termination of hexobarbital response. In the backcross progeny little correlation was found between hexobarbital oxidase activity and sleeping time. Examples were found in mice with extremely rapid metabolic rates and prolonged sleeping times; the converse was also found. Furthermore, while a large sex difference exists in response to hexobarbital, there is no difference in hexobarbital metabolism in the DBA/2 strain. In this strain the sex difference in response is related to an apparent larger volume of distribution of the drug in the female. No difference in either *in vitro* or *in vivo* rates of metabolism or in the sensitivity of the CNS to the drug (as measured by AD-50 and waking brain and plasma hexobarbital levels) is present.

HEREDITARY RESISTANCE TO COUMARIN ANTICOAGULANT DRUGS IN MAN AND RAT*

Robert A. O'Reilly, Judith G. Pool,† and Paul M. Aggeler‡

Departments of Medicine, Santa Clara Valley Medical Center, San Jose, Stanford University School of Medicine,† Palo Alto, and the University of California Medical Service, San Francisco General Hospital,‡ San Francisco; and the Institute for Medical Research of Santa Clara County, San Jose, Calif.

Introduction

The variability of the response to drugs in man is usually continuous and gives rise to a unimodal frequency distribution curve for the biologic effect measured. Such unimodal distribution curves are consistent with multifactorial inheritance and are difficult to analyze for the genetic factors involved.[1] When the responses can be segregated into clearly distinct groups, a single gene effect should be suspected and appropriate family studies should be carried out.

The coumarin anticoagulant drugs are ideal for pharmacogenetic testing because the persons receiving them usually have normal hemostatic mechanisms, and both the metabolism of the drugs and their biologic effects can be measured quantitatively. Until recently, the frequency distribution of response to a standard dose of the coumarin anticoagulant drugs was thought to be unimodal, and the variation in daily dose required to maintain therapeutic anticoagulation appeared to be continuous. In previous studies[2–4] and in this report, we have demonstrated the existence in man and the rat of a genetically determined discontinuous variation in response to drugs of this type manifested as extraordinary resistance to their prothrombinopenic effects.

Factors Influencing the Response to Coumarin Drugs in Man

Variations in response to the coumarin drugs may be either on a genetic or acquired basis, and may take the form of increased sensitivity or increased resistance to the action of the drug. These variations may be caused by differences in the capacity of the liver to produce vitamin K-dependent clotting factors, in the body stores of vitamin K, in the metabolism of the drug, or in the affinity of receptor sites in the liver for the drug and for vitamin K.

Acquired conditions that cause increased prothrombinopenic responses to the coumarin anticoagulant drugs are mostly those associated with vitamin K deficiency, impaired liver function, or increased turnover of plasma proteins. In man, vitamin K is obtained partly from the diet (vitamin K_1) and partly from bacterial action in the intestinal tract (vitamin K_2). The requirement for adults is exceedingly small, probably only about 0.03 μg/kg of body weight per day.[5] Most foods contain a small amount of vitamin K. Leafy vegetables, such as spinach, cauliflower, cabbage, kale, and dandelion leaves, have a high vitamin K content, whereas animal tissue contains little or none. The amount of vitamin K_2 absorbed from the intestine is unknown. The natural vitamins K_1 and K_2 are fat-soluble compounds and are not absorbed in the absence of bile salts. Thus, vitamin K-

* Supported by grants from the U.S. Public Health Service (HE–2754, HE–5280, HE–8058, TI–AM–5103, IK-6 HE–21,835, and AM–5239), and by the Bank of America-Giannini Foundation.

deficiency develops whenever the flow of bile salts into the gastrointestinal tract is blocked, as in patients with obstructive jaundice or biliary fistula. It can also develop in any condition associated with impaired intestinal absorption, such as sprue, steatorrhea, gastrocolic fistula, and ulcerative colitis, and after extensive surgical resection of the intestinal tract. In man, a major deficiency of vitamin K cannot be produced by either dietary deprivation or sterilization of the gastrointestinal tract. Either one of these situations alone, however, can definitely potentiate the prothrombinopenic effect of coumarin anticoagulant drugs.

All forms of liver disease, such as Laennec's cirrhosis, cancer, and viral, postnecrotic, or toxic hepatitis, may be associated with decreased ability to produce vitamin K-dependent clotting factors. These diseases therefore cause increased sensitivity to the coumarin anticoagulant drugs. Patients who have just undergone surgical procedures and those with congestion of the liver due to heart failure also may be unusually sensitive to the coumarin drugs because of impaired liver function. Both marked restriction of protein in the diet and increased metabolism of protein, such as occurs in hyperthyroidism and febrile states, can accentuate the reduction in circulating clotting factors induced by the coumarin drugs.

The concomitant administration of certain drugs can increase the prothrombinopenic response to the coumarin anticoagulant by any of several mechanisms.[6] Cinchophen and other drugs may cause liver damage, and the phenothiazines may induce cholestasis and consequent diminished absorption of vitamin K. Phenylbutazone causes a striking increase in sensitivity to the coumarin anticoagulant drugs. Our studies showed that phenylbutazone displaces warfarin from its binding to plasma albumin, thus making large amounts of free warfarin available to receptor sites in the liver.[7] Phenyramidol exerts its potentiating influence by inhibiting hepatic microsomal enzymes responsible for metabolism of the coumarin drugs.[8] The use of thyroid hormone in the treatment of hypothyroidism or as an agent to lower serum lipids may lead to increased sensitivity to the coumarin drugs because of increased turnover of blood-clotting factors. The mechanism whereby some drugs, such as benziodarone, clofibrate, and the C-17 alkylated anabolic steroids, potentiate the action of the coumarin anticoagulant drugs is not known.[6]

An occasional emotionally disturbed patient who has deliberately taken repeated large doses of a coumarin anticoagulant in order to produce a factitious hemorrhagic disease may appear to have acquired an unusual sensitivity to the drug.[9]

Increased resistance to the prothrombinopenic action of the coumarin anticoagulant drugs occurs in several conditions. For example, hyperthyroid patients treated with propylthiouracil, patients with congestive heart failure relieved by operative procedures or medications, and patients with liver disease who are being treated medically, become less sensitive to the prothrombinopenic effect of the coumarin drugs.[6] If the patient is pregnant, large doses of the coumarin drugs are required because of the increased levels of vitamin K-dependent clotting factors normally found in pregnancy.

Increased resistance to the coumarin anticoagulants can also result from simultaneous administration of other therapeutic agents, including vitamin K, the natural antidote. Barbital compounds, glutethimide, chloral hydrate, and griseofulvin appear to stimulate microsomal enzymes in the liver responsible for the metabolism of the coumarin anticoagulant drugs. The barbital preparations exert a greater effect on Dicumarol than on warfarin, perhaps because they result in increased fecal excretion of Dicumarol but not of warfarin.[10]

Normal Response to Warfarin in Man

We have used warfarin sodium throughout these investigations because of its superior pharmacologic properties. In earlier studies[11] we showed that warfarin is rapidly and completely absorbed from the gastrointestinal tract. Its apparent volume of distribution (Vd) is 12.6 percent of body weight, which is identical with that of pure albumin. Both the Vd and the biologic half-life of warfarin are independent of the amount injected. Warfarin in the plasma is entirely in the unchanged form and is 97 percent bound to plasma albumin. Metabolites of warfarin, but not the unchanged drug, appear in both the urine and stool. After administration of a standard dose of the drug, we found a highly significant correlation between the concentration of warfarin in the plasma at 48, 72, and 96 hours and the prothrombin responses at those times. A highly significant correlation was also found between the biologic half-life of warfarin in plasma and the maximum degree of prothrombin response.[11]

The response to a single oral dose of warfarin sodium, 1½ mg/kg of body weight, in 30 normal human subjects is shown in FIGURE 1. The mean biologic half-life of warfarin in plasma was 44 hours (range, 31 to 58 hours). The mean prothrombin complex activity 48 hours after administration of the drug was 18 percent of normal (range, 11 to 28 percent). These percentages differ slightly

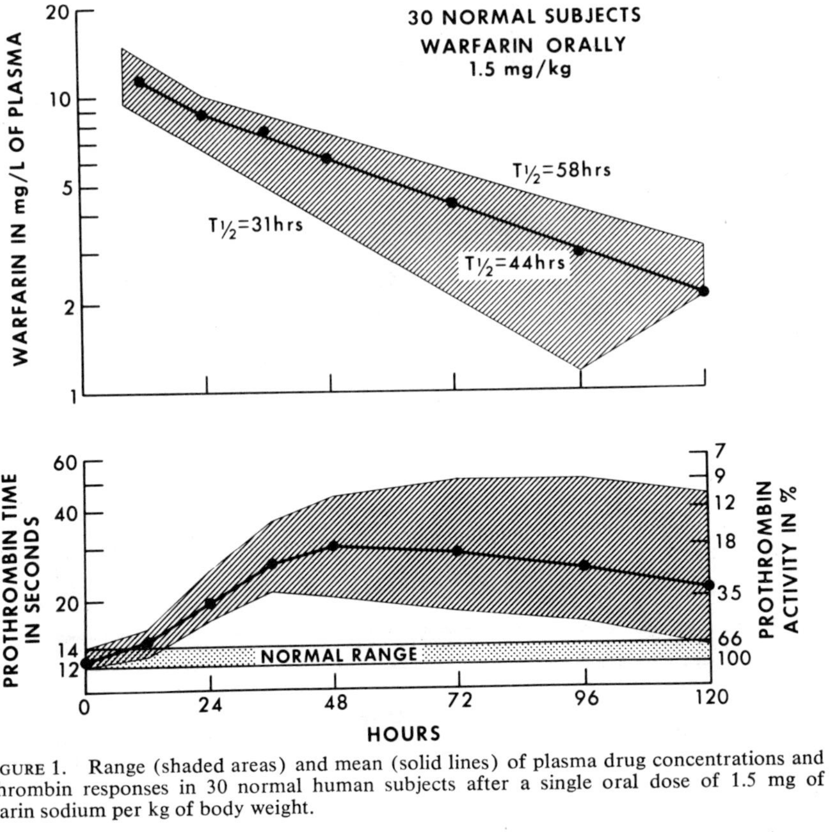

FIGURE 1. Range (shaded areas) and mean (solid lines) of plasma drug concentrations and prothrombin responses in 30 normal human subjects after a single oral dose of 1.5 mg of warfarin sodium per kg of body weight.

from the values reported earlier by us[11,12] because the group has been enlarged and the results on two subjects found to be habitual users of barbiturates have been eliminated. In these two apparently normal subjects, the biologic half-life of warfarin was rapid (15 and 28 hours) and the prothrombinopenic response was diminished.[12]

Hereditary Resistance in Man

The only known instance of hereditary resistance to the prothrombinopenic effect of coumarin anticoagulant drugs was reported from our laboratory. The results of pharmacodynamic studies on the propositus have been described in detail elsewhere[2,3] and will be reviewed only briefly here.

In 1961 the propositus, H. M., at the age of 73 years, sustained a myocardial infarction. No significant abnormalities were found by physical or laboratory examination except for a consistent reduction in the one-stage prothrombin concentration to 55 to 65 percent of normal. Because of this finding, administration of anticoagulant drugs was withheld temporarily. One month later, treatment with warfarin was instituted, and instead of being unduly sensitive to the drug, the patient was found to be resistant. He was referred to us when he failed to show any prothrombinopenic response to warfarin in a dose of 20 mg per day. We found eventually that a daily dose of 145 mg of warfarin was required to maintain reduction of the prothrombin concentration at therapeutic levels. In our series of 105 patients receiving long-term anticoagulant therapy, the mean dose of warfarin was 6.8 ± 2.8 mg per day. H. M. therefore required a daily dose that was an incredible 49 standard deviations above the mean.

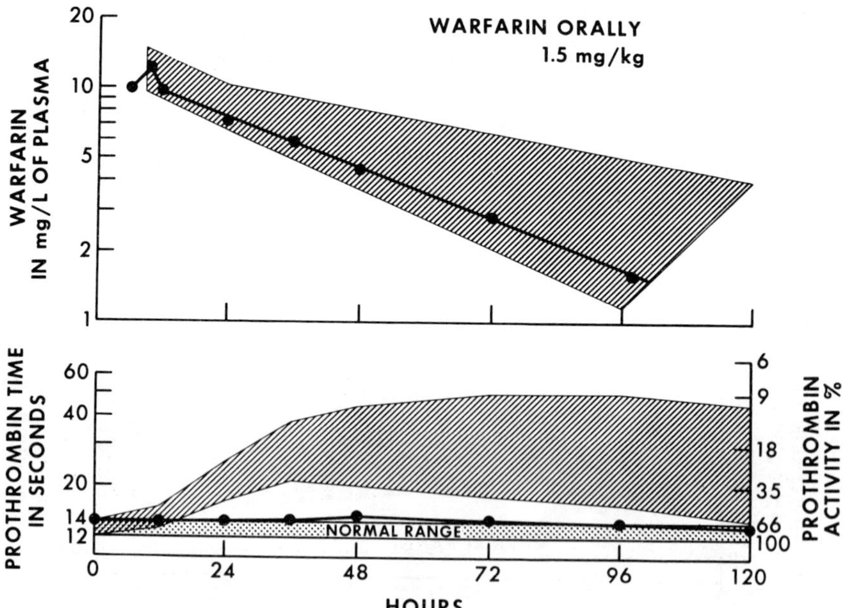

FIGURE 2. Plasma drug concentrations and prothrombin responses in the propositus after a single oral dose of 1.5 mg of warfarin sodium per kg of body weight. The data are plotted semilogarithmically. Shaded areas represent the values obtained in 30 normal subjects (See FIGURE 1).

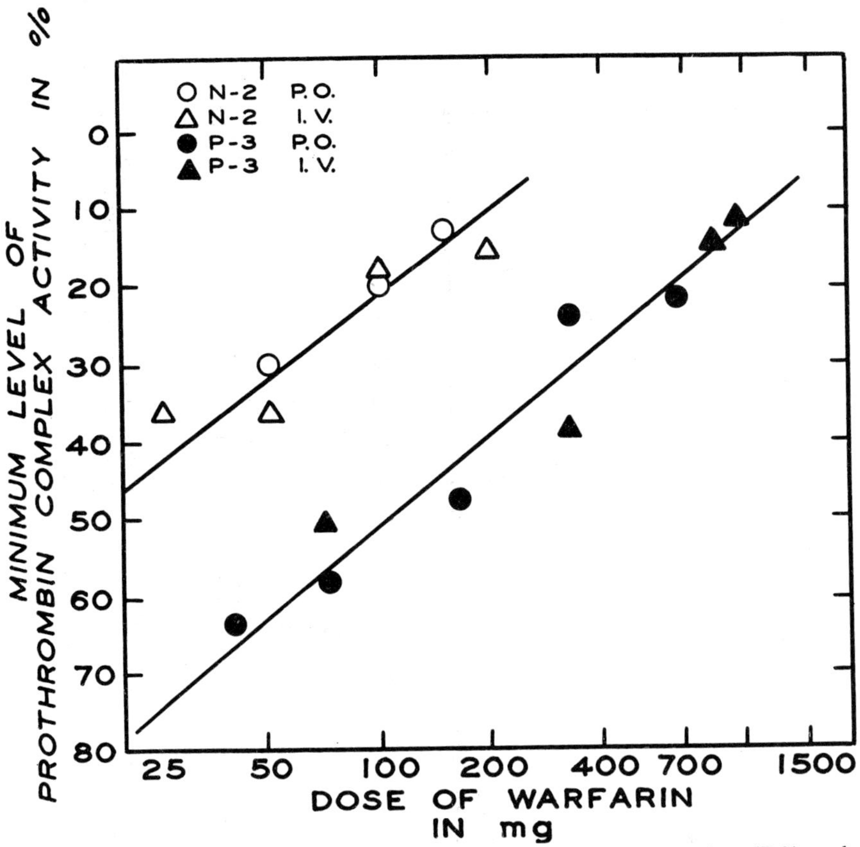

FIGURE 3. Comparison of the dose-response relationship in the propositus (P-3) and a normal subject (N-2). The result is expressed on a linear scale as the minimum level of prothrombin activity achieved (maximum effect) after the single dose administered and is plotted as a function of the log of the dose. Regression lines were fitted to the data by the method of least squares; the equation for the line of the propositus is $Y = 124 - 38X$, and for the normal subject is $Y = 95 - 37X$.

Before long-term therapy was begun, a number of pharmacodynamic studies were performed. The patient was given the standard dose of 1.5 mg of warfarin sodium per kg of body weight (82.5 mg). The concentrations of warfarin in the plasma and the prothrombin complex activity were determined serially and compared with the results obtained in the normal subjects (FIGURE 2). The rapid rise in the concentration of warfarin in the plasma indicated no difficulty in absorption of the drug; the level of warfarin achieved in the plasma and its exponential decline with time showed a normal volume of distribution and a normal rate of biotransformation of the drug. Yet, this dose of warfarin had practically no effect on the prothrombin complex activity. The propositus was then tested with a series of orally and intravenously administered doses of warfarin ranging from 40 to 1,010 mg. (FIGURE 3). In these experiments the warfarin levels in plasma and the prothrombin responses were proportional to the size of the dose ad-

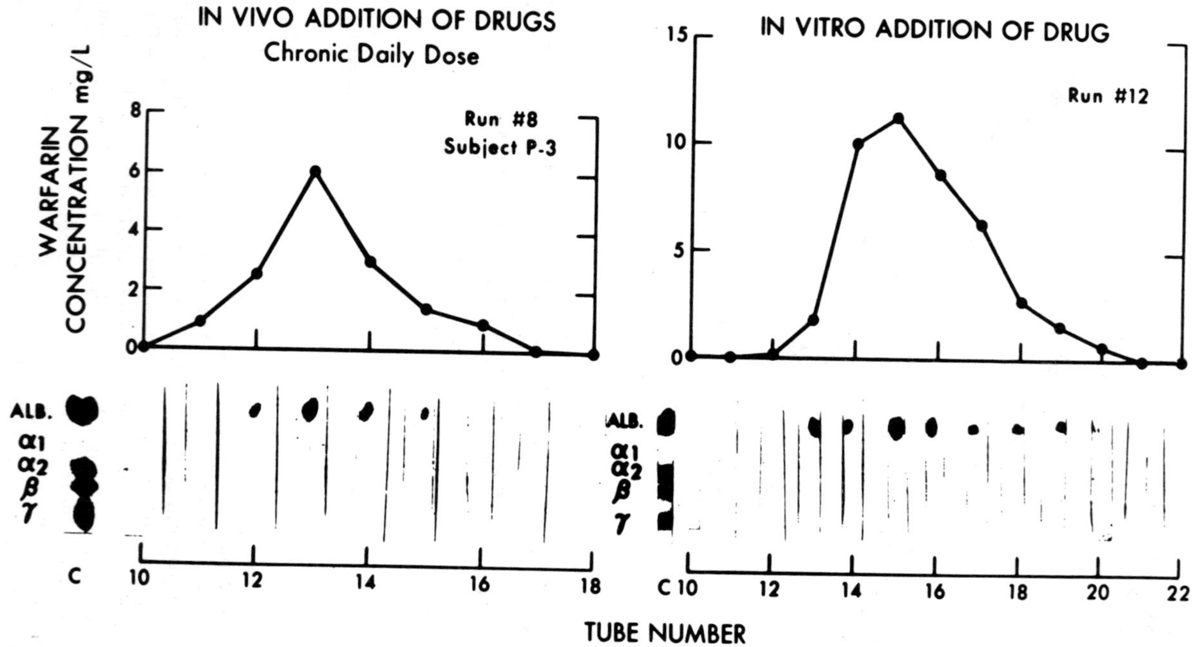

FIGURE 4. Electrochromatographic studies comparing in vitro binding of warfarin sodium to normal human plasma albumin (right) to in vivo binding of warfarin sodium to plasma of the propositus after oral administration of the drug (left). The warfarin concentration, plotted as a function of the electrochromatographic plasma fraction expressed by tube number, is shown in the upper graph. The cellulose acetate electrophoretic strips indicating the protein content of each tube fraction are shown below. C = control strip; ALB = albumin fraction.

ministered; a greater maximum depression and longer duration of effect were achieved with the higher doses. The dose-response relationship for the propositus was parallel to and considerably to the right of that of an average normal subject (nearly equal slopes for the two regression lines), indicating that he required a much larger amount of warfarin to achieve any given response. He was found to be equally resistant to the biologic action of another coumarin anticoagulant drug, Dicumarol, as well as to that of the indanedione anticoagulant phenindione; but his response to heparin, 50 mg given intravenously, was normal.

The ultraviolet absorption spectrum and countercurrent distribution pattern of extracts of the plasma of H. M. showed that, as in the normal subjects, the warfarin measured was in the form of unchanged drug. The degree of binding of warfarin to the plasma proteins, 97 percent, was identical to that found in normal subjects. Continuous flow electrophoretic analysis of the patient's plasma showed that the warfarin was bound exclusively to plasma albumin, in a pattern similar to that obtained by adding pure warfarin to normal human plasma[13] (FIGURE 4). Unchanged warfarin was not detected in the urine or stools even after administration of the largest doses. A metabolite of warfarin (probably 7-hydroxy-warfarin)[14] was recovered from the patient's urine in approximately the same amount found in the urine of normal subjects given equivalent amounts of the drug.[15]

In 1962 long-term treatment of the patient was begun with warfarin in a daily dose of 40 mg. The dose was gradually increased over a 6-month-period; a total

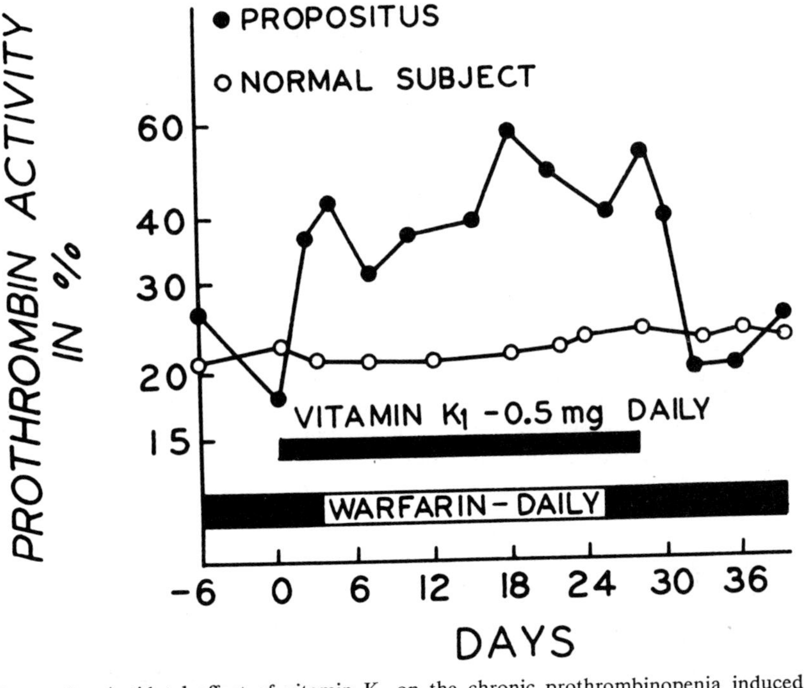

FIGURE 5. Antidotal effect of vitamin K_1 on the chronic prothrombinopenia induced by warfarin in the propositus and in a normal subject. The daily dose of warfarin was 145 mg for the propositus and 7.5 mg for the normal subject. (From O'Reilly and Aggeler,[3] by permission of Federation Proceedings **24:** 126, 1965.)

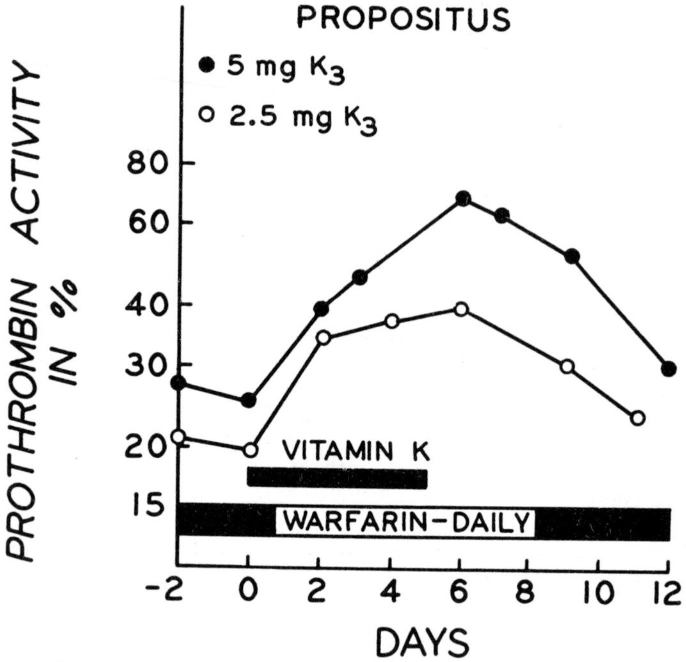

FIGURE 6. Antidotal effect of 2.5 mg and 5.0 mg of vitamin K_3 on the chronic prothrombinopenia induced by warfarin in the propositus during treatment with 145 mg of the drug per day.

of 145 mg a day was required before a satisfactory response could be achieved. This dose was continued without interruption for nine months. The patient was later maintained for many months with a dose of 140 mg a day, but recently he has required only 125 mg a day. During the treatment periods the prothrombin complex activity of the patient's plasma has been within the usual "therapeutic range" of 15 to 35 percent. The concentration of warfarin in the plasma has averaged 55 mg/liter, or about 20 times the concentration found in the plasma of the average patient with well-controlled prothrombin activity during long-term treatment with this drug. Whenever treatment has been discontinued for any length of time, the rate of elimination of warfarin from the blood has been normal. Despite the very high levels of warfarin in the plasma, the patient's liver function has remained unimpaired and no evidence of a toxic vascular effect has been seen. He has shown no evidence of bleeding or any other symptoms throughout the 6-year-period of study and has led an active life as an oil-field developer.

Since vitamin K is the therapeutic antidote to the coumarin anticoagulants, the sensitivity of H. M. to the vitamin was assessed. While receiving 145 mg of warfarin daily on a maintenance basis, he was given 1 mg of vitamin K_1 daily for seven days. The prothrombin activity rose from 20 to 57 percent. When he was given ½ mg of vitamin K_1 daily for one month, the prothrombin activity rose from a mean value of 25 percent to an average sustained level of 43 percent (FIGURE 5). A normal subject given warfarin in a dose sufficient to maintain an equal degree of hypoprothrombinemia (7½ mg a day) showed no response at all to this tiny daily dose of vitamin K_1. Administration of the vitamin K_3 analogue (menadione sodium bisulfite), 2.5 mg daily, caused a significant increase in the prothrombin complex activity in the propositus, and a dose of 5 mg a day resulted in a maximum response (FIGURE 6). A normal subject whose prothrombin activity was maintained at a therapeutic level with warfarin showed no response to a daily dose of 5 mg of vitamin K_3 (FIGURE 7); a dose of 10 to 25 mg a day was required to produce a significant rise. Similar results were obtained with another analogue, vitamin K_5 (2-methyl-4-amino-1-naphthol hydrochloride). Thus, while he was receiving 18 times as much anticoagulant as the normal subjects, the propositus showed significant prothrombin complex responses to doses of vitamin K too small to elicit any effect in normal subjects. This remarkable sensitivity to vitamin K was evaluated by the inhibition index method of Woolley[16] (TABLE 1). The amount of warfarin, in millimoles, needed daily to maintain the prothrombin activity of H. M. at 25 percent of normal was divided by the amount of vitamin K, in mmole, required daily to raise and maintain the prothrombin level above 50 percent of normal. The inhibition index for vitamin K in H. M. was 25 (K_1) to 84 (K_3) times greater than for the normal subjects.

To determine whether the basis of the resistance in H. M. could be the result of an abnormally slow turnover rate of the vitamin K-dependent clotting factors, the half-disappearance times of the factors were determined after i.v. administration of a huge dose of warfarin sodium—1,010 mg. The half-disappearance times were: factor II, 59 hours; factor VII, 8 hours; factor IX, 25 hours; and factor X, 48 hours. These values are within normal limits. During the time he was not

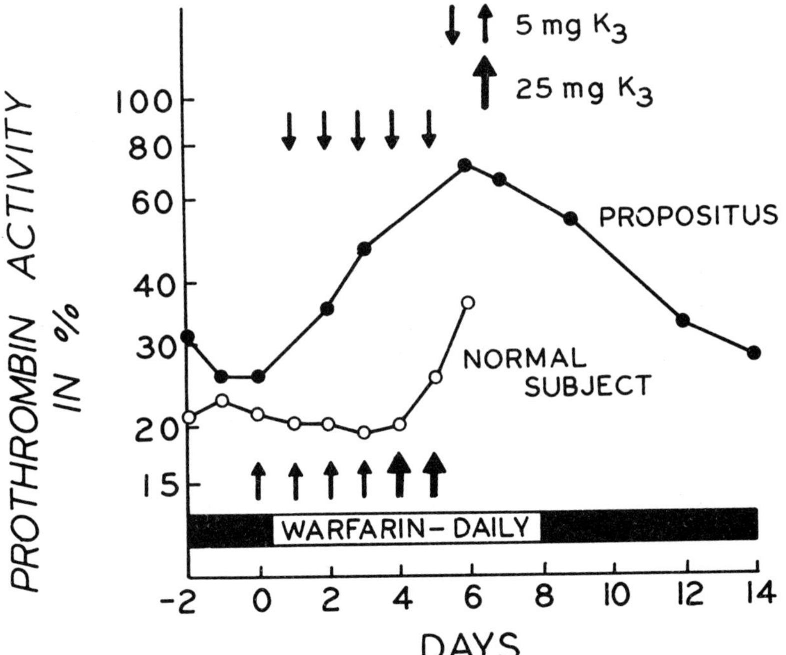

FIGURE 7. Antidotal effect of vitamin K_3 on the chronic prothrombinopenia induced by warfarin in the propositus and in a normal subject. Daily dose of warfarin was 145 mg for the propositus and 7.5 mg. for the normal subject. (From O'Reilly and Aggeler,[3] by permission of Federation Proceedings **24**: 126, 1965.)

TABLE 1

INHIBITION INDEX FOR WARFARIN AND TWO FORMS OF VITAMIN K IN PROPOSITUS AND NORMAL SUBJECTS

Subject	Dose of warfarin per day mg	Dose of warfarin per day mmole	Dose of vitamin K per day mg	Dose of vitamin K per day mmole	Inhibition Index*
		vitamin K_1			
Propositus	145.0	442	0.7	1.6	276.0
Normal subject	9.0	27	1.0	2.2	12.0
Normal subject	7.5	21	1.0	2.2	10.0
		vitamin K_3			
Propositus	145.0	442	3.5	10.6	42.0
Normal subject	7.5	21	15.0	45.6	0.5

* Millimoles of warfarin needed daily to maintain prothrombin activity of subject at 25 percent of normal divided by millimoles of vitamin K required daily to raise prothrombin activity to a mean of 50 percent.

receiving anticoagulant therapy, the propositus was given 50 mg of vitamin K_1 intravenously. No significant rise in the concentration of any of the clotting factors occurred.

We then tested members of three generations of the family of the propositus with a method based on the results of a previous study.[11] The concentration of warfarin and the prothrombin activity of plasma samples from the family members, determined 48 hours after administration of the drug in a standard dose of 1.5 mg per kg of body weight, were compared with the responses in normal subjects (FIGURE 8). The concentrations of warfarin in the plasma of all eight members of the kindred tested were within normal limits. The prothrombin responses of six of the eight members, however, were definitely reduced (FIGURE 9); the seventh (III-2) showed a normal response, whereas the eighth (III-3), a 3-year-old girl, showed an intermediate response, which exceeded the normal adult response when corrected for her body surface area.

A single gene effect cannot be proved from the available data.[17] It can be postulated, however, that a pair of allelic genes (regulator or otherwise) control the structure or amount of the substances involved in the synthesis of the clotting factors dependent on vitamin K and that resistance to the coumarin anticoagulant drugs may be a polymorphic characteristic. The transmission of a dominant allele is suggested by the fact that all the generations and most of the members of the kindred are affected. Whether the gene is located on an X or an autosomal chromosome cannot be discerned from the available data.[18] Since the wife of the propositus was not affected, her two affected daughters (II-1 and II-2) would necessarily be heterozygous. It can be assumed that the other members of the kindred were heterozygous, because with a gene as rare as this the existence of a phenotype is practically an assurance of a heterozygous genotype.[19]

Mechanism of Hereditary Resistance in Man

Coumarin anticoagulant drugs are thought to function as antimetabolites that compete with the natural metabolite vitamin K in an enzyme system that is responsible for the synthesis of clotting factors II, VII, IX, and X. In bacteria, sulfonamide drugs are thought to function as antimetabolites that compete with the natural metabolite para-aminobenzoic acid in an enzyme system that is

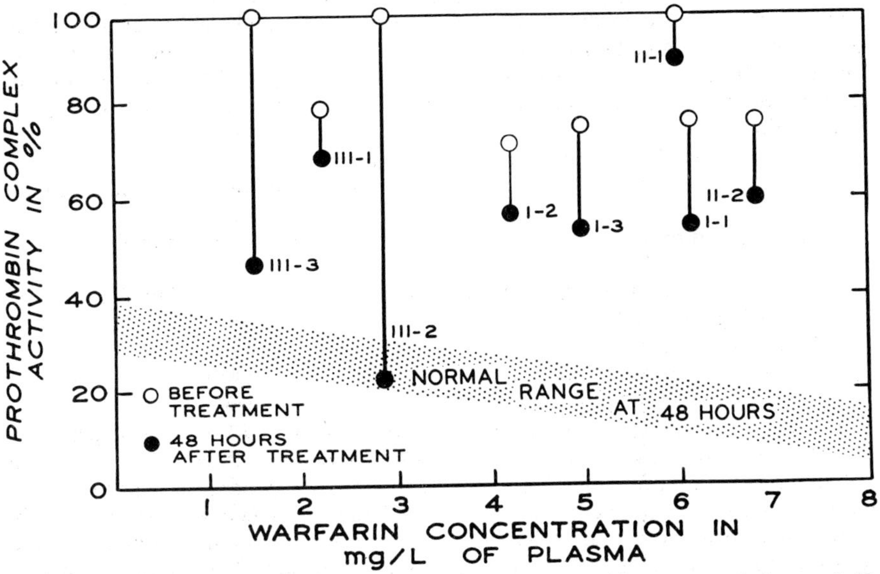

FIGURE 8. Plasma concentrations of warfarin and prothrombin response before and 48 hours after single oral doses of 1.5 mg of warfarin per kg of body weight in eight members of family M. The response of III-3, a 3-year-old girl, when corrected for her body surface area, exceeds the normal adult range at 48 hours. (From O'Reilly and Aggeler,[3] by permission of Federation Proceedings **24**: 126, 1965.)

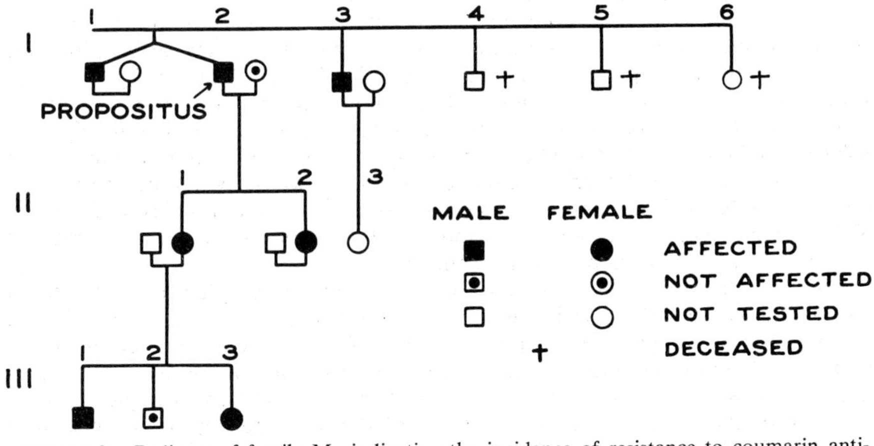

FIGURE 9. Pedigree of family M., indicating the incidence of resistance to coumarin anti-coagulant drugs. Subject III-3 is shown to be "affected," but when her response is corrected for body surface area, she falls into the "not affected" group. (From O'Reilly and Aggeler,[3] by permission of Federation Proceeding **24**: 126, 1965.)

responsible for the synthesis of folic acid.[20,21] By analogy with the possible mechanisms involved in the development of sulfonamide-resistant bacterial mutants, any of the mechanisms listed below might account for the resistance to coumarin drugs in man. Most of these mechanisms can be ruled out in this kindred. Some of the possible mechanisms for resistance to coumarin drugs in man are these:

1. Decreased absorption of anticoagulant drug
2. Increased destruction, excretion or volume of distribution of anticoagulant drug
3. Increased production of clotting factors dependent on vitamin K
4. Decreased half-life of clotting factors
5. Presence of alternate pathway for production of clotting factors, bypassing vitamin K
6. Increased concentration of vitamin K
7. Presence of enzyme or receptor site with altered affinity for vitamin K or anticoagulant drug

The pronounced resistance to the prothrombinopenic effect of warfarin was clearly not caused by decreased absorption, increased destruction, or altered volume of distribution of the drug. Nor was it caused by increased production of clotting factors, since the concentrations of factors dependent on vitamin K were either normal or reduced. The resistance to warfarin could not be attributed to a decreased turnover rate of the various clotting factors, because the rate of disappearance of each from the plasma after administration of the drug was normal. If an alternate pathway for the production of clotting factors, bypassing vitamin K, was operative in the affected members of the family, resistance to warfarin should have been complete regardless of the amount given. The resistance to coumarin drugs in the propositus was relative rather than absolute, since it could be completely overcome if sufficiently large doses were administered.

The possibility that increased concentrations or activity of vitamin K was the causative factor cannot be completely ruled out in the absence of an assay method sensitive enough to measure physiologic levels of the vitamin. Hypervitaminosis K could be produced by increased intake from food or medication, by increased production of vitamin K through bacterial action in the gut, or by a reduced rate of turnover of the vitamin. Increased intake of vitamin K is unlikely considering the number of affected persons living in several different households, and an excess of vitamin K from an endogenous source would be difficult to explain on a genetic basis. The marked response of the propositus to tiny doses of vitamin K is evidence against an increase in the size of the body pool of the vitamin, as well as against hypervitaminosis K from any source.

The final possibility is the existence of an enzyme or receptor site with altered affinity for vitamin K or anticoagulant drugs. Comparison of the dose-response relationship in the propositus and a normal subject (FIGURE 3) demonstrated that when the minimum level of activity of the prothrombin complex (the maximum response), achieved with varying amounts of warfarin, was plotted as a function of the log of the dose, the slopes of the resulting regression lines were parallel. The same data can be expressed in kinetic terms. The mass action equation has been adapted to pharmacologic problems (22) so that:

$$E + I \underset{k_2}{\overset{k_1}{\rightleftharpoons}} EI$$

where E is the number of drug receptors in the milieu of its natural metabolite vitamin K, I is the concentration or dosage of the inhibitor of the reaction, the coumarin anticoagulant, EI are the drug-receptor linkages representing the extent of the pharmacologic action of the anticoagulant drug, and k_1 and k_2 are first-order rate constants of the reaction. The Michaelis constant (K_m) represents the ratio of the two constants k_2/k_1. If the drug-receptor linkages have a great tendency to dissociate (high K_m), a very high dosage level (I) is required to achieve a pharmacologic response (EI) of average magnitude. When the data were plotted by the graphical method of Lineweaver and Burk[23] and the regression lines were fitted by the method of least squares (FIGURE 10), the K_m for the normal subject was 0.06 mmole of warfarin and for the propositus 1.63 mmole (27-fold greater). As the K_m is an inverse function of the affinity of a drug for its receptor site, the affinity for warfarin in the propositus is 27 times less than that in the normal subject. The plots, however, are also typical of a competitive inhibition process (a common ordinate point and markedly different slopes); therefore, these results are also consistent with the presence of drug-receptor sites having an increased affinity for vitamin K.

On the basis of present knowledge, it is not possible to choose between the alternatives of decreased affinity for the coumarin anticoagulant drugs and increased affinity of receptor sites for vitamin K as the theoretical mechanism for the resistance. The latter explanation is favored, however, because it would account for both the decreased responsiveness to the anticoagulants and the increased responsiveness to vitamin K, whereas the great responsiveness to vitamin K would be difficult to explain on the basis of altered affinity for the coumarin anticoagulants.

We previously suggested that the genetic defect in this family could be an abnormal regulator gene.[3] This hypothesis was based on work indicating that

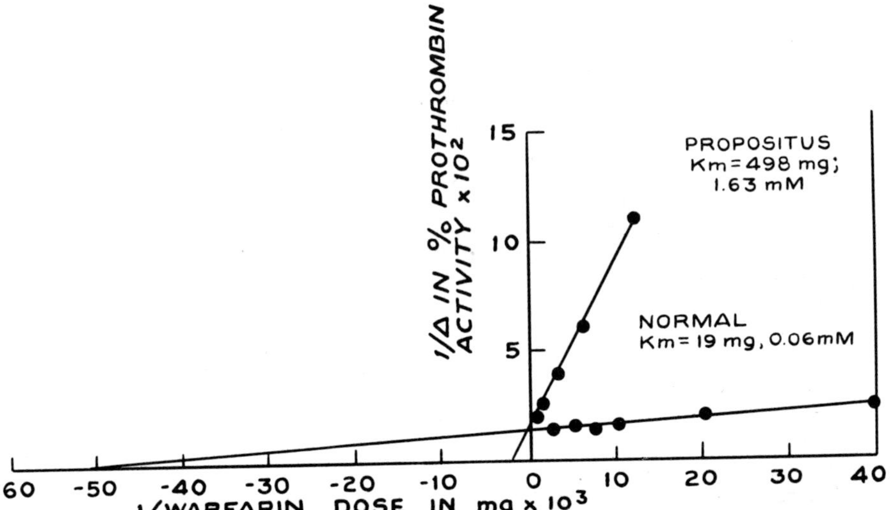

FIGURE 10. Determination of the Michaelis constant (K_m) for the propositus and a normal subject by the double reciprocal plot. The reciprocal of the maximum change in prothrombin activity for any given dose is plotted as a function of the reciprocal of single doses of warfarin. Regression lines were fitted to the data by the method of least squares.

vitamin K acts at the regulator gene level.[24] More recent studies, however, have shown that the site of action of the vitamin is at some step in protein biosynthesis subsequent to the formation of the specific messenger RNA and before the release of the complete protein from the liver.[25] Based on current theory, the following model can be proposed. Normally, the four clotting factors are synthesized in the presence of vitamin K; in its absence their synthesis is suppressed. When coumarin anticoagulant drugs are present, they competitively displace vitamin K from the synthesis sites, and the production of the four clotting factors is suppressed. In the M. family the affinity or concentration of the synthetic machinery for vitamin K is greatly increased, but the level of the vitamin K-dependent clotting factors is not augmented, perhaps because of end-product inhibition. Thus, ordinary doses of warfarin are ineffective in this kindred and only extraordinarily large doses can displace vitamin K from the synthesis sites and suppress production of the clotting factors.

Hereditary Resistance in Rats

Using the response of clotting factor VII to warfarin for selection, Pyörälä and Nevanlinna[26] selectively inbred two lines of animals from a random-bred colony of Sprague-Dawley rats: one line characterized by rapid metabolism of warfarin and the other by slow metabolism of the drug. The corrected median plasma half-life ($T\frac{1}{2}$) of warfarin in rats of the fourth generation of the non-reactor line (resistant response) was 5 hours and that of the reactor line (sensitive response) was 30 hours. In normal rats, the plasma $T\frac{1}{2}$ of warfarin was 18 hours for males and 28 hours for females. Recently, resistance to the rodenticidal effect of warfarin has been described in England, Scotland, and Denmark.[27–29] In 1965, we obtained two dozen warfarin-resistant rats from the Ministry of Agriculture, Fisheries, and Food in England.[30] The resistant wild rats (*rattus norvegicus*) were bred with normal Sprague-Dawley rats. Repeated backcrossing of resistant offspring with the normal rats resulted in five generations of animals with white coats, good handling characteristics, the behavior of Sprague-Dawley rats, and the gene trait of resistance to warfarin.[4]

We were able to segregate the resistant rats from the warfarin-sensitive normal rats by testing the level of the vitamin K-dependent coagulation factors II, VII, and X by the P & P test of Owren[31] 48 hours after the animals had ingested warfarin contained in their drinking water (250 parts per million) (FIGURE 11). Excellent separation was achieved, and backcrosses of selected resistant rats always resulted in resistant offspring in new litters. Of the 273 rats in the F_2 to F_5 generations, 53 percent were resistant. These data indicate a dominant mode of inheritance. Seven resistant and five sensitive rats from the F_1 offspring were given a single dose of 1 mg of warfarin orally. The blood warfarin levels 3 hours after administration of the drug were not significantly different in the two groups (TABLE 2). The resistance in these animals, therefore, is similar in nature to the hereditary resistance we observed in man and in the wild rats (normal drug metabolism) and is clearly different from the resistance in the non-reactor strain of rats bred by Pyörälä and Nevanlinna (rapid drug metabolism) and in the patient described by Lewis *et al.* (rapid plasma $T\frac{1}{2}$ of warfarin).[32]

The resistance in our rats was not caused by lack of gastrointestinal absorption of warfarin or its failure to reach the liver. We found no significant difference in the concentration of warfarin in the liver of normal and resistant rats given i.v. injections of the drug. When we incubated liver slices from sensitive and resistant rats with various concentrations of warfarin,[33] the synthesis of clotting factor VII

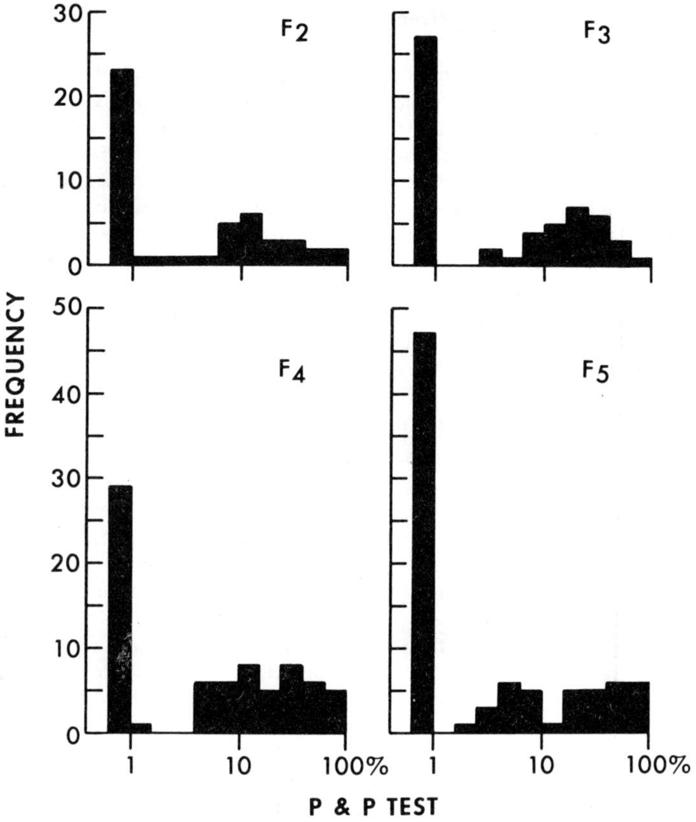

FIGURE 11. Bar histogram of the response to the P & P test of Owren in percent of normal values in 273 rats 48 hours after they had ingested warfarin from drinking water. The 2nd, 3rd, 4th, and 5th generations of backcrosses of resistant rats to normal Sprague-Dawley rats separate into a sensitive group (less than 1% P & P activity) and a resistant group (more than 1% P & P activity).

TABLE 2

PLASMA DRUG LEVEL IN FIVE WARFARIN-SENSITIVE AND SEVEN WARFARIN-RESISTANT RATS THREE HOURS AFTER ORAL ADMINISTRATION OF 1 MG OF WARFARIN

	Plasma Warfarin Concentration mg/liter	
	Sensitive rats	Resistant rats
	4.4	3.7
	4.9	4.2
	6.3	4.7
	6.7	5.8
	7.0	6.0
		6.1
		7.1
Mean	5.9	5.4

(proconvertin) by the slices from both groups was inhibited to a comparable degree.

Sheppard[34] stated that whenever resistance to anticoagulants used as rodenticides appears, it is important to determine whether the genetic control is monofactorial or multifactorial, and if monofactorial, whether the gene is fully dominant or not. If the resistance is multifactorial, other control methods can be used until genes from neighboring non-resistant stock enter the gene pool of the resistant rodents; thereafter, the population can again be controlled with anticoagulants. If the genetic control is monofactorial, this method will be ineffective unless dominance is absent and the heterozygotes are susceptible to intense anticoagulant poisoning. Our data on five generations of warfarin-resistant heterozygote rats and those of Evans and Sheppard[35] and those of Greaver and Ayres[36] indicate that the genetic control for the resistance is monofactorial and fully dominant, as in the human kindred.

Response Variation in Rabbits

Early studies in the laboratory of Professor K. P. Link[37,38] showed considerable variation in the responsiveness of rabbits to Dicumarol. The basis for the difference between animals was not determined, but the degree of sensitivity appeared to be hereditary. In 1960, we found a wide range of prothrombin complex responses in 20 rabbits given a standard dose of Dicumarol by stomach tube. Plasma Dicumarol determinations were made on two "reactor" and two "non-reactor" rabbits, representing the two ends of the distribution curve as shown in FIGURE 12. Plasma from the "non-reactor" rabbits contained far less Dicumarol than plasma from the "reactor" rabbits, perhaps because of less absorption but probably because of faster biotransformation of the drug. Studies by Link's group[37,38] suggested that Dicumarol resistance in rabbits might be inherited as a recessive mendelian character; however, the genetic data, which Link later considered to be inadequate, were never published.[39] In a study of more than 700 rabbits, Miller *et al.*[40] showed that the reactor and non-reactor responses to Dicumarol represented only the extremes of a normal distribution of responses. Unimodal frequency distribution curves of this type indicate multifactorial genetic control for the metabolism and biologic effect of the drug. Unusual variations in response, which might suggest single gene effects, have not been reported in the rabbit.

Conclusions

Hereditary resistance to the biologic action of drugs in both man and animals has been found only with the coumarin-indanedione type of oral anticoagulants. It appears that the same mechanism is responsible for the pharmacologic disorder in man and the rat. In both species the metabolism of the drugs is entirely normal. In the resistant human kindred described in this report, the lack of responsiveness to oral anticoagulants appears to be directly related to their great responsiveness to vitamin K; sensitivity to vitamin K has not yet been tested in the resistant rats. The genetic mutation appears to have no deleterious effect on the persons or rats affected. What effect resistance to the action of the coumarin anticoagulant drugs may have on survival in man is unknown. The favorable effects on survival in resistant wild rats, however, is potentially dangerous, as the genetic trait appears to be monofactorial and fully dominant in heterozygous rodents and apparently does not hinder the reproductive capacity of the affected animals. Therefore, the biochemical mechanism for this extraordinary resistance forms an important area for further pharmacogenetic research in man and rat.

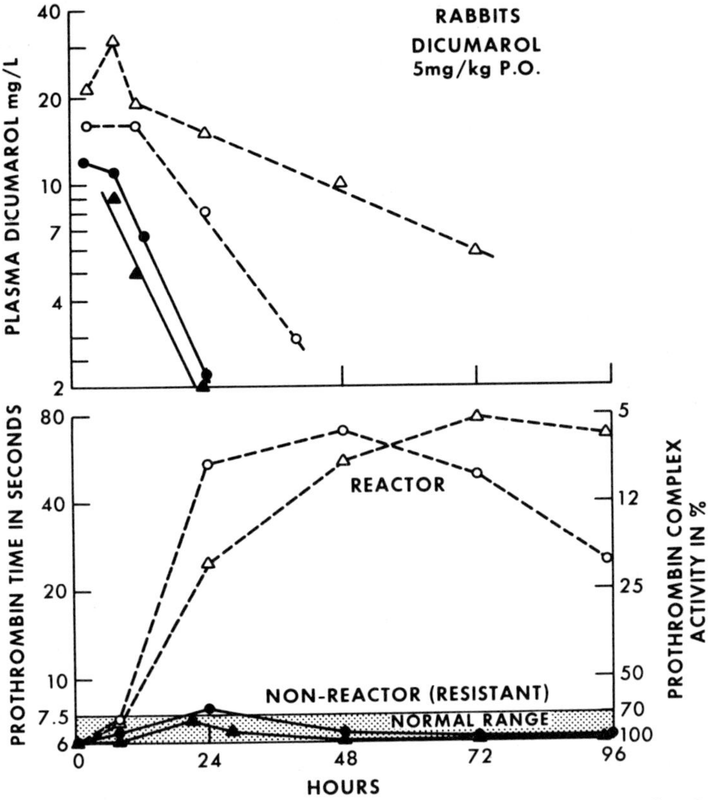

FIGURE 12. Plasma drug concentrations and prothrombin responses in 4 rabbits after single oral doses of 5 mg of Dicumarol per kg of body weight. The data are plotted semilogarithmically.

Acknowledgments

The authors are indebted to Miss Mary Morrow, Department of Medicine Editorial Office, University of California School of Medicine, for her invaluable editorial assistance. The wild rats were kindly supplied by Mr. David Drummond of the Ministry of Agriculture, Fisheries, and Food, U. K.

References

1. EVANS, D. A. P. 1963. Pharmacogenetics. Am. J. Med. **34:** 639–662.
2. O'REILLY, R. A., P. M. AGGELER, M. S. HOAG, L. S. LEONG & M. L. KROPATKIN. 1964. Hereditary transmission of exceptional resistance to coumarin anticoagulant drugs. The first reported kindred. New Engl. J. Med. **271:** 809–815.
3. O'REILLY, R. A. & P. M. AGGELER. 1965. Coumarin anticoagulant drugs: hereditary resistance in man. Federation Proc. **24:** 1266–1273.
4. POOL, J. G., R. A. O'REILLY, L. SCHNEIDERMAN & M. ALEXANDER. 1967. Studies on warfarin resistance in the rat. Am. J. Physiol. (In press).
5. FRICK, P. G., G. RIEDLER & H. BROGLI. 1967. The dose response and the minimal requirement for vitamin K in man. J. Appl. Physiol. (In press).
6. ELIAS, R. A. 1965. Effect of various drugs on anticoagulation dosage in anticoagulant

therapy. *In* Ischemic Heart Disease. Ed. E. S. Nichol. Grune & Stratton. N. Y., N. Y. 443–448.

7. AGGELER, P. M., R. A. O'REILLY, L. S. LEONG & P. E. KOWITZ. 1967. Potentiation of the anticoagulant effect of warfarin by phenylbutazone. New Engl. J. Med. **276:** 496–501.
8. SOLOMON, H. M. & J. J. SCHROGIE. 1966. The effect of phenyramidol on the metabolism of bishydroxycoumarin. J. Pharmacol. Exp. Therap. **154:** 660–666.
9. O'REILLY, R. A. & P. M. AGGELER. 1966. Surreptitious ingestion of coumarin anticoagulant drugs. Ann. Int. Med. **64:** 1034–1041.
10. AGGELER, P. M. & R. A. O'REILLY. 1967. Unpublished observations.
11. O'REILLY, R. A., P. M. AGGELER & L. S. LEONG. 1963. Studies on the coumarin anticoagulant drugs: the pharmacodynamics of warfarin in man. J. Clin. Invest. **42:** 1542–1551.
12. AGGELER, P. M. & R. A. O'REILLY. 1966. The pharmacological basis of oral anticoagulant therapy. Thromb. Diath. Haemorrhag. Supp. **21:** 227–256.
13. O'REILLY, R. A. & P. E. KOWITZ. 1967. Studies on the coumarin anticoagulant drugs: interaction of human plasma albumin and warfarin sodium. J. Clin. Invest. **46:** 829–837.
14. BARKER, W. M. 1965. The metabolism of 4-C^{14}-warfarin sodium in the rat. Ph.D. Thesis, University of Wisconsin.
15. O'REILLY, R. A., P. M. AGGELER, M. S. HOAG & L. LEONG. 1962. Studies on the coumarin anticoagulant drugs: the assay of warfarin and its biologic application. Thromb. Diath. Haemorrhag. **8:** 82–95.
16. WOOLLEY, D. W. 1952. A Study of Antimetabolites. John Wiley & Sons, N. Y., N. Y.
17. KALOW, W. 1962. Pharmacogenetics: Heredity and The Response to Drugs. W. B. Saunders, Philadelphia, Pa.
18. O'REILLY, R. A. 1965. "A medley of kindred." New Engl. J. Med. **272:** 108.
19. STERN, C. 1960. Principles of Human Genetics. W. H. Freeman. San Francisco, Calif.
20. DAVIS, B. D. & W. K. MAAS. 1952. Analysis of the biochemical mechanism of drug resistance in certain bacterial mutants. Proc. Nat. Acad. Sci. U.S. **38:** 775–785.
21. HOTCHKISS, R. D. & A. H. EVANS. 1958. Analysis of the complex sulfonamide resistance locus of pneumococcus. Cold Springs Harbor Symp. Quant. Biol. **23:** 85–97.
22. CHEN, G. & D. RUSSELL. 1950. A quantitative study of blood pressure response to cardiovascular drugs and their antagonists. J. Pharmacol. Exp. Therap. **99:** 401–408.
23. LINEWEAVER, H. & D. BURK. 1934. The determination of enzyme dissociation constants. J. Am. Chem. Soc. **56:** 658–666.
24. OLSON, R. E. 1964. Vitamin K induced prothrombin formation: antagonism by actinomycin D. Science **145:** 926–928.
25. SUTTIE, J. W. 1967. Control of prothrombin and factor VII biosynthesis by vitamin K. Arch. Biochem. Biophys. **118:** 166–171.
26. PYÖRÄLÄ, K. & H. R. NEVANLINNA. 1967. Experimental studies on genetic factors in warfarin metabolism. Scand. J. Clin. Lab. Invest. (abstract) (In press).
27. BOYLE, C. M. 1960. Case of apparent resistance of *Rattus norvegicus* Berkenhout to anticoagulant poisons. Nature **188:** 517.
28. CUTHBERT, J. H. 1963. Further evidence of resistance to warfarin in the rat. Nature **198:** 807–808.
29. LUND, M. 1964. Resistance to warfarin in the common rat. Nature **203:** 778.
30. DRUMMOND, D. 1966. Rats resistant to warfarin. New Scientist **30:** 771–772.
31. OWREN, P. A. & K. AAS. 1951. The control of Dicumarol therapy and the quantitative determination of prothrombin and proconvertin. Scand. J. Clin. Lab. Invest. **3:** 201–208.
32. LEWIS, R. J., M. SPIVACK & T. H. SPAET. 1967. Warfarin resistance. Am. J. Med. **42:** 620–624.
33. POOL, J. G. & C. F. BORCHGREVINK. 1964. Comparison of rat liver response to coumarin administered in vivo versus in vitro. Am. J. Physiol. **206:** 229–238.
34. SHEPPARD, P. M. 1966. Research on the genetic basis of anticoagulant resistance in rodents. W.H.O. Seminar on Rodents and Rodent Ectoparasites. Vector Control. **66:** 217–218.
35. EVANS, D. A. P. & P. M. SHEPPARD. 1966. Some preliminary data on the genetics of resistance to anticoagulants in the Norway rat. W.H.O. Seminar on Rodents and Rodent Ectoparasites. Vector Control. **66:** 155–160.
36. GREAVES, J. H. & P. AYRES. 1967. Heritable resistance to warfarin in rats. Nature **215:** 877–878.
37. CAMPBELL, H. A., W. K. SMITH, W. L. ROBERTS & K. P. LINK. 1941. Studies on the hemorrhagic sweet clover disease. II. The bioassay of hemorrhagic concentrates by following the prothrombin level in the plasma of rabbit blood. J. Biol. Chem. **138:** 1–20.

38. Overman, R. S., M. A. Stahmann, W. R. Sullivan, C. F. Huebner, H. A. Campbell & K. P. Link. 1942. Studies on the hemorrhagic sweet clover disease. VII. The effect of 3,3′-methylenebis(4-hydroxycoumarin) on the prothrombin time of the plasma of various animals. J. Biol. Chem. **142:** 941–955.
39. Link, K. P. 1944. The anticoagulant from spoiled sweet clover hay. Harvey Lectures **39:** 162–216.
40. Millar, G. J., L. B. Jaques & M. Henriet. 1964. The prothrombin time response of rabbits to Dicumarol. Arch. Intern. Pharmacodyn. **150:** 197–219.

COMMENT SUBSEQUENT TO THE CONFERENCE

Dr. K. Hirschhorn (*Mount Sinai Hospital, N. Y.*): The statement that if a character is normally distributed in the population, it is due to polygenic inheritance, is not true and will discourage investigators from searching for monofactorial or single gene variation. For example, Harris has shown that, although red cell acid phosphatase activity is normally distributed in the population, it is controlled by a single locus with only three common alleles. These determine three structurally different enzymes, each with different activity. The distribution of the six genotypes is such that activity is normally distributed. Such distribution therefore should not deter investigators from searching for single genes determining differences in enzyme activity or drug response.

VARIATIONS IN METABOLISM OF COUMARIN ANTICOAGULANT DRUGS

Harvey M. Solomon

Hoffmann-La Roche Special Treatment Unit
Newark City Hospital, Newark, N. J.

In man, marked variation in the response to indirect anticoagulants such as warfarin and bishydroxycoumarin has been observed.[1-3] Therapy with these compounds occasionally results in serious hemorrhage. A variety of factors including rate of metabolism of drug,[4,5] affinity of the receptor site for the drug,[6] and the vitamin K status of the subject influence the pharmacologic response to the indirect anticoagulants.[7]

Genetic factors also influence the response to indirect anticoagulants in various animal species including man. Early studies by Smith demonstrated marked variation in the susceptibility of rabbits to spoiled sweet clover hay.[8] Indeed, Link observed that susceptibility to the toxicity of bishydroxycoumarin in rabbits was inherited as a Mendelian recessive characteristic.[9] We have recently studied a population of rabbits composed of rapid and slow inactivators of bishydroxycoumarin.[5]

Genetic factors also appear to influence the response to warfarin in the rat. This compound has enjoyed widespread use as a rodenticide; however, in recent years, animals have been observed who are resistant to the drug.[10] Recent genetic studies have indicated that resistance to warfarin in the rat depends upon a single dominant autosomal gene.[11] Resistant animals may metabolize the drug more rapidly than do sensitive animals. Alternatively receptor site affinity for vitamin K may be greater in resistant animals than in sensitive animals.

In man, genetic factors also influence the response to the indirect anticoagulants. Motulsky has suggested that multiple recessive genes are involved in determining the rate of metabolism of bishydroxycoumarin in man.[12]

We recently studied a patient who was extremely sensitive to warfarin and whose family history suggested the possibility of an inherited sensitivity to the drug. His mother had been aniticoagulated with warfarin following a myocardial infarction and was maintained on a weekly dose of 2.5 to 5 mg (normal maintenance dose – 2 to 25 mg per day). On this small dose of drug she suffered a spinal cord hematoma and developed permanent paraplegia.

Our patient, who was hospitalized because of a myocardial infarction, was treated with a low dose of warfarin (15 mg). The magnitude and duration of his anticoagulant response is shown in FIGURE 1. At a later date, his plasma half-life of bishydroxycoumarin was determined following the oral administration of various doses of the drug (FIGURE 2). Characteristically, the half-life of bishydroxycoumarin increased as the dose of drug was increased. Following the administration of 150 mg of bishydroxycoumarin, the plasma half-life of the drug was 82 hours. In normal subjects, the half-life of this drug is 27 $\pm$ 5 hours. Thus the patient's marked sensitivity to this drug is due, in part, to a relatively slow rate of metabolism of the compound.

The patient's mother has, thus far, been unwilling to participate in studies designed to determine her plasma half-life of various indirect anticoagulants. Unfortunately, the patient has no siblings.

Warfarin and bishydroxycoumarin are extensively metabolized by hepatic microsomal enzymes. The major metabolites of these drugs in the rat are ring

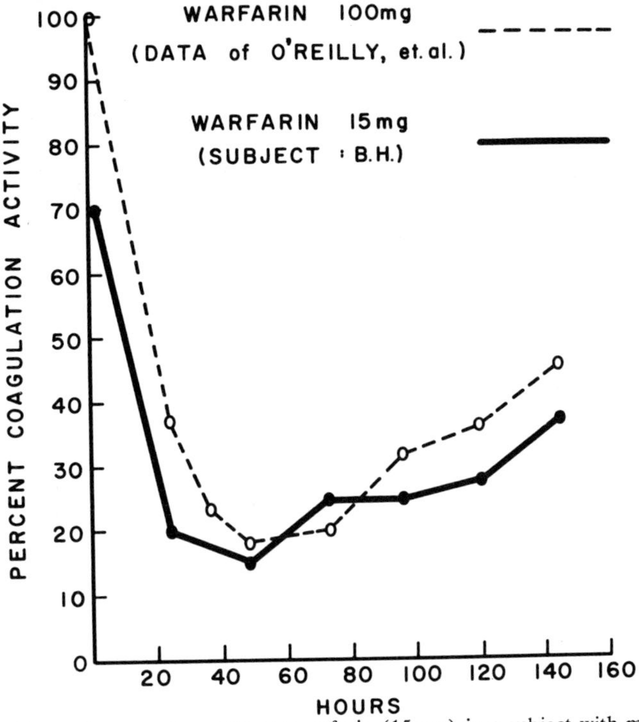

FIGURE 1. The anticoagulant response to warfarin (15 mg) in a subject with marked sensitivity to the drug. The results are compared to the average response of 14 normal subjects who received 100 mg of the drug (data of O'Reilly, R. A. *et al.* 1963. J. Clin. Invest. **42**: 1542–1551).

hydroxylated compounds;[13,14] in man, the metabolites of warfarin and bishydroxycoumarin have not been characterized. Phenobarbital induces the synthesis coumarin-like anticoagulants.[15] In contrast, phenyramidol inhibits the metabolism of these drugs by hepatic microsomal enzymes and in this way increases the magnitude and duration of the anticoagulant response.[5]

Resistance to the anticoagulant effect of warfarin has been described in subjects who metabolize the drug rapidly ($T½ = 5.5 - 6.9$ hours).[16,17] However, no information was presented concerning the drug histories of these patients. Thus the rapid rate of metabolism of warfarin in these subjects could be due to either enzyme induction or genetic factors.

In man, diphenylhydantoin also undergoes extensive metabolism by hepatic microsomal enzymes.[15] The major metabolite, p-hydroxyphenyl-5-phenylhydantoin is excreted in the urine as a glucuronide.[18,19] Phenyramidol inhibits the metabolism of both diphenylhydantoin and bishydroxycoumarin in human subjects. Moreover, we have recently observed that a patient who metabolized diphenylhydantoin slowly also metabolized bishydroxycoumarin slowly. These results suggest that both drugs may be metabolized by the same microsomal enzyme in man.

Kutt *et al.* have described a family in which the inability to hydroxylate diphenylhydantoin was genetically controlled.[20] It would be of value to determine

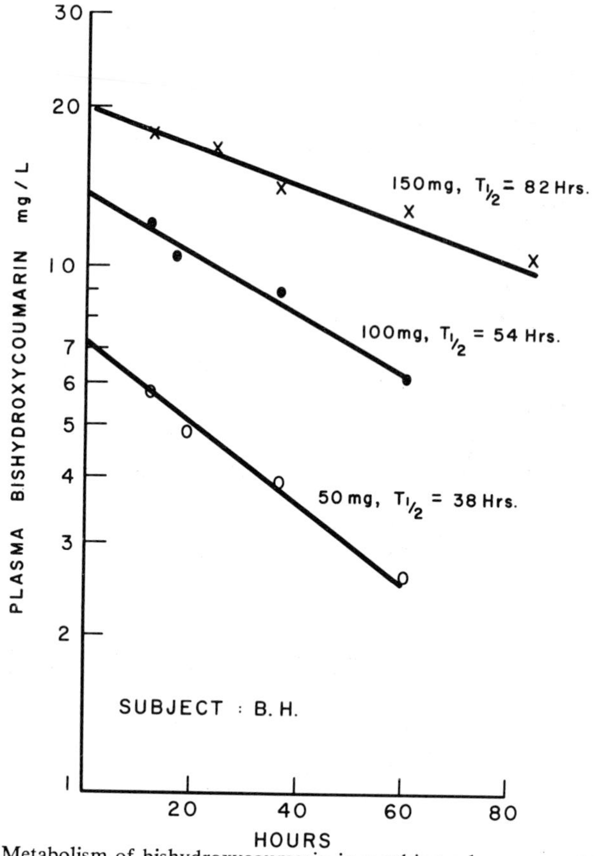

FIGURE 2. Metabolism of bishydroxycoumarin in a subject who was sensitive to the drug. Single oral doses, in the amounts indicated, were administered to the patient on three separate occasions.

if the members of this family who metabolized the anticonvulsant slowly also metabolized bishydroxycoumarin slowly.

Summary

The magnitude and duration of the pharmacologic response to various indirect anticoagulants is determined, in part, by the rate of metabolism of these compounds. In the rabbit, the rate of metabolism of the indirect anticoagulants is genetically controlled. Resistance to warfarin is inherited as a dominant characteristic in the rat. In man, exposure to various drugs and chemicals as well as genetic factors appear to influence the rate of metabolism of the coumarin-like anticoagulants.

References

1. WEINER, M., S. SHAPIRO, J. AXELROD, J. R. COOPER & B. B. BRODIE. 1950. The physiological disposition of Dicumarol in man. J. Pharmacol. Exp. Therap. **99:** 409–420.
2. SOLOMON, H. M. & J. J. SCHROGIE. 1967. The anticoagulant response to bishydroxycoumarin 1. The role of individual variation. Clin. Pharmacol. Therap. **8:** 65–69.

3. O'Reilly, R. A., P. M. Aggeler & L. S. Leong. 1963. Studies on the coumarin anticoagulant drugs: The pharmacodynamics of warfarin in man. 1963. J. Clin. Invest. **42:** 1542–1551.
4. Dayton, P. G., Y. Tarcan, T. Chenkin & M. Weiner. 1961. The influence of barbiturates on coumarin plasma levels and prothrombin response. 1961. J. Clin. Invest. **40:** 1797–1802.
5. Solomon, H. M. & J. J. Schrogie. 1966. The effect of phenyramidol on the metabolism of bishydroxycoumarin. J. Pharmacol. Exp. Therap. **154:** 660–666.
6. O'Reilly, R. A. & P. M. Aggeler. 1965. Coumarin anticoagulant drugs: Hereditary resistance in man. Feder. Proc. **24:** 1266–1273.
7. Finkel, M. J. 1961. Vitamin K_1 and the vitamin K analogues. Clin. Pharmacol. Therap. **2:** 794–814.
8. Smith, W. K. 1939. The alleged protective action of alfalfa against the hemorrhagic sweet clover disease. J. Agr. Res. **59:** 211–215.
9. Link, K. P. 1943–1944. The anticoagulant from spoiled sweet colver hay. Harvey Lectures **39:** 162–216.
10. Annon. 1966. Rats become resistant to anticoagulants. World Health Organ. Chronicle **20:** 29–31.
11. Greaves, J. H. & P. Ayres. 1967. Heritable resistance to warfarin in rats. Nature **215:** 877–878.
12. Motulsky, A. 1964. Pharmacogenetics. Progr. Med. Genet. **3:** 49–74.
13. Ikeda, M., B. Sezesny & M. Barnes. 1966. Enhanced metabolism and decreased toxicity of warfarin in rats pretreated with phenobarbital. Feder. Proc. **25:** 417.
14. Christensen, F. 1966. Crystallization and preliminary characterization of a Dicoumarol metabolite in the faeces of Dicoumarol-treated rats. Acta Pharmacol. Toxicol. **24:** 232–242.
15. Cucinell, S. A., A. H. Conney, M. Sansur & J. J. Burns. 1965. Drug interactions in man 1. Lowering effect of phenobarbital on plasma levels of bishydroxycoumarin (Dicoumarol) and diphenylhydantoin (Dilantin). Clin. Pharmacol. Therap. **6:** 420–429.
16. Lewis, R. J., M. Spivak & T. H. Spaet. 1967. Warfarin resistance. Am. J. Med. **42:** 620–624.
17. Aggeler, P. M. 1967. Blood coagulation and the coumarin anticoagulant drugs. Calif. Med. **106:** 255–271.
18. Butler, T. C. 1957. The metabolic conversion of 5-5 diphenylhydantoin to 5 (p-hydroxyphenyl)-5-phenylhydantoin. J. Pharmacol. Exp. Therap. **119:** 1–11.
19. Maynert, E. W. 1960. The metabolic fate of diphenylhydantoin in the dog, rat and man. J. Pharmacol. Exp. Therap. **130:** 275–284.
20. Kutt, H., M. Wolk, R. Scherman & F. McDowell. 1964. Insufficient parahydroxylation as a cause of diphenylhydantoin toxicity. Neurology **14:** 542–548.

ATYPICAL HUMAN LIVER ALCOHOL DEHYDROGENASE

J. P. von Wartburg and P. M. Schürch
Medizinisch-chemisches Institut der Universität Bern, Berne, Switzerland

An exceptionally active enzyme variant of human liver alcohol dehydrogenase* occurs in some individuals. This atypical human enzyme has been purified from two livers.[1]

Properties of Atypical Human Alcohol Dehydrogenase

In TABLE 1 some properties of the atypical enzyme are summarized and compared to those of normal ADH. The highest specific activity obtained for the atypical enzyme after a 200-fold purification is at least three to four times higher than that of normal ADH.[2] Livers of carriers of the variant ADH show total activities about five times higher than normal livers, when determined in biopsy samples and at physiological pH and temperature. For all the liver specimens including those obtained by autopsy this difference is even larger (FIGURE 1). The normal pH-optimum for ethanol oxidation lies at pH 10.8. It is shifted to pH 8.5 for the atypical enzyme. These enzymes are also different regarding their sensitivity toward several effectors. Thiourea activates purified human alcohol dehydrogenase as it does the isoenzymes of rhesus monkey and horse liver.[3,4] The atypical enzyme on the other hand is inhibited, as is yeast ADH.

o-Phenanthroline which chelates the zinc in the active center of human ADH[2] inhibits the normal ADH more strongly than the atypical enzyme. A similar situation pertains to the inhibitors tribromethanol and 5-hydroxymethyl furfurol. These two compounds do not serve as substrates of either the normal or the atypical ADH. Pyrazol is a specific inhibitor of alcohol dehydrogenase, and is competitive with ethanol as substrate.[5] This inhibitor has a stronger action on atypical ADH than on the normal one. Characteristic differences are also found in the relative turnover rates of various alcohols. The normal enzyme oxidizes n-butanol, benzyl alcohol and cyclohexanol faster than does the variant ADH.

Finally, no differences were detected for the Michaelis constants for ethanol, acetaldehyde and the coenzymes NAD and $NADH_2$. Within the limits of the method, identical molecular weights were found for both enzymes by gel chromatography on a Sephadex G-200.

A simple screening test was designed to detect atypical ADH in liver homogenates. According to the difference in the pH rate profiles (see FIGURE 2) the ratio of the activity at pH 10.8 to the one determined at 8.8 is greater than 1 for the normal enzyme and less than 1 for the atypical ADH. In addition to this Q_{pH} (= Quotient pH), a ratio $Q_{Thiourea}$ was determined. It represents the ratio between the activity in presence and in absence of this effector in the reaction mixture. It is lower for atypical than for normal ADH.

In order to include a parameter in the screening which is based on a difference in the turnover of some substrate, we searched for a substrate exerting some pharmacological activity. Recently, J. Raaflaub suggested that β-pyridyl carbinol (Ronicol), a vasodilator, is oxidized to the corresponding aldehyde by alcohol dehydrogenase and finally to nicotinic acid.[6] Working with human liver homog-

* The following abbreviations are used: ADH for alcohol dehydrogenase; NAD and $NADH_2$ for oxidized and reduced nicotinamide adenine dinucleotide.

TABLE 1

PROPERTIES OF NORMAL AND ATYPICAL LIVER ALCOHOL DEHYDROGENASE

Property	Normal ADH	Atypical ADH
Specific activity of purified enzyme (IU/mg protein)	ca. 3	ca. 10
Total activity in liver (IU/1350 g tissue)	3′600	17′000
pH optimum (ethanol oxidation)	10.8	8.5
Effect of 0.66 M thiourea (V_{TH}/V_c)	2.20	0.65
$I_{50\%}$ (M) for o-Phenanthroline	6.7×10^{-5}	3.3×10^{-4}
Inhibition of ethanol oxidation (%) in liver homogenates by		
5×10^{-3} M tribromethanol	52	10
3×10^{-4} M 5-hydroxymethyl furfurol	49	21
4×10^{-5} M pyrazol	50	14
Substrate specificity (%)		
1.6×10^{-2} M ethanol (= 100%)	100	100
3.3×10^{-4} M butanol	87	54
3.3×10^{-4} M benzyl alcohol	85	22
3.3×10^{-4} M cyclohexanol	82	18

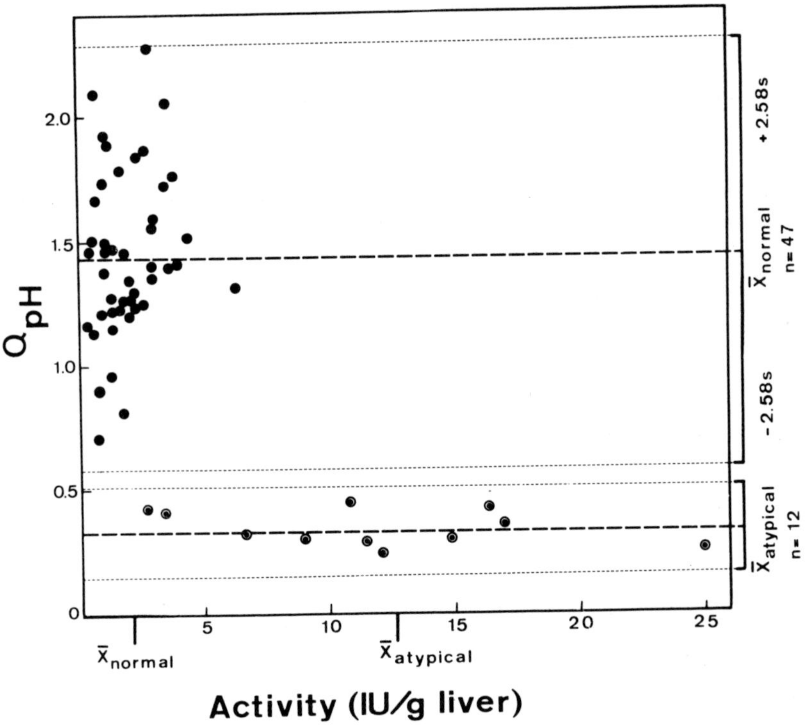

FIGURE 1. Alcohol dehydrogenase activity and Q_{pH} of 59 Swiss liver samples. Activities determined as change in A_{366} at 25° C and expressed in International Units per gram of fresh liver. Q_{pH} = ratio of activity in 3.3×10^{-2} M glycine-NaOH, pH 10.8 to activity in 3.3×10^{-2} M Na pyrophosphate, pH 8.8. Conditions: NAD, 1.6×10^{-3} M; ethanol, 1.6×10^{-2} M.

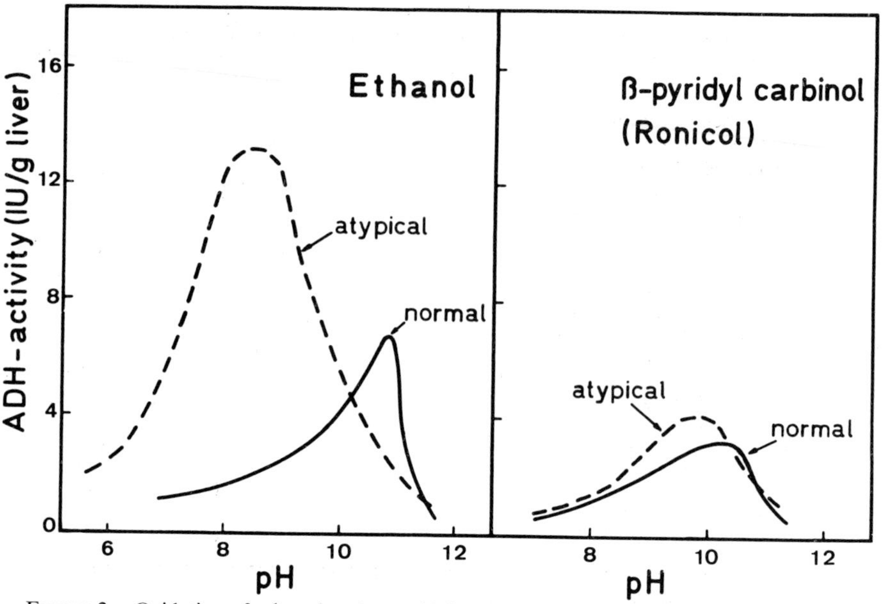

FIGURE 2. Oxidation of ethanol and β-pyridyl carbinol by normal and atypical human liver alcohol dehydrogenase; dependence on pH of the reaction mixture. Ethanol oxidation by purified enzymes; Ronicol oxidation by liver homogenates. NAD, 1.6×10^{-3} M; ethanol, 1.6×10^{-2} M; Ronicol, 1.6×10^{-3} M. Change in A_{366} determined at 25° C.

enates or with purified enzymes, we found that both the normal and the atypical human ADH can use β-pyridyl carbinol as a substrate. FIGURE 2 compares the pH dependence of the activity of the normal and of the variant enzyme with ethanol and Ronicol, respectively. The large difference in the pH optimum of the normal and the atypical enzyme observed with ethanol visibly diminishes when Ronicol is the substrate. With the normal enzyme at pH 8.8 (standard assay condition) the turnover of Ronicol is about the same as that of ethanol. With the atypical ADH the turnover of Ronicol is only about 25% that of ethanol. This difference in the ratio of Ronicol oxidation to ethanol oxidation can be used to detect atypical livers (see TABLES 2 & 3 and FIGURE 3). On the other hand, the absolute activities of both enzymes are similar, suggesting no or little difference for the in vivo turnover of this substrate in normal and atypical individuals.

TABLE 2

PROPERTIES OF ATYPICAL AND NORMAL HUMAN LIVER ALCOHOL DEHYDROGENASE IN SWISS LIVER SAMPLES*

Parameter	Normal Livers $\overline{X} \pm S$	Normal Livers N	Atypical Livers $\overline{X} \pm S$	Atypical Livers N
Q_{pH}	1.43 ± 0.33	47	0.33 ± 0.07	12
$Q_{Thiourea}$	1.07 ± 0.20	28	0.59 ± 0.20	6
$Q_{Ronicol}$	0.95 ± 0.40	22	0.26 ± 0.05	7

* For conditions see FIGURE 3 and text.

TABLE 3

PROPERTIES OF ATYPICAL AND NORMAL HUMAN LIVER ALCOHOL DEHYDROGENASE IN LONDON LIVER SAMPLES*

Parameter	Normal Livers $X \pm S$	Normal Livers Confidence Limits (99%)	Atypical Livers No. 12	Atypical Livers No. 16
Q_{pH}	1.39 ± 0.17	0.96 – 1.82	0.29	0.38
$Q_{Thiourea}$	1.14 ± 0.16	0.74 – 1.54	0.59	0.58
$Q_{Ronicol}$	0.84 ± 0.24	0.22 – 1.45	0.15	0.21
$Q_{Pyrazol}$	0.68 ± 0.10	0.43 – 0.93	0.33	0.34
$Q_{Acetaldehyde}$	14.00 ± 4.10	3.50 – 24.50	9.60	11.90
$Q_{Chloralhydrate}$	0.36 ± 0.08	0.16 – 0.57	0.17	0.15

* For conditions see FIGURES 3 and 5 and text.

Drug Metabolism

Family studies, i.e., a screening of members of families of known carriers of the variant ADH, depend on the availability of an in vivo screening test, since blood, urine etc. contain no measurable ADH activity. An in vivo test could be based upon differences between normal and atypical individuals in turnover of some pharmacologically active compounds. Such a pharmacogenetic effect could be applicable to healthy normal individuals for the determination of the characteristics of inheritance. TABLE 4 lists the substances tested in this respect so far. As mentioned before, β-pyridyl carbinol is oxidized at similar rates by atypical and normal ADH, although the turnover relative to ethanol is quite different. A similar situation pertains to 1.2-propandiol and its derivative, 3-o-Toloxy-1.2-propandiol; the latter is a muscle relaxant known as Myanesin, a substitute for curare. The findings with chloral hydrate are analogous. Normal liver reduces this substrate twice as fast as it does ethanol, whereas the rate is only one-third with the atypical liver ADH. Nevertheless, the absolute rates of reduction and hence the formation of the pharmacologically active product, trichlorethanol, are almost the same for both enzymes. Therefore, it must be concluded that the occurrence of a pharmacogenetic effect for these compounds is unlikely on the basis of the atypical human ADH.

A different situation is found for acetaldol, i.e., β-hydroxy butyraldehyde. This compound is reduced five times faster by the atypical enzyme than by normal ADH. Thus, the large difference found in the turnover of ethanol between normal and atypical ADH also pertains to this substrate. This compound has been suggested as a hypnotic and sedative. This drug is currently being investigated for use in an in vivo screening test for detection of living carriers of the atypical enzyme.

Ethanol Metabolism

The finding of an in vitro difference in the turnover of ethanol prompted an investigation of the in vivo rates of ethanol oxidation in humans with the atypical enzyme. Drinking experiments were performed on a normal and an atypical subject. The results are shown in FIGURE 4. A dose of 0.7 g of ethanol per kg body weight was given to a normal subject. As seen in curve 1 this dose led to an initial blood alcohol concentration of about 0.1%. The distribution factor r of Widmark and the rate of alcohol oxidation were calculated from the linear drop of the blood alcohol levels during a certain period of time. An ethanol oxidation of 90 mg per kg body weight in one hour was computed for this normal subject.

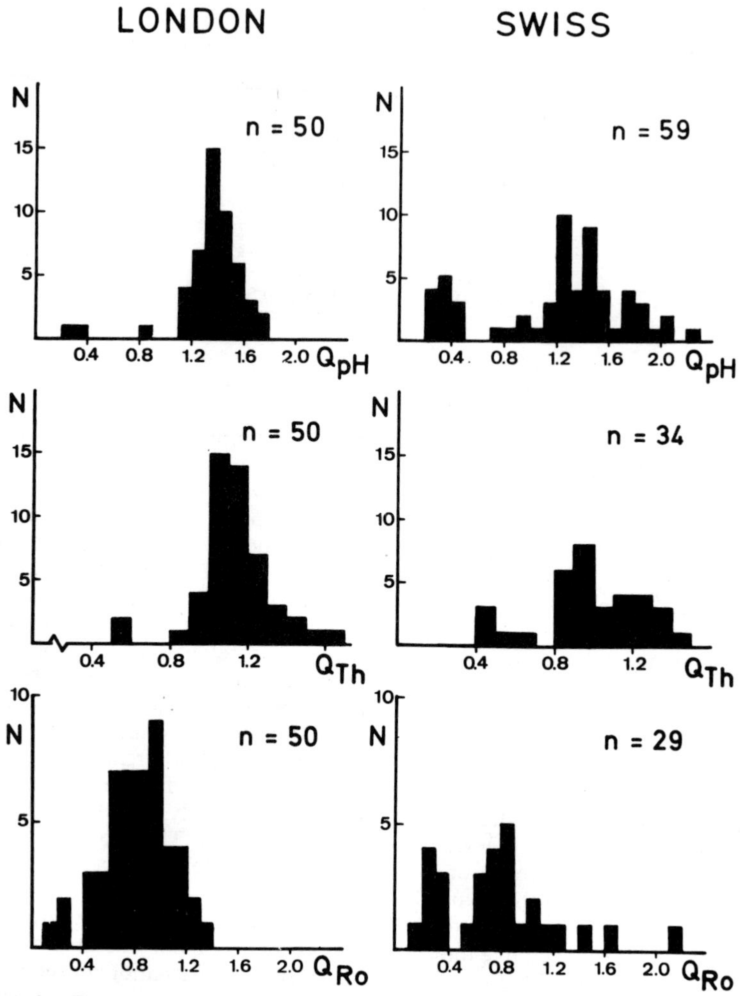

FIGURE 3. Frequency distribution patterns of liver samples from a London and a Swiss population. For the definitions of Q_{pH}, $Q_{Thiourea}$ and $Q_{Ronicol}$, and for further explanation see text. Conditions: Q_{pH} see FIGURE 1. Na pyrophosphate, 3.3×10^{-2} M, pH 8.8; NAD, 1.6×10^{-3} M; ethanol, 1.6×10^{-2} M; thiourea, 6.6×10^{-1} M; Ronicol, 1.6×10^{-3} M.

From curve 2 it can be seen that the drop in blood alcohol concentrations due to ethanol oxidation was somewhat faster in a subject who was a carrier of the atypical alcohol dehydrogenase. The corresponding value for ethanol oxidation was higher, namely 141 mg of ethanol oxidized per kg body weight per hour. This figure is above the average value of approximately 100 mg/kg/hour found in the literature and recommended for purposes of legal medicine by the expert commission of the World Health Organization. But this enhancement by 40–50% does not correspond to the five-to sixfold increase in ADH activity determined in the liver biopsy of this individual. It is probable that another factor, such as the reoxidation of $NADH_2$ formed in the alcohol dehydrogenase reaction, becomes

TABLE 4

TURNOVER OF SOME DRUGS BY LIVER HOMOGENATES CONTAINING NORMAL OR ATYPICAL HUMAN ALCOHOL DEHYDROGENASE*

Substrate	Conc. (m M)	Normal Liver IU/g	Normal Liver % of EtOH	Atypical Liver IU/g	Atypical Liver % of EtOH
Ethanol	17	2.84	100	25.60	100
β-pyridyl carbinol	1.7	2.86	101	3.71	15
1.2-Propandiol	17	0.47	16	0.46	2
3-o-Toloxy-1.2-propandiol	0.33	0.31	11	0.40	2
Chloral hydrate	3.3	6.10	214	8.70	34
Acetaldol	1.7	15.30	537	77.80	304

* Conditions: Na pyrophosphate, 3.3×10^{-2} M, pH 8.8; NAD, 1.6×10^{-2} M; substrate concentrations as indicated; change in A_{366} determined at 25° C.

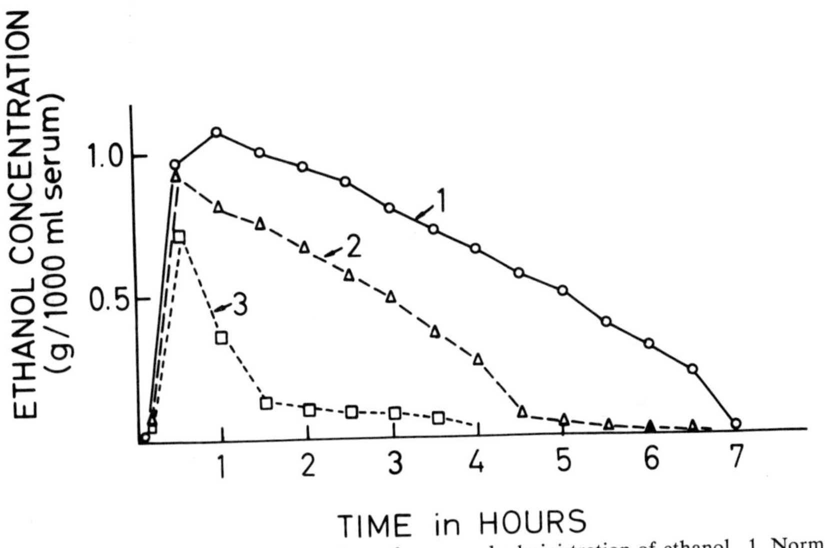

FIGURE 4. Blood alcohol concentrations after peroral administration of ethanol. 1. Normal individual; 2. individual with atypical alcohol dehydrogenase; 3. infant with glycogenosis (glucose-6-phosphatase deficiency). Ethanol dose at time = 0 : 0.7 g/kg of body weight. Blood alcohol concentration determined enzymatically (ADH–method).

rate limiting. This interpretation is supported by analogous drinking experiments carried out with children suffering from glycogen storage disease, type I, i.e., glucose-6-phosphatase deficiency.

These experiments were suggested by Prof. E. Rossi of the Dept. of Pediatrics of the University of Berne, Switzerland, and carried out in collaboration with his group. Curve 3 shows that these children are fully sober within 1–2 hours after drinking the same dose of ethanol. This is the result of a manifold increase in ethanol oxidation, namely 460 mg per kg body weight per hour. It is probable that this enhancement correlates with an increase in $NADH_2$ reoxidation due to the high pyruvate concentration found in these patients.

Population Studies

A further question of interest was, to what extent were the two livers used for the isolation of the atypical ADH representative for a variant group within the Swiss population. In the case of positive results it would prove necessary to determine the frequency of this anomaly. Using the Q_{pH} as the discriminating parameter, a screening was performed for the atypical enzyme in liver specimens obtained by biopsy or autopsy. Some samples were stored at $-20°$ C before use, others were assayed directly. Atypical liver ADH was found in all types of samples and no change in the Q_{pH} was ever observed due to storage. Thus, artifacts due to storage, as have been suspected by Blair and Vallee,[7] can be excluded. Storage of liver tissue at 4° C, however, is accompanied by a relatively fast drop in ADH activity. A slow decrease in activity can be observed in deep frozen samples.

It is likely that a genetic basis exists for the occurrence of the atypical ADH. The case histories of the individuals found to be carriers of the variant enzyme give no indication as to any kind of induction or dependence upon environmental factors. The atypical individuals ranged from 16 to 82 years of age. The causes of death were traffic accidents, death by drowning, murder, and thrombosis of both carotid arteries.

The results of the screening of 59 liver specimens from a Swiss population are shown in FIGURE 1. Twelve atypical livers with an average Q_{pH} of 0.33 were detected, thus amounting to a frequency of 20%. The confidence limits for $\pm$ 2.58 standard deviations, that is for the 99% probability of the samples, indicate that there is no overlap between the normal and atypical group. This is in contrast to the considerable overlapping of the activities of the atypical and normal livers. The average activity for the normal livers is 2.07 $\pm$ 1.25 IU per g of wet liver ($\overline{X} \pm S$) as compared to 12.6 $\pm$ 6.7 IU/g for the atypical livers. The considerable variance in these activities is due partially to the difference in storage of the samples and, on the other hand, to individual variation. Nevertheless, it becomes quite obvious that the atypical livers are unusually active.

To find out whether this anomaly occurs in a population other than the Swiss, we screened a sampling of 50 livers from a London population*. FIGURE 3 compares the frequency distribution patterns for the two populations for three parameters, namely Q_{pH}, $Q_{Thiourea}$, and $Q_{Ronicol}$. In the London population the frequency of atypical liver ADH is 2 out of 50 livers; that is, only 4% as compared to 20% in the Swiss population. The same bimodal distribution is found in both populations. However, it seems that the variance is larger in the normal Swiss livers especially for the Q_{pH} and the $Q_{Ronicol}$, where the top values are in a much higher range compared to the London livers.

The mean values for Q_{pH}, $Q_{Thiourea}$ and $Q_{Ronicol}$ of the normal and atypical Swiss livers are listed in TABLE 2. It becomes evident that $Q_{Ronicol}$ and $Q_{Thiourea}$ show a considerable overlap between the normal and atypical livers. Therefore, these two parameters seem less discriminating than Q_{pH}. However, increasing the total number of samples may disclose a logarithmic-normal distribution pattern, so that no premature conclusions should be drawn on the basis of the small number of tested specimens.

Additional kinetic properties of human alcohol dehydrogenase were investigated in the liver specimens from London. FIGURE 5 shows the frequency dis-

* We are grateful to Prof. F. E. Camps and Dr. Ann Robinson of the Dept. of Forensic Medicine at the London Hospital for providing the liver specimens.

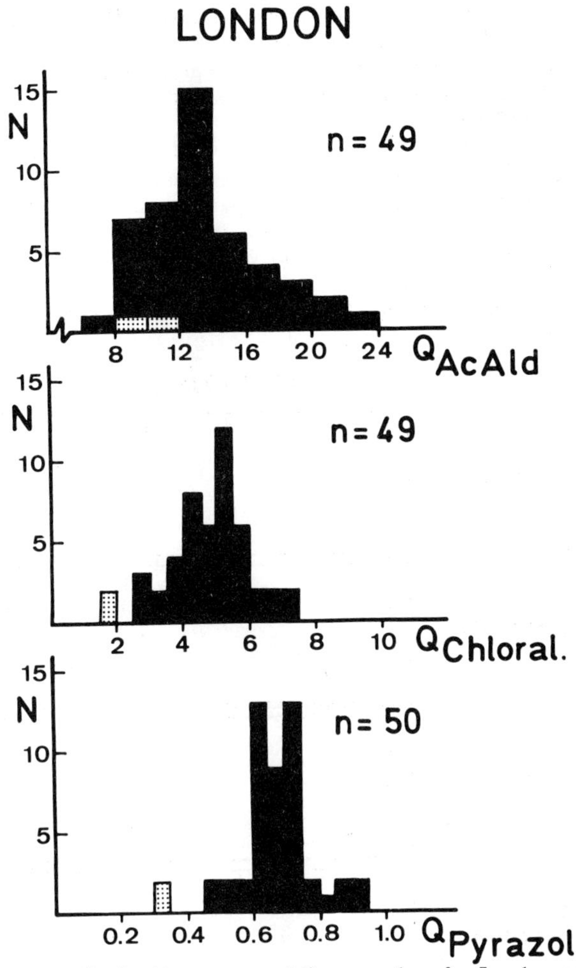

FIGURE 5. Frequency distribution patterns of liver samples of a London population. For definitions of $Q_{Acetaldehyde}$, $Q_{Chloral\ hydrate}$ and $Q_{Pyrazol}$, and for further explanation see text. Conditions for Q_{AcAld} and $Q_{Chloral}$. : Na phosphate, 3.3×10^{-2} M, pH 7.0; $NADH_2$, 3.3×10^{-4} M; acetaldehyde, 3.3×10^{-2} M; chloral hydrate, 3.3×10^{-2} M. Conditions for $Q_{Pyrazol}$: Na pyrophosphate, 3.3×10^{-2} M, pH 8.8; ethanol, 1.6×10^{-2} M; NAD, 1.6×10^{-3} M; pyrazol, 3.0×10^{-4} M. Dotted fields = atypical livers.

tribution patterns for these further parameters. $Q_{Acetaldehyde}$ represents the ratio of the acetaldehyde reduction to the ethanol oxidation, the forward and backward reactions being determined under standard conditions. $Q_{Chloral\ hydrate}$ represents the ratio of the reduction of trichloroacetaldehyde to ethanol oxidation. Finally, $Q_{Pyrazol}$ is the ratio of activities with and without this substance. Pyrazol is a specific inhibitor of alcohol dehydrogenase, which is competitive with the substrate ethanol.

It becomes evident that there is no difference in the $Q_{Acetaldehyde}$ between normal and atypical livers. This finding would indirectly confirm the formerly reported one, that there are no differences between the normal and the variant enzyme regarding the Michaelis constants for these substrates and the coenzymes. Chloral hydrate is reduced more slowly by the atypical enzyme than by the normal enzyme. Finally, pyrazol is a considerably better inhibitor of the variant enzyme than of the normal one.

TABLE 3 summarizes the results obtained with the liver samples from London. The confidence limits for 99% of all observations were calculated as the mean value ± 2.58 standard deviation. A comparison of the parameters of the two atypical livers, numbers 12 and 16, with the confidence limits shows that the values for Q_{pH}, $Q_{Thiourea}$, $Q_{Ronicol}$ and $Q_{Pyrazol}$ all lie outside the 99% range. The figures for $Q_{Chloral\ hydrate}$ are around the limit and, therefore, perhaps less discriminating than the others. $Q_{Acetaldehyde}$ of the atypical livers lies within the

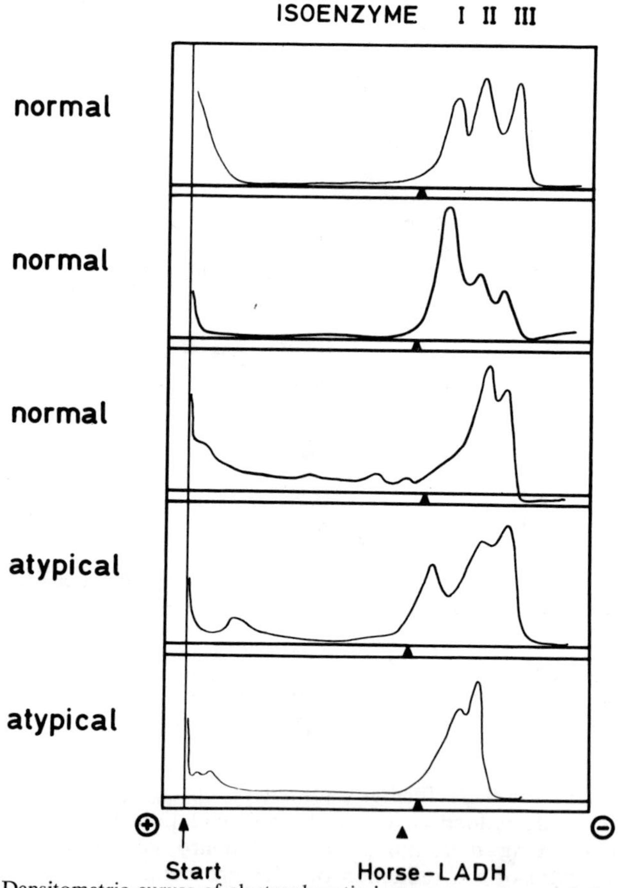

FIGURE 6. Densitometric curves of electrophoretic isoenzyme patterns of alcohol dehydrogenase in normal and atypical human liver homogenates. Electrophoresis in agar gel at pH 9.0. Activity visualized with 2.5×10^{-2} M ethanol; 1.25×10^{-3} M NAD; 33 μg/ml phenazine methosulfate; 0.4 mg/ml nitro tetrazolium blue chloride. ▲ Reference enzyme = horse liver alcohol dehydrogenase, main fraction.

normal range. It is important to note, that all the parameters of the atypical livers are abnormal in the London samples although these ratios were designed on the basis of atypical livers from Switzerland. Furthermore, it is noteworthy to mention that besides the values of the atypical livers only 2 normal livers showed one parameter each outside the 99% range. Hence, we can conclude that the same anomaly observed in Switzerland occurs at a diminished frequency in London.

Multiple Forms of Alcohol Dehydrogenase

In addition to the polymorphism discussed above, both normal and atypical human liver alcohol dehydrogenase exist in multiple forms. The number of alcohol dehydrogenase isoenzymes depends on the species. This is in contrast to the findings with lactic dehydrogenase, where five isoenzymes are found in practically all species. They can be separated by electrophoresis on agar gel or by chromatography on ion exchange cellulose. Rhesus monkey liver contains two isoenzymes, which have been purified and characterized.[2] Horse liver reveals five fractions.[2,8,9-11] Human liver alcohol dehydrogenase can be separated into three bands on agar gel electrophoresis.[8,9,12] Recently, Blair and Vallee have observed three fractions of human liver alcohol dehydrogenase upon chromatography on Carboxymethyl cellulose.[7] Preliminary results in our laboratory show that these chromatographic fractions probably correspond to those demonstrated by electrophoresis.

FIGURE 6 shows the densitometric curves of some isoenzyme patterns after electrophoresis on agar gel of normal and atypical human liver extracts. Horse liver alcohol dehydrogenase (main fraction) was run in each electrophoresis as a reference enzyme. It becomes evident that the isoenzyme patterns of individual livers vary considerably in respect to the proportion of total activity contributed by single isoenzymes. Some livers contain only two isoenzymes. But the three normal and the three atypical isoenzymes have identical electrophoretic mobilities within the accuracy of this method. It is likely that the three isoenzymes are formed by all possible combinations of two distinct polypeptides with different primary structure. Hence, the question arises as to how many of the isoenzymes in atypical liver differ from the normal one. This is subject to current research in our laboratory and the results should show whether one or two structural genes are mutant. It is also conceivable that a more discriminating screening test than the one used would uncover a trimodal distribution within the apparent bimodal one. However, such a trimodal distribution may be difficult to find because it could be masked by differences in the properties of the isoenzymes and variable isoenzyme patterns.

Summary

An exceptionally active atypical liver alcohol dehydrogenase variant occurs in 20% of a Swiss and 4% of a London population. Both populations reveal a bimodal distribution for several parameters discriminative for the atypical and the normal enzyme. The in vitro turnover for some drugs and the in vivo oxidation of ethanol by both enzymes have been investigated. Normal and atypical human liver alcohol dehydrogenase exist in multiple molecular forms.

Acknowledgments

The authors are indebted to Dr. H. Aebi for his continuous interest in this work, and for valuable suggestions and discussions. They greatly appreciate the excellent technical assistance of Miss. L. Steiner. They are grateful to Dr. R. Bigley for valuable editorial suggestions. This work was supported by the Fritz Hoffman-La Roche-Stiftung zur Förderung wissenschaftlicher Arbeitsgemeinschaften in der Schweiz, Basle, Switzerland.

References

1. Von Wartburg, J. P., J. Papenberg & H. Aebi. 1965. An atypical human alcohol dehydrogenase. Canad. J. Biochem. **43:** 889–898.
2. Von Wartburg, J. P., J. L. Bethune & B. L. Vallee. 1964. Human liver alcohol dehydrogenase. Kinetic and physicochemical properties. Biochem. **3:** 1775–1782.
3. Papenberg, J., J. P. von Wartburg & H. Aebi. 1965. Die Heterogenität der Alkoholdehydrogenase aus Rhesusaffenleber. Biochem. Z. **342:** 95–107.
4. Von Wartburg, J. P. & J. Papenberg. 1966. Alcohol dehydrogenase in ethanol metabolism. Psychosom. Med. **28:** 405–413.
5. Theorell, H. 1964. The role of proteins in biological oxido-reduction. Bull. Soc. chim. biol. **46:** 1533–1553.
6. Raaflaub, J. 1966. Zur Umwandlung von β-Pyridyl-carbinol in Nicotinsäure im tierischen Organismus. Experientia **22:** 258–259.
7. Blair, H. A. & B. L. Vallee. 1966. Some catalytic properties of human liver alcohol dehydrogenase. Biochem. **5:** 2026–2034.
8. Aebi, H., R. Richterich & J. P. von Wartburg. 1966. The isoenzyme pattern: Some comparative-biochemical and developmental aspects. Helgoländer wiss. Meeresunters. **14:** 343–351.
9. Von Wartburg, J. P. 1966. Isoenzymes of various Alcohol Dehydrogenases. 3rd Meeting Fed. Europ. Biochem. Soc., Warsaw, April 1966. Abstracts, F 180.
10. Pietruszko, R., A. Clark, J. M. H. Graves & H. J. Ringold. 1966. The steroid activity and multiplicity of crystalline horse liver alcohol dehydrogenase. Biochem. Biophys. Res. Comm. **23:** 526–534.
11. Von Wartburg, J. P., J. Papenberg & H. Aebi. The heterogeneity of horse liver alcohol dehydrogenase. In preparation.
12. Von Wartburg, J. P. 1966. Alcohol dehydrogenase distribution in tissues of different species. Internatl. Symposium Alcohol and Alcoholism. Santiago de Chile, Aug. 1966. Proceedings. In press.

HYPERRIGIDITY AND HYPERTHERMIA ASSOCIATED WITH ANESTHESIA

B. A. Britt* and W. Kalow†

University of Toronto, Toronto, Canada

INTRODUCTION

A number of reports have recently appeared which describe the occurrence of extreme hyperthermia during or immediately after general anesthesia often associated with rigidity.[1–18] One of us has had firsthand experience with two such cases in the operating theatre. Several patients have been described to us by personal communication, so that we are aware of about 75 cases. However, sufficient information to permit summarization was available to us for only 39 patients to whom 42 anesthetics were administered.[2–4, 6–18] Cardiac arrest and death occurred in 25 of the 39 patients. Even in these cases the available information was often incomplete, particularly in regard to the sequence of events. Nevertheless an attempt at a synopsis of all available material appears to be worthwhile.

Epidemiology and Classification of Patients

The incidence of hyper-rigidity and hyperthermia is undoubtedly rare, but apparently not as rare as the anesthetic literature to date might lead one to think. During the past two or three years, the frequency of cases being reported has been increasing. This is probably due to the growing awareness of the problem by anesthesiologists.

A rough estimate of incidence in one section of a population may be obtained from the following data. In the Hospital for Sick Children in Toronto, Canada, four cases were observed. The first of these, which occurred about three years ago, resulted in the introduction of routine continuous thermometry during anesthesia in the hospital. Thus there is some assurance that no hyperthermic patients have been overlooked since. The total number of general anesthetics from that time was approximately 43,000 so that a crude estimate would be 1 in 10,000. The 95% confidence limits of this estimate in round figures are between 1:5,000 and 1:70,000 (binomial limits; for the calculation of the lower limits of this estimate, the initial attention-drawing case has not been counted in). It must be recognized, of course, that incidence figures based on records of a children's hospital are not necessarily representative of a whole population since the occurrence is not confined to children.

The age distribution of the cases is shown in TABLE 1. The ages ranged from 3 to 47 but the highest incidence was found in the younger age groups. The majority of patients are known to be Caucasian but at least three Negroes have also been reported. Males were affected nearly twice as commonly as were females (25 males and 14 females).

Rigidity was associated with the hyperthermia in 28 of the 42 anesthetics (TABLE 2). In 22 of these 28 cases succinylcholine was employed. In all cases its administration was followed not by the usual sequence of fasciculation and paralysis but rather by a sudden and prolonged rigidity which tended to pass into rigor mortis. In the remaining six cases the onset of the rigidity was somewhat

* Departments of Anesthesia and Pharmacology.

† Department of Pharmacology.

TABLE 1

CASES OF HYPERTHERMIA SORTED BY AGE, OCCURRENCE OF RIGIDITY, DEATH AND SURVIVAL

Age (years)	Rigidity Present		Rigidity Not Present	
	D*	S†	D*	S†
1 – 5	1	7	1	0
6 – 10	1	2	0	1
11 – 15	3	1	1	0
16 – 20	3	0	2	0
21 – 25	3	1	2	1
26 – 30	1	0	0	0
31 – 35	0	0	2	0
36 – 40	0	1	1	1
41 – 45	3	1	1	0
46 – 50	0	0	0	1
Totals	15	13	10	4

* Died.
† Survived.

TABLE 2

CLASSIFICATION OF HYPERTHERMIA PATIENTS BY OCCURRENCE OF RIGIDITY, SURVIVAL, AND USE OF SUCCINYLCHOLINE

		Died	Survived	Totals
Rigidity	with succinylcholine	13	9	22
	without succinylcholine	2	4	6
No Rigidity	with succinylcholine	10	4	14
	without succinylcholine	0	0	0

TABLE 3

SURGERY IN CASES OF HYPERTHERMIA

Type of Operation	Rigidity Present	Rigidity Not Present
Ophthalmological	3	1
Otolaryngological	3	0
Genito-Urinary	3	0
Gynecological	0	1
Orthopedic	12	2
Plastic	1	3
General	3	6
Unknown	3	1
Total	28	14

delayed and its development gradual. As will be seen, the cases characterized by rigidity differed in several other features from those not associated with rigidity.

The patients were anesthetized for a large variety of operations (TABLE 3). While in the "rigidity" group the greatest number of operations were classified as orthopedic; this was not so with the "nonrigidity" group. A considerable number of patients, twelve, were found to have preexisting musculo-skeletal disease. In all of these patients rigidity developed during the course of their anesthetic (TABLE

4). Thus it seems worthwhile to continue to look for a possible connection between musculo-skeletal disease and hyperpyrexia.

A possible allergic or immunological involvement has been noted in five patients. That is, an elevated eosinophil count (10%) was found in one, urticaria in the arm into which succinylcholine was injected in another, polymyositis in a third, a chronic maculo-papular rash aggravated by sun in a fourth, and red blotches following probathine administration in a fifth. Allergies were not observed in 7 other patients and no record was available for the remaining 27 patients.

Nine of the 39 patients had had previous general anesthetics for a variety of conditions, four on more than one occasion. In two patients the anesthetic was a rather long one which would make one suspect that these patients did not have a prior tendency to hyperpyrexia. Furthermore, neither of these two patients displayed rigidity when they reacted with hyperthermia.

Three patients showed a hyperthermic reaction associated with rigidity on two different occasions. The second anesthetic technique in each case was essentially similar to the first one. A fourth patient who exhibited rigidity as well as hyperthermia and was also reanesthetized a second time did not have a recurrence. However, the type of anesthesia was purposely changed. The anesthetic technique employed for this patient on the second occasion involved intermittent i.v. injection of pethidine, local laryngeal anesthesia, and administration of a mixture of nitrous oxide and oxygen, while volatile anesthetics and muscle relaxants were avoided.

Five patients showed familial involvement.[2,3,8,9,16] Two patients who both expired on the operating room table within three months of each other were an aunt and a niece. The brother of one of the patients described here has recently died under the same circumstances in another city. Two of the cases reported by Carpenter were siblings. Denborough and his collaborators in Australia reported some years ago a large family tree indicating that 10 out of 38 patients at risk had died following general anesthesia (FIGURE 1). Exact records were not available in all cases but hyperthermia played a role in at least some of them.[2,3] All patients with a positive family history displayed rigidity during anesthesia. On the other hand, none of the patients who did not develop rigidity had a positive family history.

Since there is this evidence of an hereditary factor in man it is interesting to note that two families of pigs are known to suffer from what appears to be a similar

TABLE 4

PRESENCE OR ABSENCE OF RIGIDITY IN HYPERTHERMIC PATIENTS WITH PREVIOUS MUSCULOSKELETAL DISEASE*

Previous Musculoskeletal Disease	Rigidity: Present	Rigidity: Not Present
Idiopathic Kyphoscoliosis	5	0
Herniated nucleus pulposus	2	0
Arthrogryposis	1	0
Equinovarus	1	0
Pes Excavatum	1	0
Umbilical hernia	1	0
Strabismus	3	0
Polymyositis	1	0

* Two or more musculo-skeletal diseases were present in 3 patients.

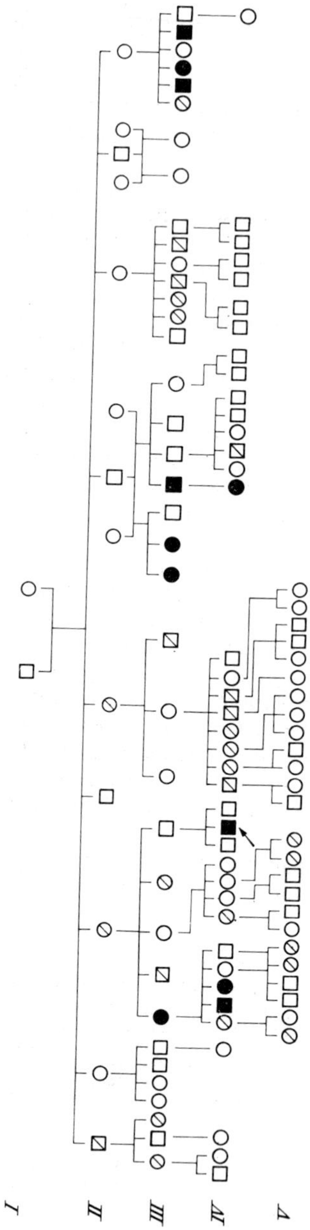

FIGURE 1. Pedigree indicating fatal reaction (hyperthermia) to general anesthesia. Square shapes = males; round shapes = females; black areas = fatal reaction; area with diagonal line = normal reaction; blank areas = not exposed, i.e., no anesthetic received. Courtesy of Denborough *et al.*[3] and Brit. J. Anaesthesia.

condition. In one family[19] three 6-month-old male littermates all died during a succinylcholine-halothane anesthesia with rigidity and temperatures of 111°F. All the remaining littermates were subsequently found to be affected. When the sow was then rebred to a different and presumably normal boar, one out of the ten littermates was still affected. There would thus, in the case of this pig family at least, appear to be a dominant inheritance of an abnormal responsiveness to general anesthesia.

Drugs and Laboratory Findings

The following material is a summary of as many clinical data as were available and seemed to be pertinent. Unfortunately, it took considerable time to prepare this summary; on the other hand, it was recognized only in recent days that the cases with hyperthermia could be divided profitably into those with and without rigidity. We have, therefore, not been able to apply the criterion of rigidity uniformly during the following analysis of data.

Let us first consider the agents used in preparation for or in the conduction of anesthesia. A considerable variety of preoperative atropine-like agents, sedatives, and induction agents were employed. The frequency of use of different types of agents does not seem to be unusual (TABLE 5).

Succinylcholine was given to assist intubation in 36 anesthetics. Prolonged rigidity ensued in 22, 13 of whom succumbed (TABLE 2). Further increments of succinylcholine injected into eight patients intensified muscle stiffness in all cases. Four of the six patients who are known not to have received succinylcholine survived. The administration of repeated doses of curare in four patients and of gallamine in one patient in all instances aggravated the rigidity.

Because of inability to open the jaws, intubation was difficult in 13 out of the 18 cases in which the matter was commented upon.

Inhalational agents more potent than N_2O were administered in all except two anesthetics (TABLE 5). Five patients received more than one agent. Halothane was the most usual, being given to 35 patients, 22 of whom died. All three patients who received methoxyflurane expired. Nonfluorinated substances such as ether and cyclo-propane were also employed in a few cases. Two patients received no inhalational agent other than N_2O and both of these recovered.

Prior to operation, the temperature was normal in eleven patients and slightly elevated in two in whom infection was present. Between 10 minutes and 4½ hours after the induction of the anesthetic, the temperature was found to be elevated in all 42 cases, though exact records are not available for four patients. The maximum level attained varied from 100.1°F to 112°F with a median maximum temperature of 108°F (TABLE 6). In the two cases in which the maximum temperature was less than 102°F, anesthesia was discontinued within 3 or 4 minutes of the induction and both of these patients recovered. All patients with temperatures higher than 109°F died.

Tachycardia occurred in 30 patients–the rate varied from 110 to 190 per minute. The heart rate was apparently not recorded in the other anesthetics. In many of the reports the time relationship of onset of tachycardia to temperature rise is not clearly stated.

A variety of observations were made about the skin. The most common comment (in 14 cases), as might be expected, was that the skin was hot. Four authors noted that the skin was flushed while three considered it to be pale. Five reports mentioned dryness of the skin, but two others conversely noted sweating. Cyanosis of the skin or darkness of the blood was noted during 12 anesthetics, in spite of

TABLE 5

PREOPERATIVE AND ANESTHETIC AGENTS

Atropine-Like Agent	No. of Cases	Sedative Agent	No. of Cases	Induction Agent	No. of Cases	Inhalational Agent Other than N_2O	No. of Cases
Atropine	22	Pethidine	19	Thiopentone	28	Halothane	31
Scopolamine	11	Morphine	4	Methohexitone	1	Methoxyflurane	2
Promethazine	1	Secobarbital	3	Halothane	6	Cyclopropane	1
No Record	6	Phenobarbital	1	Cyclopropane	3	Halothane and Ether	2
None	2	Pentobarbital	8	No Record	4	Halothane and Cyclopropane	1
		Hydroxyzine Pamoate	3			Halothane, Ether and Cyclopropane	1
		Promethazine	1			Ether and Cyclopropane	1
						Methoxyflurane and Cyclopropane	1
		No Record	7			None	2
		None	6				

TABLE 6

MAXIMUM TEMPERATURES

°F	Died	Survived
99.0 – 101.9	0	2
102.0 – 104.9	1	1
105.0 – 107.9	7	7
108.0 – 110.9	15	3
> 111.0	2	0

adequate artificial ventilation with an oxygen-enriched mixture. Rigidity was present in all except one of these latter cases.

Arterial CO_2 tension was elevated in six anesthetics—the maximum level varying between 54 and 179 mm Hg. In one of these cases an elevation to 100 mm Hg was detected within 5 minutes of the induction and prior to any temperature rise. Arterial CO_2 tension was normal in two patients, low in one patient and the test was apparently not performed during the 33 other anesthetics (TABLE 7).

The pH was measured in nine patients and found to be low in all nine, the minimum point reached varied from 6.80 to 7.32 (TABLE 7). Metabolic acidosis as determined by base deficit calculation was noted in seven patients. The deficit varied from −6 to −24.5 mEq/L. A base excess of +3mEq/L was present in one patient. No record was available for the remaining cases (TABLE 7).

Serum potassium was measured in six patients. In three, all of whom displayed rigidity and all of whom died, it was elevated to between 8.0 and 19 mEq/L. In the other three, none of whom were rigid, and all of whom survived, it was within normal limits (TABLE 7). Because of the small sample size chi-square estimation is not warranted.

Hemo- or myoglobinuria was present in seven patients, four of whom failed to recover (TABLE 7). Prothrombin time was prolonged in both of the two patients in whom it was measured (21 and 35 seconds) and both expired (TABLE 7).

TABLE 7

LABORATORY FINDINGS

	Numbers of Patients				Range of Measurements
	High	Low	Normal	No Record	
Arterial CO_2 tension	6	1	2	33	high – 54–179 mm Hg low – 21 mm Hg
pH	0	9	0	33	6.8 – 7.32
Base Excess	1	7	0	34	low = −6 to −24.5 mEq/L high = +3 mEq/L
Serum Potassium	3*	3†	0	36	high = 8 – 19 mEq/L low = 3.1 – 4.7 mEq/L
Hemo- or Myoglobinuria	7	–	0	35	++++ (no quantity)
Prothrombin Time	0	2	0	40	21 – 35 seconds

* Rigidity present
† Rigidity absent

Miscellaneous arrhythmias were recorded by EKG monitoring in six patients. They included atrial and ventricular tachycardia and extrasystoles and changes characteristic of hyperkalemia.

Muscle biopsies carried out on three patients[8] showed normal staining with hematoxylin and eosin but round densities in sections fixed with osmic acid. Under the electron microscope, these appeared to be dense globules of lipid resulting from mitochondrial degeneration. SGOT* and CPK† levels were markedly elevated in the same three patients for several days. All these patients had developed rigidity immediately following succinylcholine administration and all had muscle weakness and tenderness for several days following operation.

None of the many drugs employed appear to have significantly improved the survival rate of 35.9% with the possible exception of buffers (TABLE 8), though they were not used often enough to permit a conclusion. Buffers (sodium bicarbonate or THAM) were given in 11 cases, 6 of whom died. Whether the amounts of buffer administered were adequate is an open question. Seven out of the eight patients to whom vasopressors were administered expired; these drugs either have worsened the chance of recovery or they may have been terminal and futile treatment. All three patients who were known to have received calcium salts also failed to recover, but in one of these the author reported that calcium gluconate injection was followed by a transient lessening of rigidity and improvement of the cardiovascular status.[16] Four of the five patients who received steroids succumbed. Four other patients to whom steroids were not given all survived.

* SGOT = serum glutamic oxalic transaminase.
† CPK = pyruvate kinase.

TABLE 8

DRUG TREATMENT

		Died	Survived
Buffers			
	Used	6	5
	Not used	0	2
	No record	18	13
Vasopressors			
	Used	7	1
	Not used	0	2
	No record	17	15
Tranquilizers			
	Used	1	0
	Not used	0	2
	No Record	23	16
Potassium salts			
	Used	2	0
	Not used	0	4
	No record	22	14
Calcium Salts			
	Used	3	0
	Not used	0	4
	No record	21	14
Steroids			
	Used	4	1
	Not used	0	4
	No record	20	13

TABLE 9

TREATMENT BY COOLING

	Cooling Used		Cooling Not Used		No Record		
	D*	S†	D*	S†	D*	S†	Total
Rigidity	9	9	2	4	4	0	28
No Rigidity	8	3	2	1	0	0	14
Total	17	12	4	5	4	0	42

* died
† survived

Hypothermia was applied to 29 patients, 12 of whom survived (TABLE 9). Its use appears to be somewhat more effective in the "rigidity" group of cases.

Speculations on Possible Aetiology

It seems that most efforts to reach some understanding of the causes of hyperthermia after general anesthesia took account of the rigidity which, however, does not always accompany hyperthermia. Nevertheless, a brief report recording possible causes may still be warranted.

Fifteen patients were autopsied and apart from changes characteristic of anoxia, nothing of note was detected.

The cause or causes could be central[20–30] or peripheral. Clinical findings do not favor a central cause. The rigidity appears to be a continuous muscle stiffness, without visible fasciculations and without a following paralytic phase; in other words, it appears clinically, at least, to be a myotonia rather than a tetanic contraction, but to date no work has been carried out to delineate this point. The early rise in arterial CO_2 tension preceding temperature rise that has been noted in one patient would also favor a peripheral cause. Moreover, patients who have received trauma to the hypothalamic temperature regulating center do not display the extreme metabolic acidosis and hyperkalemia that has been observed in this syndrome. Furthermore, while patients suffering from severe heat stroke with irreversible damage to the temperature regulating center do manifest metabolic acidosis and potassium intoxication, their muscles are frequently found to be flaccid, and rigidity occurs only as a terminal rather than an initial event.[31–34]

In favor of a peripheral cause several authors such as Wilson[35] have drawn attention to some similarities between these patients and poisoning by dinitrophenol. Snodgrass[36] has shown that halothane and other halogenated hydrocarbons are true uncouplers of oxidative phosphorylation. However, his work was done in vitro and at very high concentrations of halothane in mitochondria.

Experimental results obtained in our laboratory have tended to deemphasize these similarities. Intraperitoneal dinitrophenol administration, while certainly elevating temperature, is not associated with rigidity in the living rat as measured by myography, nor does the addition of halothane heighten muscle tone. These findings agree with a similar study carried out on chickens by Viguera.[37]

In another study we determined the dose response curves for halothane and dinitrophenol using batches of 10 male rats each. These curves were found not to be parallel (FIGURE 2) (TABLE 10). When we then administered a half LD50 of both halothane and dinitrophenol to batches of ten male rats, the mortality

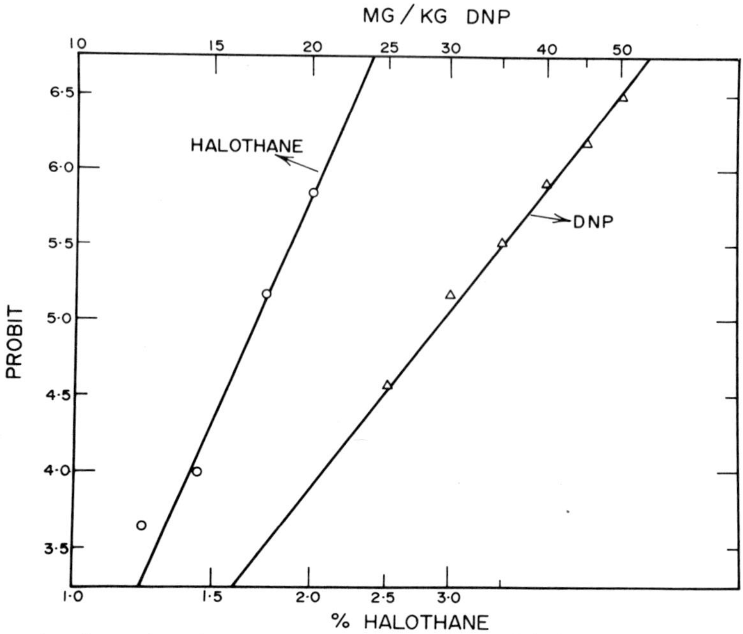

FIGURE 2. Comparison between dose-response curves of halothane and dinitrophenol (DNP) in rats. Each symbol indicates groups of 10 adult male rats; their response measured as percent dead is expressed in probit units. The lower scale of the abscissa indicates concentration of halothane vapor in the air to which the rats were exposed for 3 hours. The upper scale of the abscissa indicates milligrams of dinitrophenol injected i.p. per kg of body weight. In each case, rates of death were counted after 24 hours. See TABLE 10 for statistical parameters.

TABLE 10

RESPONSE CURVES FOR HALOTHANE AND DINITROPHENOL

	Slope	S.E. (Slope)	LD50	95% Limits	Homogeneity of Data	Test for Parallelism of Lines
Halothane	12.01	0.90	1.72%	1.68 – 1.77	$^{2}_{(6)} = 6.52$ n.s.	$^{2}_{(1)} = 18.55$ (P 0.001)
DNP	6.59	0.94	30.3 mg/kg	28.3 – 32.1	$^{2}_{(7)} = 7.34$ n.s.	

rate was found to be 78%—a moderate but not an overwhelming increase above the mortality of 50% which would have been expected if the two agents had had the same mode of lethal action. Thus, dinitrophenol appears to act in a different manner from halothane, and dinitrophenol only moderately potentiates the action of halothane.

Obviously many other working hypotheses remain to be tested. If an experimental model such as a strain of affected pigs could be obtained, it would be of interest to see if rigidity and hyperthermia developed in a denervated or occluded limb after succinylcholine and halothane administration.

Conclusion

We have collected information on those rare patients who respond to general anesthesia with malignant hyperthermia. It seems possible to bring some order into the complex set of data by dividing the cases into those characterized by rigidity and those characterized by absence of rigidity. In the former group there is not infrequently preexisting musculoskeletal disease, familial involvement, recurrence during subsequent anesthetics, arterial desaturation and occasionally hyperpotassemia, elevated SGOT, CPK and muscle biopsy abnormalities. None of these features have been observed in the latter group. Thus more than one entity appears to be represented among these cases. Some may be genetic and some may be acquired.

With regard to treatment, the best treatment is undoubtedly prevention. In the selection of an anesthetic technique for affected patients or patients with a known positive family history, the limited experience suggests that regional or conduction anesthesia or a narcotic-N_2O/O_2 mixture may be safe. Continuous temperature monitoring cannot be too highly recommended. If rigidity develops following succinylcholine administration, anesthesia should be immediately discontinued. If hyperthermia does occur, vigorous cooling, preferably by intragastric and rectal lavage has been instituted at some local hospitals, apparently with good success. Very large doses of buffers would appear to be warranted since the ideal intracellular pH for maximum enzyme activity has been said to increase with increasing temperature.[38] Hyperventilation with 100% O2 should be maintained till consciousness has fully returned. Finally, we can only hope that these precautions will help to prevent further deaths from this obscure syndrome.

References

1. Inhalation Anaesthesia. 1952. Guedel, 2nd ed. Macmillan Co. N. Y.
2. Denborough, M. A. & R. H. Lovell. 1960. Anaesthetic Deaths in a Family. Lancet **II:** 45.
3. Denborough, M. A., J. F. A. Forster & P. A. Maplestone. 1962. Anaesthetic Deaths in a Family. B.J.A. **34:** 395.
4. Ruttle, L. D. 1962. Case Report 247. Death occurred in the operating room following extreme hyperthermia during an elective cholecystectomy. American Society of Anesthesiologists' Newsletter July 1962 : 21.
5. Comment on Case Report No. 247. 1962. American Society of Anesthesiologists' Newsletter August 1962 WAC (Calif.) : 30.
6. Comment on Case Report No. 247. 1962. American Society of Anesthesiologists' Newsletter November 1962 PSM (Mass.) : 11.
7. Saidman, L. J., E. S. Havard & E. I. Eger. 1964. Hyperthermia During Anesthesia. J.A.M.A. **190:** 1029.
8. Carpenter, G. G., V. H. Auerbach, A. M. DiGeorge, B. W. Mayer & H. S. Schutta. 1966. Rhabdomyolysis after routine administration of succinylcholine in children. The Society for Pediatric Research Apr. 29–30, 1966 : 175.
9. Relton, J. E. S., D. A. Pelton & A. W. Conn. 1966. Hyperpyrexia in association with general anaesthesia in children. C.A.S.J. **13:** 419.
10. Thut, W. H. & H. T. Davenport. 1966. Hyperpyrexia associated with succinylcholine-induced muscle rigidity: A case report. C.A.S.J. **13:** 425.
11. Hogg, S. & W. Renwick. 1966. Hyperthermia during anaesthesia. C.A.S.J. **13:** 429.
12. Cullen, W. G. 1966. Malignant hyperpyrexia during general anaesthesia: A report of 2 cases. C.A.S.J. **13:** 437.
13. Lavoie, G. 1966. Hyperpyrexia during general anaesthesia: A case report. C.A.S.J. **13:** 444.
14. Davies, L. E. & H. B. Graves. 1966. Hyperpyrexia and death associated with general anaesthesia. C.A.S.J. **13:** 447.
15. Relton, J. E. S., R. E. Creighton, A. W. Conn & S. Nabeta. 1967. Generalized muscular hypertonicity associated with general anaesthesia: A suggested anaesthetic manage-

ment. C.A.S.J. **14:** 22.
16. Purkis, I. E., O. Horrelt, G. deYoung, R. A. P. Fleming & G. R. Langley. 1967. Hyperpyrexia following anaesthesia in a second member of a family, with associated coagulation defect. Canad. Anaesth. Soc. **14:** 183.
17. Stephen, C. R. 1967. Fulminant hyperthermia during anesthesia and surgery. J.A.M.A. **202:** 178.
18. Wilson, R. D., T. E. Dent, D. L. Traber, N. R. McCoy & C. R. Allen. 1967. Malignant hyperpyrexia with anesthesia. J.A.M.A. **202:** 183.
19. Hall, L. W., N. Woolf, J. W. Bradley & D. W. Jolly. 1966. Unusual reaction to suxemethonium chloride. B.M.J. **26:** 1305.
20. Clark, G., H. W. Magoun & S. W. Ranson. 1939. Hypothalamic Regulation of Body Temperature. J. Neurophysiol. **2:** 61.
21. Burton, A. C. 1956. The clinical importance of the physiology of temperature regulation. C.M.A.J. **75:** 715.
22. Pickering, G. 1958. Regulation of body temperature in health and disease. The Lancet **II:** 59.
23. Domer, F. R. & W. Feldberg. 1960. Tremor in cats: The effect of administration of drugs into the cerebral ventricles. Brit. J. Pharmacol. **15:** 578.
24. Hardy, J. D. 1961. Physiology of temperature regulation. Physiol. Rev. **41:** 521.
25. Carmichael, E. A., W. Feldberg & K. Fleischhauer. 1962. The site of origin of the tremor produced by tubocurarine acting from the cerebral ventricles. J. Physiol. **162:** 539.
26. Feldberg, W. & R. D. Myers. 1963. A new concept of temperature regulation by amines in the hypothalamus. Nature **28:** 1325.
27. Feldberg, W. & R. D. Myers. 1964. Temperature changes produced by amines injected into the cerebral ventricles during anesthesia. J. Physiol. **175:** 464.
28. Feldberg, W. & R. D. Myers. 1965. Changes in temperature produced by microinjections of amines into the anterior hypothalamus of cats. J. Physiol. **177:** 239.
29. Cranston, W. I. 1966. Temperature Regulation. B.M.J. **II:** 69.
30. Nielsen, B. 1966. Regulation of body temperature and heat dissipation at different levels of energy and heat production in man. Acta Physiol. Scand. **68:** 215.
31. Daily, W. M. & R. H. Tinsley. 1948. A study of the mechanism and treatment of experimental heat pyrexia. Am. J. Med. Sc. **215:** 42.
32. Baxter, C. R. & P. E. Teschan. 1958. Atypical heat stroke with hypernatremia, acute renal failure and fulminating potassium intoxication. Arch. Int. Med. **101:** 1040.
33. Kumar, P., C. K. Rathore, A. M. Nagar & M. P. Mehrotra. 1964. Hyperpyrexia with special reference to heat stroke. J. Indian Med. Ass. **43:** 213.
34. Wakim, K. G. 1964. Bodily reactions to high temperature. Anaesthesiology **25:** 532.
35. Wilson, R. D., T. J. Nichols, T. E. Dent & C. R. Allen. 1966. Disturbances of the oxidative-phosphorylation mechanism as a possible aetiological factor in sudden unexplained hyperthermia. Anaesthesiology **27:** 232.
36. Snodgrass, P. J. & M. M. Piras. 1966. The effects of halothane on rat liver mitochondria. Biochemistry **5:** 1140.
37. Viguera, M. G. & A. W. Conn. 1967. An investigation of general anaesthesia and hyperpyrexia in chickens. C.A.S.J. **14:** 193.
38. Morris, L. E. Personal communication.

Part IV. Pharmacogenetics and Drug Toxicity

VARIATION OF DRUG METABOLISM IN ANIMALS AND THE PREDICTION OF DRUG ACTION IN MAN

J. J. Burns

Hoffmann-La Roche Inc.
Nutley, N. J.

Species differences in response to drugs must be considered in the extrapolation of pharmacological and toxicological data obtained in experimental animals to man. Many factors can explain species differences in drug response and they have been reviewed in the recent International Symposium on Comparative Pharmacology.[1] The most important factor appears to be the variation in the rate and pattern of drug metabolism in different animal species, but species differences may exist in renal excretion, binding to plasma proteins, tissue distribution and response of the drug at its "receptor site." It is the purpose of this paper to discuss the importance of drug metabolic studies in accounting for species differences in drug response.

Studies with the antirheumatic agent, phenylbutazone, have demonstrated in a striking way the importance of species differences in drug metabolism. Phenylbutazone is metabolized in man at a very slow rate with a half-life averaging three days.[2] However, in the monkey, dog, rabbit, rat, guinea pig and horse the drug is metabolized at a very rapid rate (TABLE 1). Knowledge of the rapid rate of metabolism of phenylbutazone in the horse is of practical importance in view of the fairly wide use of the drug in the treatment of arthritis in racehorses.

Information on the marked species differences in the metabolism of phenylbutazone has made it possible to demonstrate its anti-inflammatory and sodium-retaining effects in experimental animals. Phenylbutazone exerts an anti-inflammatory effect in patients with rheumatoid arthritis comparable to cortisone[3] and, like the steroid, is capable of blocking the inflammatory effect produced by glycerin injected into the anterior chamber of the rabbit eye.[4] However, in order to show this effect in the rabbit it was necessary to take into account the fact that the drug is metabolized much more rapidly in this species than in man (TABLE 1). When phenylbutazone was administered intramuscularly to the rabbit in a dose of 100 mg/kg every 8 hours, plasma levels ranged from 100–175 mg/l. which are comparable to those obtained in humans receiving a total daily dose of about 10 mg/kg. Similarly, in order to demonstrate sodium retention with phenylbutazone in the rat, it was also necessary to administer the drug at a high dosage (150 mg/kg orally) to achieve plasma levels of the same order as those which gave sodium retention in man.[3]

A striking species difference was noted in the metabolism of the experimental oxybarbiturate derivative, 5-allyl-5(2-bromo-2-cyclohexenyl)-2-barbituric acid. In the dog this drug disappeared at a very rapid rate (half-life less than one hour) and had a fleeting duration of action. However, when the drug was given to man, it disappeared at an extremely slow rate and its effects persisted for many hours (FIGURE 1).

In studies carried out in collaboration with Dr. Richard Welch of The Wellcome Research Laboratories, Tuckahoe, New York, the rate of metabolism of several representative drugs has been compared in the rhesus monkey, dog and man (TABLE 2). It was found that antipyrine, phenylbutazone, oxyphenbutazone and

TABLE 1

SPECIES DIFFERENCES IN THE METABOLISM OF PHENYLBUTAZONE

Species	Half-life hours
Man	72
Monkey	8
Dog	6
Rabbit	3
Rat	6
Guinea pig	5
Horse	6

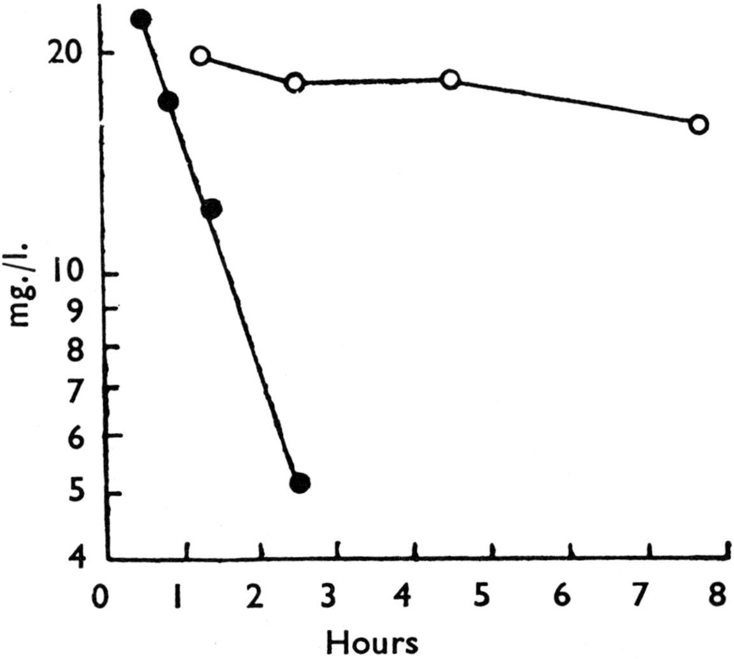

FIGURE 1. Plasma levels of 5-allyl-5(2-bromo-2-cyclohexenyl)-2-barbituric acid in man and dog.

TABLE 2

COMPARATIVE HALF-LIFE OF DRUGS IN VARIOUS SPECIES

	Man hr	Rhesus Monkey hr	Dog hr
Phenylbutazone	72	8	6
Oxyphenbutazone	72	8	0.5
Antipyrine	12	1.8	1.7
Meperidine	5.5	1.2	0.9

meperidine are metabolized at a considerably slower rate in man than in the rhesus monkey. In the case of all the drugs, except oxyphenbutazone, their rate of metabolism is about the same in the rhesus monkey as in the dog. It is of interest to note that oxyphenbutazone is metabolized at an extremely rapid rate in the dog with a biological half-life of less than one hour. In general, these data show that the rhesus monkey metabolizes phenylbutazone, meperidine and antipyrine more like the dog than like man. It would appear from these results and from those presented at a recent conference[5] that more research must be carried out before metabolic data in monkeys can be accepted as predictable for drug action in man.

There are unusual differences in the manner in which animal species metabolize the anticoagulant drug, ethyl biscoumacetate.[6] Man and rabbit both metabolize the drug rapidly with a biological half-life of about two hours, and in both species it exerts a brief anticoagulant effect. The dog, on the other hand, metabolizes ethyl biscoumacetate extremely slowly, so slowly in fact that pharmacological studies of the drug in the dog would have given little indication of its short action in man. Although man and rabbit metabolize ethyl biscoumacetate at about the same rapid rate, they do so by different mechanisms (FIGURE 2). The rabbit metabolizes the drug by hydrolysis of the ester group to form an inactive acid derivative. In contrast, man inactivates ethyl biscoumacetate by introduction of a phenolic group into the benzene ring. Thus, it is possible to have qualitative as well as quantitative differences in drug metabolism among animal species.

Marked species differences have also been observed in the metabolic fate of the analgesic drug, N-acetyl-*p*-aminophenol (APAP).[7] In man and dog the drug is mainly excreted in the urine as a glucuronide conjugate (TABLE 3). However, no detectable glucuronide of the drug was found in the urine of cats receiving the drug. The nature of conjugates formed by the cat is not known. The failure of this species to form glucuronides can be explained by the absence of the neces-

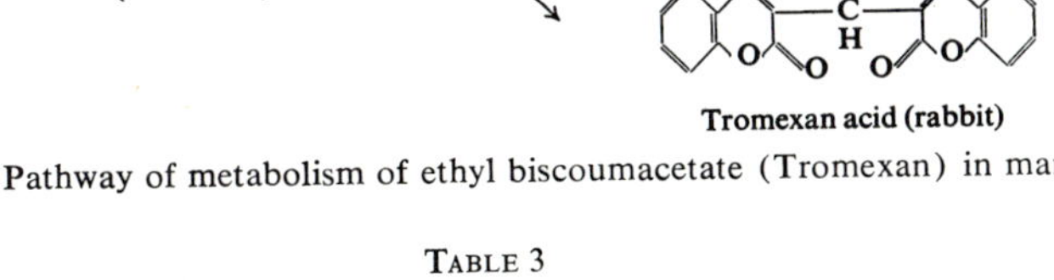

FIGURE 2. Pathway of metabolism of ethyl biscoumacetate (Tromexan) in man and rabbit.

TABLE 3

METABOLISM OF N-ACETYL-P-AMINOPHENOL (APAP) IN DIFFERENT ANIMAL SPECIES

	Percent of APAP dose in urine		
Species	Total Conjugates by Acid Hydrolysis	APAP Glucuronide	APAP Sulfate
Man	90	58	4.4
Dog	78	54	4.1
Cat	78	<3	<2

sary liver enzyme required for the conjugation reaction. It is possible that the altered metabolism of APAP in the cat explains the sensitivity of this species to the drug.

Marked species differences also exist in the metabolism of L-ascorbic acid.[8] Man, monkey and guinea pig, unlike all other species studied, cannot synthesize L-ascorbic acid; vitamin C must be included in the diet to prevent scurvy. These animal species lack an enzyme system in their liver microsomes required for the oxidation of L-gulonolactone to L-ascorbic acid. Differences also exist in the fate of L-ascorbic acid in man and guinea pig (FIGURE 3). The rate of metabolism of L-ascorbic acid in the guinea pig (half-life 4 days) is much faster than that in man (half-life 16 days). The persistence of L-ascorbic acid in man is correlated with the much longer time it takes human subjects to show signs of scurvy. For instance, it requires about four months for humans on a vitamin C free diet to develop scurvy, while guinea pigs on such a diet become markedly scorbutic in about three weeks.

Two important factors which must be considered in the evaluation of species differences in drug metabolism are as follows: (1) Intraspecies differences in drug metabolism; (2) Effect of drugs, insecticides and other environmental chemicals to stimulate drug metabolism.

Marked individual differences exist in the metabolism of drugs within the same species which has been explained on a genetic basis by other papers in this Annal. Thus, a sufficient number of animals in a given species must be studied before conclusions concerning interspecies differences can be made. This is well illustrated from data in FIGURE 4 which indicate considerable variation in the metabolism

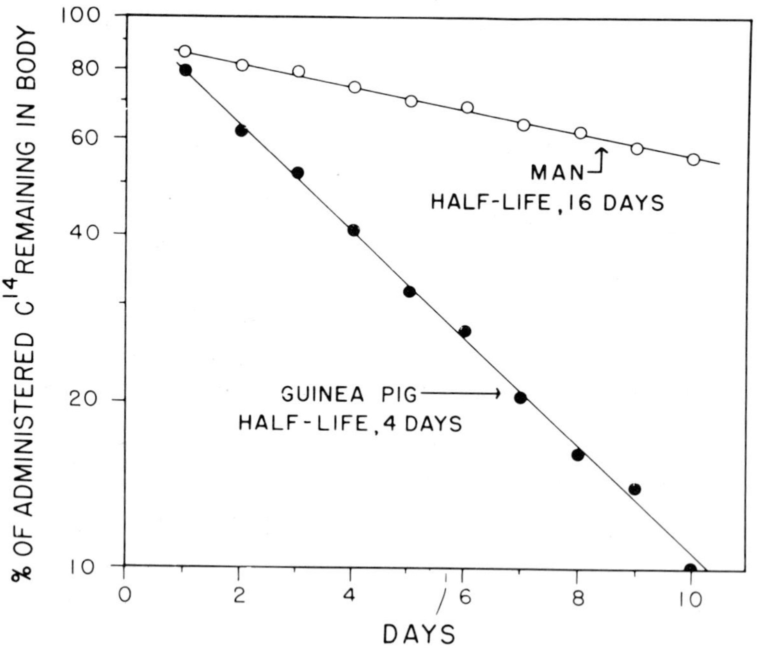

FIGURE 3. Disappearance of L-ascorbic acid-1-C^{14} after its administration to man and guinea pig.

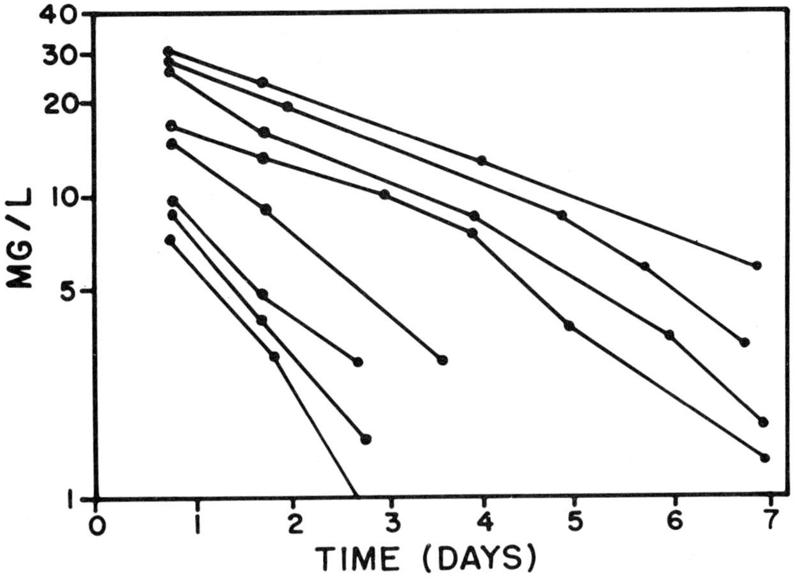

FIGURE 4. Plasma levels of Dicumarol after i.v. administration of 5 mg/kg to various subjects.

in man of the anticoagulant drug, bishydroxycoumarin (Dicumarol). The rate of metabolism of this drug may vary from a biological half-life of 7 to 100 hours. In some subjects, levels remain elevated for more than seven days, while in other subjects negligible levels were reached in less than three days. The wide individual differences in the metabolism of this drug are an important factor in explaining why it is difficult to predict the dosage needed to obtain a desired prothrombin response.

Considerable individual variations have been noted in the metabolism of ascorbic acid in man, rat and guinea pig. Conclusions to be drawn on species differences must be considered in light of these intraspecies differences in the metabolism of the vitamin. These differences can explain why individual needs in requirement for the vitamin can vary over a wide range. A discussion of individual requirements for vitamin C in man and guinea pig has recently been presented.[9]

Studies in recent years have shown that pretreatment of animals with various drugs, insecticides, food additives and carcinogenic hydrocarbons can increase the ability of the animal to metabolize both the administered chemical as well as other related and unrelated compounds. It is now well established that this enhancing effect on drug metabolism results from increased activity of drug-metabolizing enzymes in liver microsomes, which is referred to as enzyme induction.[10,11]

In studying species differences in drug metabolism, it is important to know whether environmental factors, such as prior administration of another drug or exposure to an insecticide or other chemical, may influence the metabolism of the drug under study. The marked stimulatory effect of chronic phenobarbital administration on the metabolism of antipyrine in the dog and monkey is shown in FIGURE 5.[12] In FIGURE 6 the stimulatory effect of the insecticide, Chlordane, on antipyrine metabolism in the dog is shown. It is apparent that conclusions concerning the metabolic rate of antipyrine in these species would be erroneous if one were not aware that the animals had been exposed to another drug or to the insecticide. Thus, such environmental factors always must be considered in the interpretation of genetically controlled inter- and intraspecies differences in drug metabolism.

Enzyme induction has been observed in many species including rat, dog, mouse, rabbit, monkey and man. However, there are examples where a drug will stimulate its own metabolism in one species but not in another. For instance, a marked stimulation in the metabolism of phenylbutazone occurs following its chronic administration to dogs.[12] The data in TABLE 4 show a marked fall-off in plasma levels of the drug when dogs received 100 mg/kg/day for a period of 20 days. However, a similar effect does not occur in humans who receive the drugs chronically. As shown in FIGURE 7, the plasma level of phenylbutazone remains fairly constant for each individual over a period of 4 to 14 days after administration of 800 mg/day of the drug.[2] In other studies, no decline in plasma levels of phenylbutazone was observed when patients continuously received 400 mg/day for periods up to six months. A similar species difference in enzyme induction has been reported to occur with the hypoglycemic agent, tolbutamide.[13] Chronic administration of the drug to dogs results in marked stimulation of its metabolism, but this effect has not been observed in patients receiving the drug for many months.

Summary

Knowledge of species differences in drug metabolism aids in extrapolating and relating pharmacological and toxicological data from experimental animals to man. Examples of such species differences have been given in this paper from studies with antirheumatic, anticoagulant, analgesic and hypnotic drugs. Species

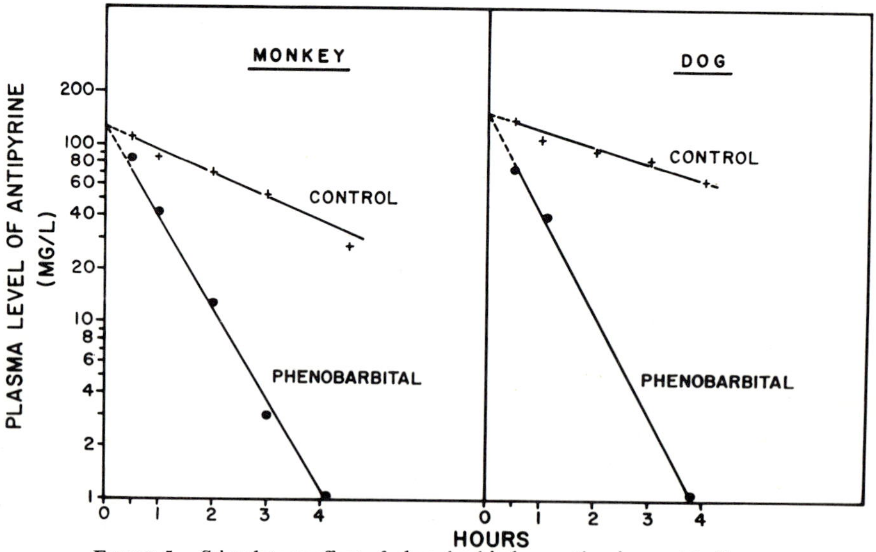

FIGURE 5. Stimulatory effect of phenobarbital on antipyrine metabolism.

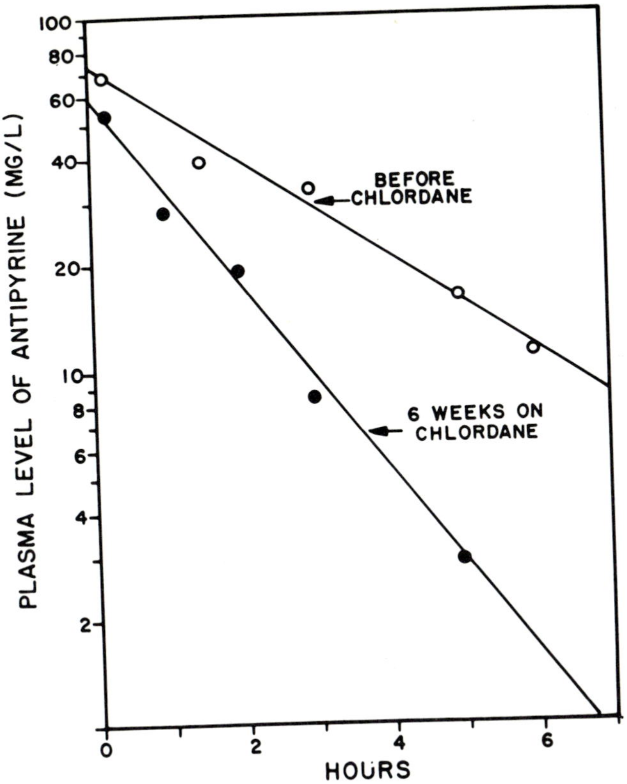

FIGURE 6. Stimulatory effect of Chlordane (5 mg/kg p.o. 3 times weekly) on antipyrine metabolism in the dog.

TABLE 4

PLASMA CONCENTRATION AFTER DAILY ADMINISTRATION OF PHENYLBUTAZONE TO DOGS*

	Plasma Concentration (mg/l)		
Day	Dog 1	Dog 2	Dog 3
1	100	146	118
2	—	—	—
3	—	—	—
4	71	69	55
5–7	—	—	—
8	28	15	14
9–19	—	—	—
20	30	19	18

* Daily dose – 100 mg/kg

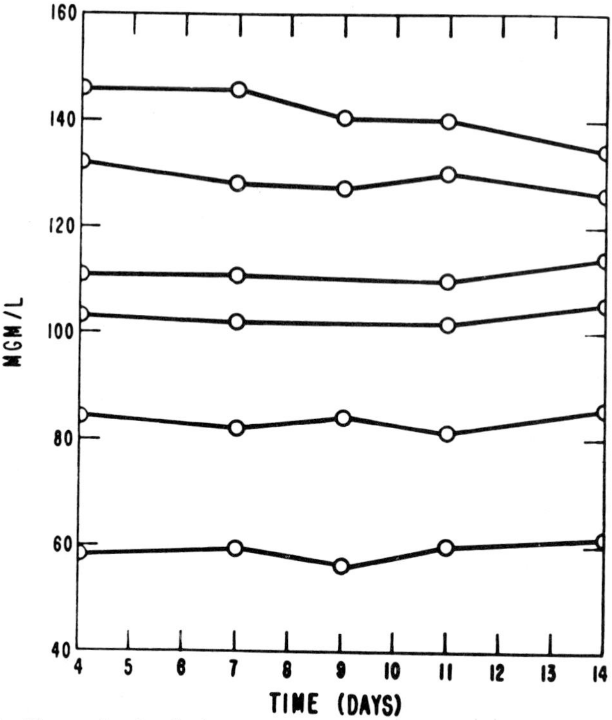

FIGURE 7. Plasma levels of phenylbutazone after oral administration of 800 mg/day of drug. Time indicates period from first day of drug administration.

differences in the metabolism of ascorbic acid were also discussed in terms of their importance in understanding the nutritional basis for the use of the vitamin. The importance of intraspecies differences in drug metabolism was discussed in terms of interpreting observed interspecies differences. In addition, it was also pointed out that exposure of experimental animals and man to drugs, insecticides and other environmental chemicals must be considered in drawing conclusions about the way any single species metabolizes the drug.

References

1. PROC. INTERNATIONAL SYMPOSIUM ON COMPARATIVE PHARMACOLOGY. 1967. Wash., D. C. Fed. Proc. **26:** No. 4.
2. BURNS, J. J., R. K. ROSE, T. CHENKIN, A. GOLDMAN, A. SCHULERT & B. B. BRODIE. 1953. The physiological disposition of phenylbutazone (Butazolidin) in man and a method for its estimation in biological material. J. Pharmacol. Exp. Ther. **109:** 346–357.
3. BRODIE, B. B., E. W. LOWMAN, J. J. BURNS, P. R. LEE, T. CHENKIN, A. GOLDMAN, M. WEINER & J. M. STEELE. 1954. Observations on the antirheumatic and physiologic effects of phenylbutazone (Butazolidin) and some comparisons with cortisone. Amer. J. Med. **16:** 181–190.
4. YOURISH, N., B. PATON, B. B. BRODIE & J. J. BURNS. 1955. Effect of phenylbutazone (Butazolidin) on experimentally induced ocular inflammation. Amer. Med. Assoc. Arch. Ophthalmology **53:** 264–266.
5. CONFERENCE ON NON-HUMAN PRIMATE TOXICOLOGY. 1966. FDA. In press.
6. BURNS, J. J., M. WEINER, G. SIMSON & B. B. BRODIE. 1953. The biotransformation of ethyl biscoumacetate (Tromexan) in man, rabbit and dog. J. Pharmacol. Exp. Ther. **108:** 33–41.

7. WELCH, R. M., A. H. CONNEY & J. J. BURNS. 1966. The metabolism of acetophenetidin and N-acetyl-p-aminophenol in the cat. Biochem. Pharmacol. **15:** 521–531.
8. BURNS, J. J. 1959. Biosynthesis of L-ascorbic acid; basic defect in scurvy. Amer. J. Med. **26:** 740–748.
9. WILLIAMS, R. J. & G. DEASON. 1967. Individuality in vitamin C needs. Proc. Natl. Acad. Sci. **57:** 1638–1641.
10. BURNS, J. J., S. A. CUCINELL, R. KOSTER & A. H. CONNEY. 1965. Application of drug metabolism to drug toxicity studies. Ann. N. Y. Acad. Sci. **123:** 273–286.
11. CONNEY, A. H. 1967. Pharmacological Implications of Microsomal Enzyme Induction. Pharmacological Reviews **19:** No. 3. The Williams & Wilkins Co., Balto., Md.
12. WELCH, R. M., Y. E. HARRISON & J. J. BURNS. 1967. Implications of enzyme induction in drug toxicity studies. Toxicol. Appl. Pharmacol. **10:** 340–351.
13. REMMER, H. 1962. *In* Ciba Foundation Symposium on Enzymes and Drug Action : 276. Little Brown & Co., Boston, Mass.

DISCUSSIONS OF THE PAPER

DR. H. W. GOEDDE (*Institute of Human Genetics, University of Hamburg*): Concerning the incidence of inter- and intraspecies variability in primates regarding pseudocholinesterase polymorphism: We found large qualitative and quantitative interspecies differences between man, *M. mulatta* (rhesus) and *C. aethiops sabaeus* (green cat). Great similarity was found between man and chimpanzee. An intraspecific polymorphism was found in *M. mulatta*. The methods used for these studies were spectophotometric measurements of specific activity, dibucaine number and fluoride number, electrophoresis in agar gel, diffusion in agar gel, immunoelectrophoresis and immunotitration.*

DR. F. F. FOLDES (*Montefiore Hospital, Bronx, N. Y.*): Dr. Burns in his excellent presentation emphasized that differences in the rate and pathways of metabolic transformation are primarily responsible for the marked species variation in the potency, duration of action and toxicity of drugs in man and other mammals. He also pointed out that the majority of drugs metabolized by the microsomal enzymes of the liver are detoxified more rapidly in most mammals, than in man. In this connection it may be worthwhile to mention that in contrast to drugs metabolized by the microsomal enzymes of the liver, those hydrolyzed by plasma butyrylcholinesterase (e.g. ester-type local anesthetic agents and muscle relaxants) are detoxified more rapidly in man, than in other mammals. Because of this the intensity and duration of action of ester-type muscle relaxants and the relative toxicity of hydrolyzable local anesthetic agents is less in man than in other mammals. Failing to take into consideration that local anesthetic agents metabolized by the microsomal enzymes of the liver are detoxified relatively more rapidly, and those hydrolyzed by plasma butyrylcholinesterase are detoxified relatively more slowly in laboratory animals than in man, led to unwarranted claims regarding the relative safety of the nonhydrolyzable local anesthetic agents in man. The uncritical acceptance of these claims resulted in severe toxic reactions, and even caused fatalities in patients to whom relatively large doses of these agents were administered.

Dr. Burns also mentioned the intra-species (individual) variation of drug metabolism. A good example of this is decreased metabolism of ester-type muscle relaxants (e.g. succinylcholine) in subjects with atypical plasma butyrylcholinesterase which results in the excessive prolongation of their duration of action. It should also be noted that in such individuals the toxicity of hydrolyzable relaxants is also increased.

* Goedde, H. W., *et al.* 1967. Pseudocholinesterasen – Pharmakogenetik, Biochemie, Klinik. Springer-Verlag, Berlin, N. Y.

PHARMACOGENETICS IN THE DETECTION OF THE HYPERSUSCEPTIBLE WORKER

H. E. Stokinger, J. T. Mountain and L. D. Scheel
U.S. Dept. of Health, Education and Welfare
Public Health Service
Bureau of Disease Prevention and Environmental Control
National Center for Urban and Industrial Health
Cincinnati, Ohio

Introduction

Our reason for making this presentation at a conference on pharmacogenetics is that as industrial toxicologists our interest in preventing disease from industrial chemicals among workers has led us to recommend predictive tests based on genetic errors in metabolism to detect the hyperreactor in industry, the worker not presently covered by the threshold limit values for industrial air contaminants.[1] Thus our contribution can be included in a conference on pharmacogenetics if one is willing to extend the definition to include chemicals as well as drugs, or alternatively, to consider toxicology as a part of pharmacology. The most common basis for the hypersensitive response is genetic – alteration or deficiency of genic structure, its cistron or operon, leading to alteration or deficiency of a specific enzyme, which in turn leads to a defective metabolic system that ultimately appears as a disease under the superimposed stress of toxic chemicals. The tests that we recommend simply depend upon measuring the extent of the defect or deficiency of an enzyme system, or its product, that is related to the hyperreactive condition. Some 120 such defects have been discussed by Stanbury *et al.*[2]

Four general types of such genetic errors in metabolism are now recognized: (a) a missing essential substance as in agamma-globulinemia and α_1-antitrypsin deficiency; (b) a deficiency in or absence of an enzyme system, e.g., glucose-6-phosphate dehydrogenase; (c) the presence of an abnormal protein, e.g., hemoglobin S in sickle cell anemia; and (d) the alteration in cellular transport of a metabolite, e.g., cystinuria and carbon disulfide sensitivity. A subgroup could be added to (c) to include the genetic variation that leads to the production of reaginic antibodies to pollen antigens, e.g., the "spread" in sensitivity to certain industrial chemicals.

We would like to present some tests based on hereditary variations in metabolism that find application in screening the hypersusceptible worker to a variety of industrial chemicals and to show how the genetic abnormalities have been used to develop these tests.

Familial Pulmonary Emphysema (FPE) and the Serum Antitrypsin Deficiency Test

Although antitrypsin activity has been used for decades[3] as a measure of the inflammatory process and pancreatitis, and the familiar aspects of emphysema have been long recognized,[4] only recently has a deficiency in serum α_1-antitrypsin been found associated with FPE. Laurell and Eriksson[5] in 1963 described five patients with degenerative pulmonary disease and diminished serum α_1-antitrypsin concentrations, Eriksson[6] later reported that 23 of 38 patients with greatly reduce α_1-antitrypsin (12% of normal) had chronic obstructive pulmonary disease as shown by reduced pulmonary function, radiographic changes, and clinical findings. Briscoe, Kueppers, Davis, and Bearn[7] in 1966 described the first such case outside Scandinavia (from the Chest Service, Bellevue Hospital, New York City), quickly followed by a report from the Harvard Medical School by Talamo, Blennerhassett, and Austen of 2 families with 12 individuals showing chronic pulmonary disease and associated reduced serum antitrypsin levels.[8]

Clinical Characteristics

According to Talamo *et al.*[8] pulmonary emphysema characterized by familial incidence differs from other variants in onset usually early in life (the earliest reported case at 27 years), death occurring as early as 55 years, a higher than usual incidence in females, absence of clinical chronic bronchitis in the early phases, and an essentially panlobular form.

Recognition of Familial Form

The serum of individuals with FPE characteristically shows the absence of a visible band in the α_1-region in paper or gel electrophoresis. The immunoelectrophoretic mobility of α_1-antitrypsin is reduced. The antitrypsin deficiency states are bimodal; the mean trypsin inhibitor capacity (TIC) in families is either 0.24 mg or 0.67 mg trypsin inhibited per ml serum. Normal TIC values are 1.07 mg/ml as determined in a Swedish population.[6]

Clinical recognition of the cases is made from roentgenologic examinations, pulmonary function tests, and dyspnea.

Heredity

Eriksson[6] determined the pedigrees of 24 families (representing 35 cases that included 213 relatives) with pulmonary emphysema associated with serum antitrypsin deficiency. Two typical pedigrees are reproduced in FIGURES 1a and 1b. FIGURE 1a shows three successive generations with the deficiency that was discovered when the male proband in generation II began to be dyspneic on exertion and on exposure to dust. This occurred in his 29th year. Lung function tests indicated obstructive ventilatory impairment without signs of reversibility. Chest x-ray showed a pattern of reduced peripheral vascularity. FIGURE 1b is included because it illustrates the rather unusual instance in which a heterozygote (11_3), as determined by the TIC index, exhibited primary bullous emphysema without known unusual environmental stimuli, the characteristic of a homozygote. Homozygotes, the only form in which emphysema is commonly expressed, is defined as a TIC value less than 0.4 mg/ml; normal family members, 1.10 mg/l.

Gene Frequency

Of 6,995 individuals studied in Sweden,[6] 25 individuals showed antitrypsin deficiency; of these, 4 individuals, 2 males and 2 females, met the criterion for homozygosity. Thus we arrive at the frequency of 0.057% for homozygotes for α_1-antitrypsin deficiency. Because the sex distribution in those with the deficiency was about equal and the atypical allele was transmitted from father to son (FIGURE 1a) and therefore was not sex-linked, and because the level of the deficiency was uninfluenced in homozygotes by external factors, it is believed that α_1-antitrypsin deficiency is transmitted by a single, autosomal recessive gene. If the Hardy-Weinberg law for recessive heterozygotes is applied, the frequency is 4.7%. Whether this frequency for Sweden is too low in view

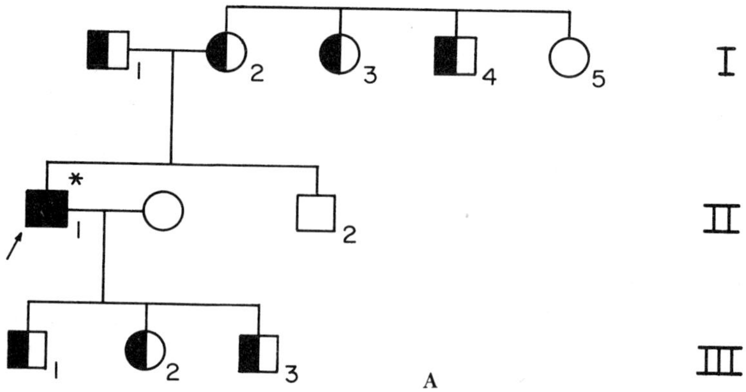

A

FIGURE 1A. Pedigrees of three generations showing serum antitrypsin deficiency. (Eriksson, 1965).

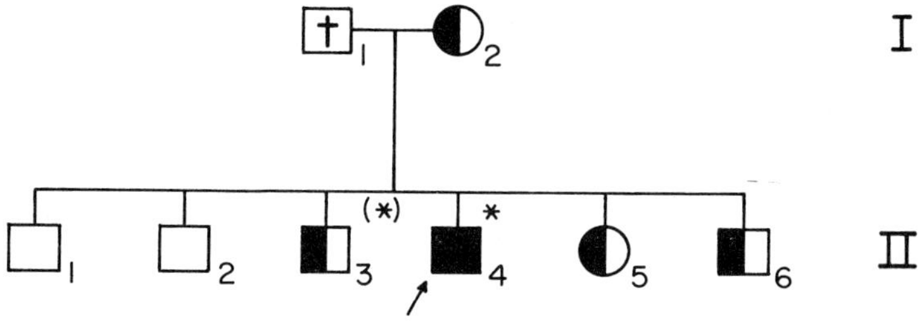

B

FIGURE 1B. Pedigree of family showing serum antitrypsin deficiency (Eriksson, 1965).

of the small number of homozygotes found and the short life expectancy of those with FPE remains a question for further study.

A limited study of 193 whites in Georgia (U.S.A.) for antitrypsin deficiency by Kueppers, Briscoe, and Bearn[9] revealed a frequency of 2.1% and a provisional estimate of homozygotes of 0.01%, values somewhat lower than those found in Sweden.

Application of Test to Industry

Because at least one cause of pulmonary emphysema can be detected in adult populations with simple tests, it seemed to us that the industrial physician could employ to advantage such tests to distinguish heredity-based disease from job-claimed disability. The hypersusceptibility being genetic in origin, the test can be made in the pre-employment examination since no prior exposure to industrial chemicals is necessary to reveal the potential. Other factors favoring the adoption of the test are the high frequency (2–5%) of heterozygotes, the number of individuals susceptible to emphysema, the evidence that repeated trauma caused by the inhalation of respiratory irritants can precipitate the expression of the genetic aberration,[6,10] and the simplicity of the tests.

Role of Antitrypsin

Experimental evidence[11] suggests that the antitrypsin factor, a glycoprotein normally comprising 90% of the α_1-globulin fraction of serum, when present in subnormal amounts is unable to counteract proteolytic activity in lung tissue. In time, this activity destroys delicate alveolar walls and results in emphysema.

Tests for Serum Antitrypsin Deficiency

A number of tests are now available for estimating serum antitrypsin deficiency. The simplest, and most useful for screening purposes, is that of James *et al.*[12] The test depends upon the capacity of the individual's serum to counteract three gradations of standard tryptic activity on the gelatin film of a used x-ray plate. A more quantitative test involves a colorimetric assay of serum trypsin inhibitor capacity using benzoyl-arginine p-nitroaniline.[7] The test used by Eriksson to screen the Swedish population involved paper electrophoresis.[6]

Hypersusceptibility to Hemolytic Chemicals

Inherited defects in red cell enzymes of pharmacogenetic interest are discussed by several other participants in this program (Kirkman, Carson, and Fraser & Vesell). A number of *in vitro* tests are available for the detection of individuals with deficiencies in glucose-6-phosphate dehydrogenase (G-6-PD). Among these are the quantitative assay for G-6-PD activity by the method of Capps *et al.*,[13] the glutathione stability test of Beutler,[14] and the methemoglobin reduction test by Brewer *et al.*[15] The quantitative assay procedure of Capps *et al.* is convenient. The method simply measures the increase in optical density as a measure of change of $TPN \rightleftharpoons TPNH$ as a function of G-6-PD activity of the red blood cell of the particular specimen. One-half milliliter of blood is required. The total time for the test is 30 minutes. To obtain the full predictive value, the test should be made at the time of job preplacement examination. It is very important that the blood sample should be kept refrigerated. In this way specimens may be stored for seven days at 4°C without deterioration.

For screening purposes, where the object is simply to detect the atypical individual, tests relying on visual indicators, i.e., dye decoloration, color development, or fluorescence, are convenient for screening industrial populations. Sets of reagents and materials for such tests are available from clinical laboratory suppliers. To avoid the need for maintaining anaerobic conditions, to lessen time and manipulations, and to avoid complications introduced when anemia is involved, Beutler[16] developed a procedure that obviates these difficulties. In his test, normal bloods, which readily generate NADPH, yield spots that fluoresce under long-wave ultra-violet light, whereas the blood-reagent spots from enzyme-deficient specimens are characterized by no, or very weak, fluorescence.

In addition to hemolytic reactions from a number of compounds, there may be other types of unusual responses of individuals with an inherited deficiency of G-6-PD. It has been suggested by Beaconsfield *et al.*[17] that they may be less likely to develop malignant disease, and the relative incidence of cancer at various tissue sites may be different. However, rigorous statistical analysis of the data has not yet been made.

Predictive Test of Carbon Disulfide (CS_2) Response

Another simple test has been developed that gives promise of detecting the abnormal responder to CS_2 exposure. First proposed by Yoshida in 1955, the test was applied by Djuric *et al.*[18] to viscose-rayon workers in Yugoslavia. A bimodal response was found with a small percentage (about 5%) responding more sensitively than the general population of workers.

The test is based on the rate at which distinct color change appears in the sodium azide-iodine reaction as modified by a urinary metabolite of CS_2 that serves as a catalyst for the reaction according to the equation:

$$\underset{\text{Color}}{2NaN_3 + I_2} \xrightarrow[\text{of } CS_2]{\substack{\text{Catalytic} \\ \text{Urinary Metabolite}}} \underset{\text{No Color}}{2NaI + 3N_2}$$

Simultaneous creatinine determinations permit account to be taken of fluctautions in urine volume and avoid the need for 24-hour urine specimens. Because the rate of disappearance of the iodine color is not linear, but is related exponentially to the degree of exposure index, E is expressed as $E = C \log t$ where C is the concentration of creatinine in milligrams/milliliter* and t is time in seconds to the disappearance of iodine color. Comparative tests made at the beginning and end of the work day show whether the worker has been overexposed; the sensitivity of the test is just below the U.S.A. recommended hygienic limit of CS_2 in air of 60 mg/m^3. The test becomes predictive of potential injury when comparative tests are made at the end of the work week and at the beinning of the new work week because hypersusceptible workers will not show a return to normal values at the beginning of the new week. The test predicts that if exposure is continued, such workers will develop overt signs (polyneuritis) of CS_2 injury. FIGURE 2 attempts to depict the situation. The general pattern of response to overexposure to CS_2 is a steady decrease in E-values throughout the work week. A normally reactive worker returns to normal E-values, 8 or above, (Yugoslavia) by the start of the new week. A hyperactive worker does not, but starts the work week showing only partial recovery in E-values. It is these responders who predictably show signs of CS_2 injury if exposure is continued. E-values were somewhat lower when the test was applied to viscose-rayon workers in Argentina (FIGURE 2).

Sufficient work has been claimed to have been done[18] on healthy nonexposed workers to show that diets unusually high in sulfur do not lead to false positive interpretations, but that administration of disulfuram leads to low values.

The heredity of the response has not yet been investigated, but the distinctly bimodal response indicates a genetic basis.

Predictive Test of Hypersensitivity to Isocyanates

The rapidly expanding application of the aromatic isocyanates, toluene diisocyanate (TDI) and methylenebisphenylisocyanate (MDI), in the production of polyurethane foams (FIGURE 3) has resulted in increased exposure of ever-increasing numbers of workers to these compounds. A not uncommon response from the inhalation of these mists and vapors is allergic sensitization of the respiratory tract, with symptoms rather like those of asthma. Such responses can occur in some individuals at extremely low concentrations of the order of a few tenths of a milligram per cubic meter of air. Because it is not possible at all times to control the isocyanate exposure below the permissible industrial air limits of 0.14 mg/m^3 and 0.2 mg/m^3 for TDI and MDI respectively, it would be of considerable advantage to have a method for detecting those individuals hypersensitive to these chemicals prior to exposure.

* The original article[18] erroneously refers to milligrams/liter.

Tests for Detecting the Allergic Reactor

These tests are based on the hypothesis that the allergic reactions to the isocyanates are mediated through reaginic, *fixed* tissue antibodies, whereas the toxic reactions result in *precipitating* (circulating) antibodies. In testing for reaginic antibodies, the serum of an individual is injected into the skin of a monkey in the Prausnitz-Kustner test for passive cutaneous anaphylaxis(PCA)

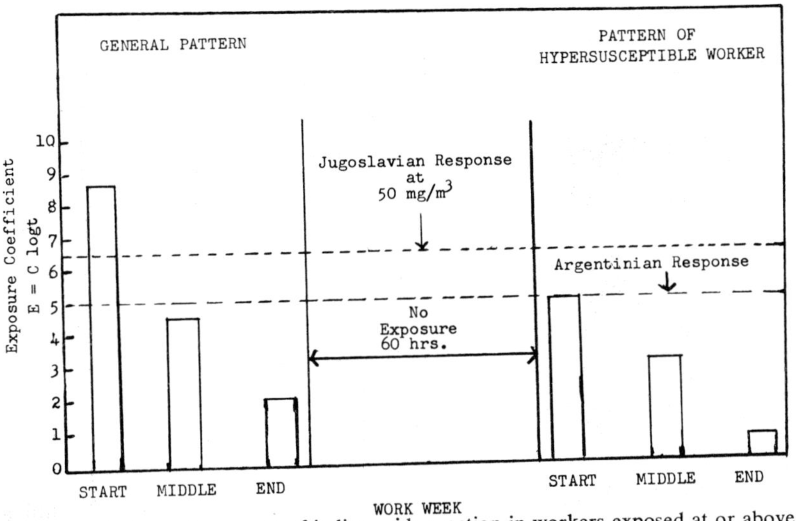

FIGURE 2. Pattern of response of iodine-azide reaction in workers exposed at or above TLV for CS_2 (60 mg/m^3). (After Djuric *et al.*, Brit. J. Ind. Med. **22**: 321).

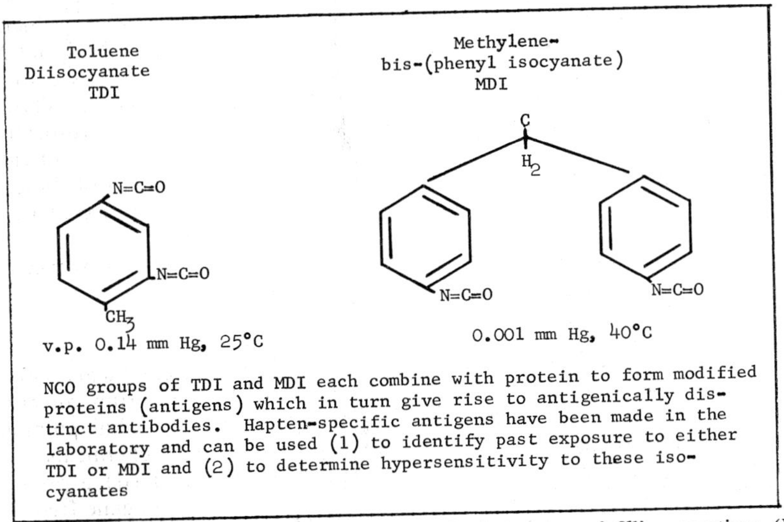

FIGURE 3. Industrially important isocyantes in plastic coating of fillin operations (Polyurethane foam).

according to Layton *et al.*[19] Twenty-four hours later the monkey is intravenously injected with either isocynanate antigens made from TDI or MDI reacted with serum globulin according to Scheel *et al.*[20] or polygen, an allergen composed of several pollen extracts. Although too few individuals have been tested to be certain, there appears to be a good correlation between those individuals who show a positive reaction to the polygen and also to the isocyanates. This correlation indicates that those allergic to the polygen may also become hypersensitive to the isocyanates (TABLE 1).

TABLE 1

PATTERN OF IMMUNOCHEMICAL RESPONSE OF WORKERS EXPOSED TO ISOCYANATES WHEN TESTED FOR CIRCULATING AND FIXED ANTIBODIES BY THE PCA TEST

Worker No.	Guinea Pig		Monkey		
	TDI N*	MDI N	TDI N	MDI N	Polygen N
C15KE†	+	+	+	+	+
UT1KE	−	+	−	−	−
UT–16KE	+	−	−	−	−
C–16KH‡	+	+	NS¶	+	+
C–14SH§	+	+	+	+	+

* N = Native serum.
† KE = Known exposure.
‡ KH = Known hypersensitive.
§ SH = Suspected hypersensitive.
¶ NS = No serum.

To determine circulating antibodies and hence to establish that a significant exposure has occurred to either TDI or MDI, the PCA test is similarly performed as above, but in guinea pigs, according to the method of Ovary.[21] The specificity of the TDI and MDI antigens, prepared according to the method of Scheel,[20] in the guinea pig, permits positive identification of that isocyanate to which the worker had significant exposure. Typical responses of workers to TDI and MDI are given in TABLE 1. Line 1 shows the response of a worker exposed to both isocyanates; line 2, of a worker exposed only to MDI; line 3, only to TDI; and lines 4 and 5, a known and a suspected hypersensitive responder, respectively.

Immunoelectrophoresis technics are being applied to the sera of the individuals having the PCA tests in an effort to provide a biologic explanation of these tests in terms of the different serum protein fraction, e.g. the appearance of gamma globulin g.

The genetics of hypersensitivity to allergenic pollens has yet to be worked out.

SUMMARY

Four predicitive tests for hypersusceptibility to industrial chemicals based on pharmacogenetic principles have been presented: (a) the serum antitrypsin deficiency test for detecting the potential development of familial pulmonary emphysema, (b) a test for hypersusceptibility to hemolytic chemicals, (c) a predictive test for abnormal response to carbon disulfide, and (d) a predictive test for hypersensitivity to isocyanates. The mode of inheritance, gene frequency, incidence, and family pedigrees have been presented for the first two, but the genetics of the last two have yet to be determined.

References

1. Threshold Limit Values for 1967. 1967. American Conference of Governmental Industrial Hygienists. Andrew Hosey, Secy-Treas. 1014 Broadway, Cincinnati, Ohio.
2. Stanbury, J. B., J. B. Wyngaarden & D. S. Fredrickson. 1966. The Metabolic Basis of Inherited Disease. 2nd Ed. McGraw-Hill, N. Y.
3. Bayer, J. & Z. Reich. 1909. The antitryptic action of urine. Biochem. Zentralbl. **9:** 510.
4. West, S. 1902. Diseases of the Organs of Respiration. C. Griffin & Co., Lond. : 205.
5. Laurell, C. B. & S. Eriksson. 1963. Electrophoretic α_1-globulin pattern of serum in α_1-antitrypsin deficiency. Scandinav. J. Clin. & Lab. Invest. **15:** 132.
6. Eriksson, S. 1965. Studies in α_1-antitrypsin deficiency. Acta Med. Scand. Suppl. to **177.**
7. Briscoe, W. A., F. Kueppers, A. L. Davis & A. G. Bearn. 1966. A case of inherited deficiency of serum alpha antitrypsin associated with pulmonary emphysema. Am. Rev. Resp. Dis. **94:** 529.
8. Talamo, R. C., J. B. Blennerhassett & K. F. Austen. 1966. Familial emphysema and alpha$_1$-antitrypsin deficiency. N. E. J. Med. **275:** 1301.
9. Kueppers, F., W. A. Briscoe & A. G. Bearn. 1964. Hereditary deficiency of serum α_1-antitrypsin. Science **146:** 1678.
10. Hole, B. V. & K. Wasserman. 1965. Familial emphysema. Ann. Internal Med. **63:** 1009.
11. Kueppers, F. & A. B. Bearn. 1966. A possible experimental approach to the association of hereditary α_1-antitrypsin deficiency and pulmonary emphysema. Proc. Soc. Exptl. Biol. & Med. **121:** 1207.
12. James, K., M. L. Collins & H. H. Fudenberg. 1966. A semiquantitative procedure for estimating serum antitrypsin levels. J. Lab. Clin. Med. **67:** 528.
13. Capps, F. P. A., H. M. Giles, H. Jolly & S. M. Worlledge. 1963. Test for glucose-6-phosphate dehydrogenase activity. Lancet **2:** 382.
14. Beutler, E. 1966. A series of new screening procedures for pyruvate kinase deficiency, glucose-6-phosphate dehydrogenase deficiency and glutathione reductase deficiency. Blood **28:** 553.
15. Brewer, G. J., A. R. Tarlov & A. S. Alving. 1960. Methemoglobin reduction test – a new simple in vitro test. Bull. WHO **22:** 633.
16. Beutler, E. 1956. In vitro studies on the stability of red cell glutathione: a test for drug sensitivity. J. Clin. Invest. **35:** 690.
17. Beaconsfield, P., R. Rainsbury & G. Kalton. 1965. Glucose-6-phosphate dehydrogenase deficiency and cancer. Oncologia **19:** 11.
18. Djuric, D., N. Surducki & I. Berkes. 1965. Iodine-azide test on urine of persons exposed to carbon disulfide. Brit. J. Ind. Med. **22:** 321.
19. Layton, L. L., S. Lee & F. de Eds. 1961. Diagnosis of human allergy utilizing passive skin-sensitization in the monkey. Proc. Soc. Exptl. Biol. & Med. **108:** 623.
20. Scheel, L. D., R. Killens & A. Josephson. 1964. Immunochemical aspects of toluene diisocyanate toxicity. Am. Ind. Hyg. Assoc. J. **25:** 179.
21. Ovary, Z. 1958. *In* Progress in Allergy V : 459, S. Karger, Basle, Switzerland.

DISCUSSIONS OF THE PAPER

Dr. E. R. Jaffe (*Albert Einstein College of Medicine, N.Y., N.Y.*): In connection with the reported observations of Beaconsfield on the association of a decreased incidence of cancer with an increased incidence of glucose-6-phosphate dehydrogenase deficiency, it is of interest that the synthesis of pyridine nucleotides for which pentose phosphate is required is not decreased in erythrocytes deficient in glucose-6-phosphate dehydrogenase activity. As was mentioned before, mature human erythrocytes can synthesize considerable amounts of DPN when incubated with suitable substrates. This biosynthetic activity requires a source of ribose-5-phosphate. The results of the studies described by Professor Bonsignore and his associates* would appear to indicate that pentose phosphate shunt activity is not essential for the formation of ribose-5-phosphate. Rather, it seems that this pentose phosphate can and does arise from the metabolism of glucose by way of the Embden-Meyerhof pathway. Thus, it well may be that

* Bonsignore, A., *et al.* 1961. Italian J. of Biochem. **10:** 212–220.

pentose phosphate shunt pathway activity would not be required for the synthesis of the pentose moiety of the nucleic acids.

DR. STOKINGER: Dr. Jaffe has pointed out that Italian scientists* have shown that the pentose-shunt pathway is but one of several possibilities of interconversion of phosphorylated sugars with a different number of carbon atoms, and thus, although Beaconsfield's correlation of strikingly lowered incidence of cancer in a population group with a very high incidence of G-6-PD deficiency is attractive, it has yet to be shown to be valid. Certainly, further investigation of the problem is indicated, for although Bonsignore, *et al.* showed adequate amounts of pentose for pyridine nucleotide synthesis under normal circumstances, in cases of tissue cellular proliferation (cancer) G-6-PD activity increases *pari passu,* a condition that may not be met in G-6-PD deficiency.

DR. MOTULSKY (*University of Washington School of Medicine, Seattle*): I think we must be careful not to assume that a given patient, who might have a G-6-PD deficiency, would prove by appropriate testing, to respond to oral medication for the hemolytic response, particularly if taken in a non-oral form. I think before advocating wholesale use of these tests, or the removal of workers from certain environments, that you should have good proof that these people actually would get into trouble.

DR. STOKINGER: To Dr. Motulsky's question of concern that the finding of a G-6-PD deficient individual may not always indicate hypersusceptibility to industrial chemicals, one answer is that the new Beutler fluorescence screening test is so simple to apply and company liability so great if a hypersusceptible were overlooked, that it is considered the better part of good judgment to utilize this test in the pre-placement job examinaion in those industries producing chemicals with potential effects on the red blood cell.

DRUG-INDUCED CHROMOSOMAL ABERRATIONS

Kurt Hirschhorn

Division of Medical Genetics, Department of Pediatrics
Mount Sinai School of Medicine, N. Y.

Maimon M. Cohen

Division of Human Genetics, Department of Pediatrics, State University of New York at Buffalo School of Medicine and the Buffalo Children's Hospital
Buffalo, N. Y.

Induced mutagenesis has long been an area of active genetic interest; however, the technical advances in tissue culture and chromosomal preparation have greatly increased the number of cytogenetic investigations. Those classes of exogenous agents capable of producing chromosomal damage include irradiation, viruses, and chemicals. This last group of compounds can be subdivided into those affecting DNA and RNA synthesis; DNA precursors and related substances; antibiotics; alkylating agents; nitroso-compounds; and a heterogenous miscellaneous group. To attempt a compilation of all those chemical agents causing chromosome breakage is beyond the scope of this paper and the reader is referred to several excellent reviews of the subjects.[1–5]

In this presentation we shall concentrate on the procedures used to assay the activity of compounds of pharmacologic interest relevant to their effect on chromosomes and the possible significance of these findings. Although the experiments to be described were carried out with antibiotics, as well as the hallucinogen lysergic acid diethylamide (LSD), they can serve as model systems for other drugs as well. The test system most frequently employed is phytohemagglutinin-stimulated peripheral lymphocytes which are incubated for a 72-hour period in commercially available "microculture kits" (Chromosome Medium 1A, Grand Island Biological Co., Grand Island, N. Y.). In addition, fibroblastic cell cultures derived from various tissues can be used as readily as the leukocytes. The test compound is added to these cultures at various concentrations and for different lengths of exposure. In this way a response curve can be ascertained with regard to both time and dose.

One of the first parameters testable in this system is the effect of the drug, if any, on cell division. Mitotic indices can be derived and a treated versus control comparison may demonstrate an effect on mitosis. Most often this is observable as a marked decrease in mitotic activity of the treated cells.

Scoring of chromosomal abnormalities may be done with relative ease by a competent cytogeneticist. The greatest difficulty encountered in this regard is the definition of aberrations. These can be divided into several clearly distinguishable classes as demonstrated in FIGURE 1. The most frequent anomaly is a chromatid break which is defined as a clear discontinuity of the chromatin material in a single chromatid with an obvious nonalignment of the distal fragment (FIGURE 1a). An isochromatid break is defined identically except that the break occurs at the same "locus" in both chromatids with a distal displacement of the "double fragment" (FIGURE 1a). Although chromatid and isochromatid breaks may be construed as occurring post- and pre-DNA synthesis respectively, they may be scored together for the following reasons: lymphocyte cultures are not synchronous populations of cells; furthermore, cells observed after 72 hours of culture are not infrequently in the second or third division and breaks that would have

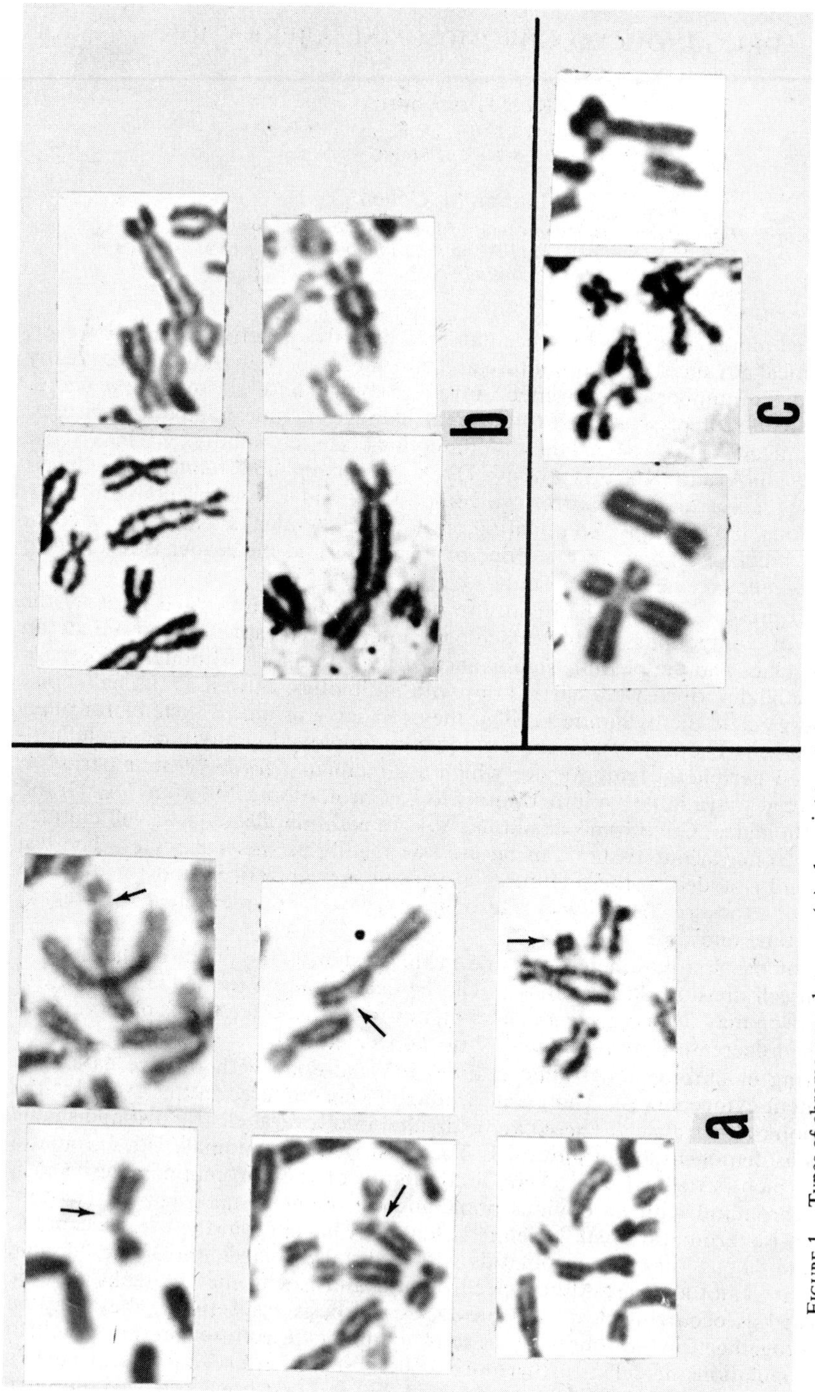

FIGURE 1. Types of chromosome damages. (a) chromatid and chromosome breaks; (b) dicentrics; (c) translocation rearrangements.

been isochromatid (chromosome) at the first division may appear as chromatid breaks due to partial restitution. In fact, 95% of chromosome damage induced by radiation is indeed restituted. Often the problem arises of a "gap" or a clear chromatin discontinuity without displacement of the fragment. Such gaps are usually noted but not included in the total frequency of abnormalities, since the criterion of nonalignment is unfulfilled. Another class of chromosomal abnormalities is that resulting in structural rearrangements, notably dicentric chromosomes (FIGURE 1b), ring chromosomes or translocation figures (FIGURE 1c). These almost invariably result from a "two-hit" phenomenon and yield morphologically unique elements. Other cytological parameters which can be quantitated in this system are the incidence of polyploidy and/or endoreduplication.

Many chromosome-breaking agents (viruses and antimetabolites) demonstrate a nonuniform or localized effect. That is, the chromosomal damage appears to occur in certain chromosomes or chromosomal segments.[6] Although the significance of such specificities is poorly understood, some general inferences may be drawn. Most of the specific effects have been localized in the heterochromatic or heteropycnotic regions of the chromosomes, e.g., the centromeres and secondary constrictions. These effects, however, may not be direct responses to the specific agents being tested since the enhancement, exaggeration and, possibly, breakage of the secondary constrictions may be intensified by various physical and chemical manipulations, e.g., fixation treatment,[7] the use of calcium-free medium,[8] and cold shock.[9–11] The similarity of effects induced by nonspecific treatment and by "specific" agents casts some doubt upon the specificity of these agents. Since most of the compounds thus far tested affect mainly heterochromatic regions, one must consider the possibility that the specificity may not reside in the agent but may reflect a specific response of the chromosome to nonspecific environmental alteration.

In addition to the chromosome-breaking potential of these agents, other profound effects are sometimes observed. Mitomycin C (MC), is a streptomyces-derived antitumor antibiotic which is known to disrupt DNA synthesis[12] and to cause cross-linking of the complementary strands of DNA.[13] In addition to extensive chromosome damage,[14,15] MC also produces cytologically detectable exchange figures which are suggestive of "translocation configurations" (FIGURE 2). Such figures are rarely observed in untreated leukocyte cultures.[16] An analysis of 220 exchange figures induced by MC[17] shows the homologous exchanges occur far in excess of what might be expected by chance, and that the genetic consequences of some of these exchanges may be analogous to somatic crossing over. Therefore, Mitomycin C represents a pharmacologic agent that not only can cause chromosomal breakage but also may be used as an extremely important tool in somatic cell genetics. FIGURE 3 depicts the four classes of two chromosome exchanges seen in the leukocyte cultures after mitomycin treatment.

The genetic consequences of these exchanges are quite different. In Class I, homologous exchange occurs and all of the daughter cells should be genetically balanced and viable unless the exchange results in homozygosity for a recessive lethal gene. In Class II, the exchange produces one dicentric, one acentric, and two normal monocentric chromosomes. If alternate segregation of the quadriradial occurs, one daughter cell receives two genetically unchanged monocentric chromosomes while the other daughter cell, though genetically balanced, would probably not survive because the acentric fragment is lost at a subsequent cell division, producing nullisomy for a block of genes. If adjacent segregation occurs, all daughter cells are genetically unbalanced (duplications and deficiencies) and

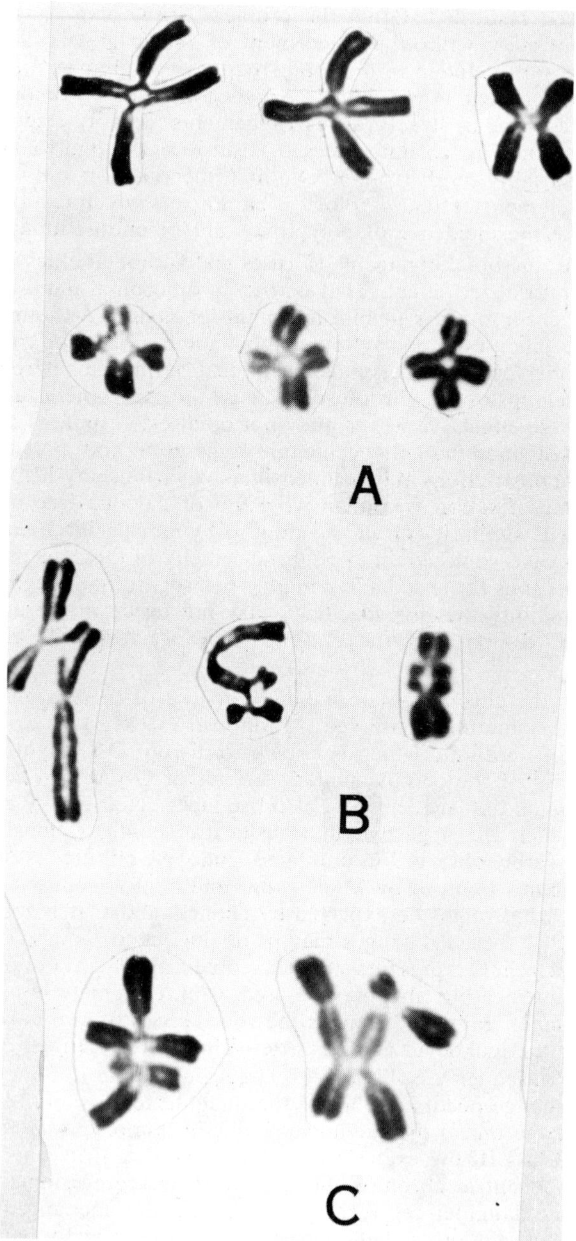

FIGURE 2. Chromosomal exchanges observed as "translocation" configurations. Group A, exchanges between apparent pairs of homologues; second row demonstrates exchanges at secondary constrictions in chromosome pair No. 9; Group B, exchanges between non-homologous chromosomes; Group C, exchanges involving more than two chromosomes.

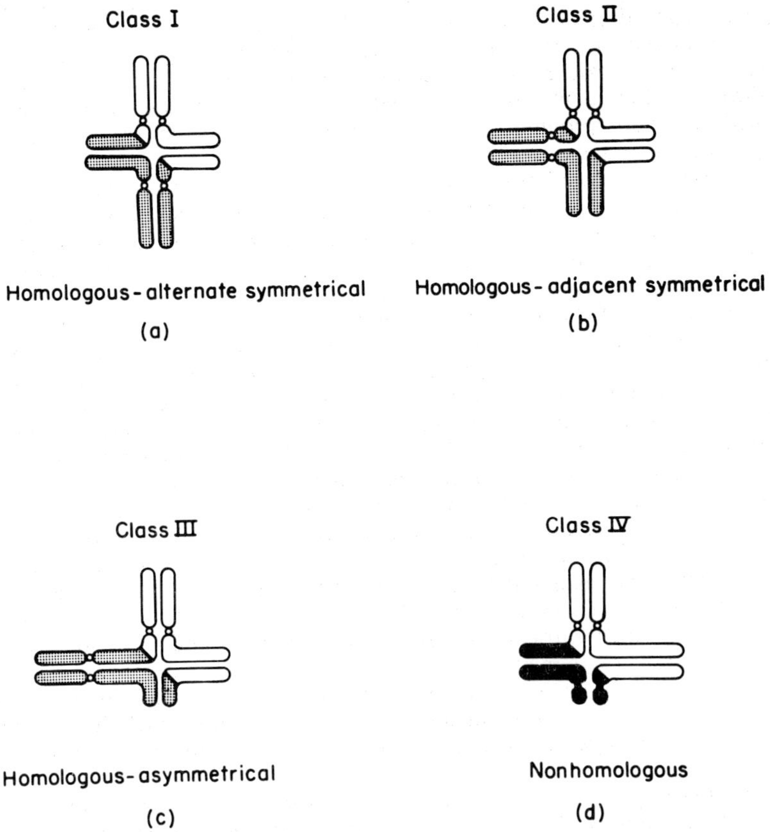

FIGURE 3. Chromosome exchanges Classes I to IV. Note that symmetry in (a) occurs in both vertical and horizontal planes while the axis of symmetry in (b) is only in one diagonal plane through the exchange points.

probably lethal. Class III exchanges would produce, if alternate segregation of opposite centromeres occurs, an unequal pair of autosomes, one carrying a duplication and the other a deficiency. The genome should be balanced, however, and the cells should be viable. Adjacent segregation of opposite centromeres leads to unbalanced daughter cells. Class IV exchanges correspond to a reciprocal translocation between two nonhomologues resulting in new linkage groups and possibly position effects. There are three classes which are genetically significant. Class I exchanges result in homozygosity for a block of genes; Class III exchanges produce unequal homologues with duplications and deficiencies; and Class IV exchanges lead to reciprocal translocations and new linkage groups.

The phenomena of somatic pairing and crossing over in Drosophila and several lower organisms, particularly fungi, have been well demonstrated.[18,19] The findings in Drosophila may be pertinent to an interpretation of the exchanges seen in the human material induced by Mitomycin C. Chromosomes 1, 9 and 16 of man contain large segments of proximal heterochromatin in the secondary constriction regions of their long arms. These chromosomes, especially numbers 1 and 9, are most frequently broken by MC[14] and most frequently take part in the exchange figures, suggesting highly localized sites of action of the drug. These points emphasize the statement made earlier that most agents and drugs apparently have their effect at the heterochromatic region of the chromatin. If such exchanges can be induced in diploid fibroblast cultured in vitro from tissues of individuals with genetic markers, problems in human somatic cell genetics may be amenable to experimental attack.

The type of drug discussed until now is generally used in terminal patients for a fatal disease. Potentially there is much greater danger of chromosome breakage and rearrangements caused by drugs in common use by an essentially normal population, particularly individuals before or during the reproductive period. That this in fact may occur is evident from recent studies with lysergic acid diethylamide (LSD) an agent in common use by a sizable proportion of the younger generation. It was found and previously reported that addition of LSD to cultures of normal human lymphocytes will produce chromosome damage.[20]

We wish to report here an extension of the in vitro studies, as well as the results of chromosome studies on the cultured lymphocytes of a series of individuals exposed to the drug in vivo.[21] The in vitro studies are summarized in TABLE 1.

Lymphocytes from six normal individuals were stimulated to divide by the addition of phytohemagglutinin, and LSD was added to the cultures in concentrations ranging from 0.001 to 10 μg/ml from 4 to 48 hours prior to the harvest of the cells. Duplicate cultures were performed for each treatment and 100 cells per treatment per individual were examined. Cultures from the same individuals without LSD served as controls. All studies were coded and evaluated without knowledge of the treatment. It is evident that all doses and all periods of exposure produced an increase in abnormalities which ranged to over four times the control values of 3.9% of chromosomally abnormal cells. The LSD-induced abnormalities, in addition to chromatid and isochromatid breaks, included a number of chromatid exchanges and dicentric chromosomes, neither of which was found in the controls.

The study of patients ingesting the drug is summarized in TABLE 2. Lymphocytes were obtained from the subjects and from age-matched controls and cultured in the presence of phytohemagglutinin. Slides again were coded and examined without knowledge of the source. About 100 metaphases were scored for each individual. Twelve normal "drug-free" controls, some of them studied more than once, showed a range of break frequencies of 2.0–5.5% with a mean of 3.8%, based on the scoring of 2,674 metaphases. This frequency is identical to that found in the controls for the in vitro studies. Eighteen adults with a history of LSD ingestion demonstrated in their lymphocytes a break frequency of from

TABLE 1

DISTRIBUTION OF CHROMOSOMAL BREAKS INDUCED IN CULTURED HUMAN LEUKOCYTES BY VARIOUS DOSAGES AND EXPOSURE TIMES TO LSD-25*

Hours prior to harvest	Dosage (μg/ml)				
	10	1	0.1	0.01	0.001
48	12.6%	7.7%	17.5%	10.7%	12.5%
24	11.5%	15.8%	13.0%	15.4%	10.8%
4	17.1%	10.6%	13.1%	15.2%	11.2%
Control	65/1680 = 3.9%		—	—	—

* Figures denote percent of cells with breaks.

TABLE 2

CHROMOSOMAL DAMAGE IN PATIENTS INGESTING LSD

	No. of Individuals	Age	Sex	Percent breaks
LSD	18	19–29 one 52	12 Male 6 Female	13.2 (5.3–25.1)
Control	12	22-39	9 Male 3 Female	3.8 (2.0–5.5)

5.3–25.1% with a mean of 13.2% based on 4,282 metaphases scored. Some of these individuals were also studied more than once. There was excellent consistency between results from the same individual, between different culture tubes, and between different culture times from the same individual. There was no apparent correlation between the number of doses, amount per dose and interval between last dose and time of culture and the frequency of chromosome breaks. The longest interval was eight months in an individual who still demonstrated a high break rate. Again, most of the abnormalities are chromatid and isochromatid breaks but a number of dicentrics and exchange figures were observed in the LSD group but not in the controls. Although a number of the subjects had taken a variety of other drugs, there seemed to be no correlation in this group with any combination of drugs to the exclusion of LSD and the rate of chromosome breaks.

We also had the opportunity to examine the chromosomes of four children exposed to LSD in utero. The results are shown in TABLE 3. Two of the children whose mothers had taken the usual doses of LSD (300–600 μg/dose) showed highly elevated frequencies of breaks, while the two children born to the mother who took only 50–100 μg showed either no or only a mild elevation in breaks. One of the children whose mother had taken large doses of the drug and who was exposed to no other drugs during pregnancy and had not been exposed to LSD since birth still showed 13% breaks two and one-half years after birth. This long-lasting retention of cells with broken chromosomes is quite similar to that found following radiation.

In view of the fact that other drugs were taken by the subjects under study, we decided to investigate individuals exposed to similar drugs but not to LSD. We found that exposure to chlorpromazine on the day of bleeding also was associated with high rates of chromosome breakage. The one individual who had stopped taking chlorpromazine one month prior to bleeding did not show such damage.

TABLE 3

CHROMOSOMAL DAMAGE IN OFFSPRING OF MOTHERS WHO INGESTED LSD DURING PREGNANCY

No. of Patient	No. of Mother	Age	Sex	No. of Doses in utero	Percent breaks
1	2	11 months	Female	4	19.0 (57/300)
15	14	2.5 yr	Male	1	13.0 (39/300)
12	9*	5.5 yr	Female	2	7.5 (15/200)
11	9*	2 months	Male	4	4.0 (8/200)
					11.9 (119/1000)

* Low dose (50–100 μg).

It was of interest that while chlorpromazine produced an increase in chromatid and isochromatid breaks, no rearrangements, that is dicentric or translocations, were seen. Although much work needs to be done on this problem, it is possible to speculate that chlorpromazine exerts only a transient effect as opposed to that seen with LSD, which is long-lasting. This could be an analogy to the difference between the transient effect observed with measles virus[22] as opposed to the long-lasting effect of radiation.[23] One patient taking diphenylhydramine up to the day of testing showed a mild increase in chromosome breakage, but it is too early to evaluate the significance of this finding. Preliminary studies by Miller indicate that this agent may be a mitotic inhibitor as has also been demonstrated with LSD in vitro.[24]

The mechanism of chromosome damage is unknown. It is quite possible and even probable that different agents may act by way of different mechanisms. Among the postulated mechanisms are the following: free radical formation due to ionizing radiation; incorporation of nucleotide analogues into DNA; cross-linking of the DNA molecule by agents such as Mitomycin C; faulty ATP and protein synthesis needed for repair; and release of lysosomal DNAase and catheps-sins by agents incorporated into lysosomes. Many of these are amenable to study with relation to the drugs in question.

The most pertinent problem is of course whether these changes are potentially dangerous either to the individual taking the drugs or to his progeny. At this early stage of investigation there are no answers. We may, however, discuss such potential dangers from our knowledge of other situations in which similar types of chromosome breakage and rearrangement are found.

Similar chromosome aberrations have been noted to occur spontaneously in three autosomal recessive diseases, Bloom's syndrome, Fanconi's anemia and ataxia telangiectasia.[25–32] Patients with these syndromes also show a high propensity to develop leukemia and other neoplasms. In this context, cells of neoplastic origin also invariably illustrate a variety of chromosomal aberrations, many of which are not unlike those seen after LSD or mitomycin exposure. Additionally, many agents known to produce similar chromosome aberrations (e.g., radiation in man and other species, viruses in experimental animals) are known carcinogens. One of the obvious potential dangers, therefore, of exposure to chromosome-breaking agents is the possible future increase in the incidence of leukemia and other neoplasms in the exposed individuals. We have, in fact, previously suggested that the conversion from chronic myelogenous leukemia to acute leukemia may be a result of additional chromosome damage produced by the agents used in the therapy of chronic myelogenous leukemia.[33]

In addition, other less evident dangers exist. In view of the demonstration of transplacental transport of LSD, as evidenced by chromosome damage in the exposed fetuses, the production of congenital defects by this and possibly other drugs is a distinct possibility. In fact the teratogenic properties of LSD through the production of congenital anomalies and increased abortions has been observed in pregnant rats or mice injected with LSD.[34,35] Mitomycin has also been reported to be a teratogen in chickens.[36]

One of the well-documented dangers of LSD exposure is prolonged or acute behavioral derangement. Recurrence of psychiatric disorders has been observed at least a year after the last exposure to the drug.[37] There seems to be no direct correlation between behavioral disorders, dosage, frequency of ingestion or time since last dose and the incidence of chromosomal damage in the group studied. There were also no obvious physical or behavioral abnormalities noted as yet in the four children exposed in utero. A larger sample of mother-child pairs has already been assembled for further assessment of in utero chromosome damage.

Perhaps the greatest danger of such agents lies in potential chromosome damage to the gametes. Since LSD appears in the circulation, it presumably has free access to germ cells. Another agent, streptonigrin, known to cause chromosomal damage in human leukocytes[38,39] and teratogenic effects in rats[40] has recently demonstrated the ability to inflict damage on the meiotic chromosomes of the ova of the mouse.[41] The existence of chromosome damage in these cells can only be ascertained through direct observation of germinal cells from gonadal biopsies. As described for mitomycin, chromosome rearrangements produced by breaks and subsequent incorrect healing can result in structural anomalies including balanced reciprocal translocations. Ample evidence already exists that segregation of such translocations results in chromosomal imbalance leading to fetal wastage and a high percentage of offspring with congenital anomalies and mental retardation. Since the carrier of such balanced translocations is clinically normal, as are many of his offspring, the consequences of the chromosomal imbalance may not appear for several generations.

Summary

A variety of pharmacological agents are capable of producing chromosome breaks and rearrangements in vitro and in vivo in human material. Such chromosome damage could be produced by a variety of mechanisms and could result in an increased incidence of neoplasia in the exposed individual, abortions and malformations of his offspring if exposed in utero and chromosomal rearrangements in future generations, again resulting in fetal wastage and damage. Which of these drugs is, in fact, capable of producing such effects will only be determined by the use of large scale epidemiologic studies.

Acknowledgments

This work was supported in part by grants from U. S. Public Health Service (HD-02552), the American Heart Association and the U. S. Children's Bureau (Project No. 417) and the N. Y. City Health Council (I-513). We wish to acknowledge the excellent technical assistance of Susan Verbo, Michelle Marinello, Maryann Solberg and Jess Sedita.

References

1. Lea, D. E. 1955. Actions of Radiations on Living Cells. 2nd Ed. University Press, Cambridge.
2. Revell, S. H. 1953. Chromosome breakage by X-rays and radiomimetic substances in *Vicia. In* Symposium on Chromosome Breakage. Heredity (Suppl.) **6:** 125.
3. Kihlman, B. A. 1961. Biochemical aspects of chromosome breakage. Advances Genet. **10:** 1.
4. Ostertag, W. 1966. Chemische Mutagenese an menschlichen Zellen in Kultur. Abh. Math.-naturw. Kl. **1:** 5.
5. Kihlman, B. A. 1966. Actions of Chemicals on Dividing Cells. Prentice-Hall, Inc., Englewood Cliffs, N. J.
6. Cohen, M. M. & M. W. Shaw. 1965. In Vitro. Vol. **1:** 50. Waverly Press, Baltimore, Md.
7. Saksela, E. & P. S. Moorhead. 1962. Enhancement of secondary constrictions and the heterochromatic X in human cells. Cytogenetics **2:** 225.
8. Sasaki, M. S. & S. Makino. 1963. The demonstration of secondary constrictions in human chromosomes by means of new techniques. Amer. J. Hum. Genet. **15:** 24.
9. Darlington, C. D. & L. F. La Cour. 1938. Differential reactivity of the chromosome. Ann. Botan. **2:** 615.

10. DARLINGTON, C. D. & L. F. LA COUR. 1940. Nucleic acid starvation of the chromosomes in Trillium. J. Genet. **40**: 185.
11. HAMPEL, K. E. & A. LEVAN. 1964. Breakage in human chromosomes induced by low temperature. Hereditas **51**: 315.
12. SHIBA, S., A. TIRAWAKI, T. TAGUCHI & J. KAWAMATA. 1959. Selective inhibition of formation of DNA in E. coli by mitomycin C. Nature **183**: 1056.
13. IYER, V. N. & W. SZYBALSKI. 1963. A molecular mechanism of mitomycin action: Linking of complementary DNA strands. Proc. Natl. Acad. Sci. **50**: 355.
14. COHEN, M. M. & M. W. SHAW. 1964. Effects of mitomycin C on human chromosomes. J. Cell Biol. **23**: 386.
15. NOWELL, P. C. 1964. Mitotic inhibition and chromosome damage by mitomycin in human leukocyte cultures. Exptl. Cell Res. **33**: 445.
16. GERMAN, J. 1964. Cytological evidence for crossing over *in vitro* in human lymphoid cells. Science **144**: 298.
17. SHAW, M. W. & M. M. COHEN. 1965. Chromosome exchanges in human leukocytes induced by mitomycin C. Genetics **51**: 181.
18. STERN, C. 1936. Somatic crossing over and segregation in *Drosophila melanogaster*. Genetics **21**: 625.
19. HOLIDAY, R. 1964. The induction of mitotic recombination by mitomycin C in ustilago and saccharomyces. Genetics **50**: 323.
20. COHEN, M. M., M. J. MARINELLO & N. BACK. Chromosomal damage in human leukocytes induced by lysergic acid diethylamide. Science **155**: 1417.
21. COHEN, M. M., K. HIRSCHHORN & W. A. FROSCH. 1967. *In vivo* and *in vitro* chromosomal damage induced by LSD-25. New Engl. J. Med. **277**: 1043.
22. HARNDEN, D. G. 1964. Cytogenetic studies on patients with virus infections and subjects vaccinated against yellow fever. Amer. J. Human Genet. **16**: 204.
23. COURT BROWN, W. M., K. E. BUCKTON & A. S. MACLEAN. 1965. Quantitative studies on chromosome aberrations in man following acute and chronic exposure to X-rays and gamma rays. Lancet **i**: 1239.
24. MILLER, O. J. 1967. Personal communication.
25. SCHROEDER, T. M., F. ANSCHUETZ & A. KNOPP. 1964. Spontane Chromosomenaberrationen bei familiaerer Panmyelopathie. Humangenetik **1**: 194.
26. SCHMID, W., K. SCHARER, T. BAUMANN & G. FANCONI. 1965. Chromosomenbruchigkeit bei der familiaeren Panmyelopathie (Typus Fanconi). Sch. Med. Woch. **95**: 1461.
27. BLOOM, G. E., S. WARNER, P. S. GERALD & L. K. DIAMOND. 1966. Chromosomal abnormalities in constitutional aplastic anemia. New Eng. J. Med. **65**: 496.
28. SWIFT, M. R. & K. HIRSCHHORN. 1966. Fanconi's anemia: inherited susceptibility to chromosome breakage in various tissues. Ann. Int. Med. **65**: 796.
29. GERMAN, J., R. ARCHIBALD & D. BLOOM. 1965. Chromosomal breakage in a rare and probably genetically determined syndrome of man. Science **148**: 506.
30. SAWITSKY, A., D. BLOOM & J. GERMAN. 1966. Chromosomal breakage and acute leukemia in congenital telangiectatic erythema and stunted growth. Ann. Int. Med. **65**: 487.
31. GERMAN, J. & L. P. CRIPPA. 1966. Chromosomal breakage in diploid cell lines from Bloom's syndrome and Fanconi's anemia. Ann. de Genet. **9**: 143.
32. HECHT, F., R. D. KOLER, D. A. RIGAS, G. S. DAHNKE, M. P. CASE, V. TISDALE & R. W. MILLER. 1966. Leukemia and lymphocytes in ataxia telangiectasia. Lancet **ii**: 1193.
33. HIRSCHHORN, K. 1967. Cytogenetic alterations in leukemia. : 113–122. *In* Perspectives in Leukemia. W. Dameshek, Ed.
34. ALEXANDER, G. J., B. E. MILES, G. M. GOLD & R. B. ALEXANDER. 1967. LSD: injection early in pregnancy produces abnormalities in offspring of rats. Science **157**: 459.
35. AUERBACH, R. & J. A. RUGOWSKI. 1967. Lysergic acid diethylamide: Effect on embryos. Science **157**: 1325.
36. KURY, G. & J. M. CRAIG. 1967. The effect of mitomycin C on developing chicken embryos. J. Embryol. exp. Morph. **17**: 229.
37. FROSCH, W. A., E. S. ROBBINS & M. STERN. 1965. Untoward reactions to lysergic acid diethylamide (LSD) resulting in hospitalization. New Eng. J. Med. **273**: 1235.
38. COHEN, M. M., M. W. SHAW & A. P. CRAIG. 1963. The effects of streptonigrin on cultured human leukocytes. Proc. Nat. Acad. Sci. **50**: 16.
39. COHEN, M. M. 1963. The specific effects of streptonigrin activity on human chromosomes in culture. Cytogenetics **2**: 271.
40. WARKANY, J. & E. TAKACS. 1965. Congenital malformations in rats from streptonigrin. Arch. Path. **79**: 65.
41. JAGIELLO, G. 1967. Streptonigrin: effect of first meiotic metaphase of the mouse egg. Science **157**: 453.

DISCUSSION OF THE PAPER

DR. W. W. WEBER (*N.Y.U. School of Medicine, N.Y.*): Since vitamin B_{12} is apparently involved in DNA synthesis, is there any evidence for an association between vitamin B_{12} deficiency and chromosome breakage—and perhaps thereby with carcinoma which develops in pernicious anemia?

DR. HIRSCHHORN: Chromosome damage has been reported in pernicious anemia, but it is mostly seen following vitamin B_{12} treatment of untreated pernicious anemia. The question can be raised whether one actually sees the chromosome damage in those cells that have been just "sitting there" as stem cells resting in the absence of vitamin B_{12}, which are now observed following B_{12} stimulation. This aspect of the problem has been discussed since Charles Ford demonstrated chromosome breakage following B_{12} in the treatment of pernicious anemia.

GENETIC FACTORS IN HYPERSENSITIVITY REACTIONS TO DRUGS

Bernard B. Levine
New York University School of Medicine
New York, N. Y.

Introduction

For the most part allergic drug reactions occur in only a small percentage of patients treated with a given drug. For example, allergic reactions to penicillin occur in about 2% of patient courses of this drug. The incidence of adverse reactions of the allergic type to aspirin is in the order of 0.01% to 0.1% It would seem that many factors, both environmental and genetic, are involved in determining which individuals of a random population will develop allergic reactions to a given drug. If one considers that a long sequence of separate molecular events (concerning drug metabolism, the induction of antibody synthesis, etc.) must cumulate in order to result in a clinical allergic reaction, it is clear that the number and interplay of genetic factors involved in drug allergy must be enormous. To further complicate matters, there is a large number of different clinical varieties of allergic drug reactions (e.g., exanthematic, anaphylaxis, hemolytic anemia, etc.), each with different physiological mechanisms, and, accordingly, different kinds of genetic controls.

At present there is little or no data concerning the genetic controls in drug allergy other than the many clinical observations that anaphylactic reactions to various drugs occur more frequently among atopic patients.[1,2]

The purpose of this paper is to discuss the kind of genetic controls which may operate in various drug allergies. I will describe briefly the various clinical varieties of allergic drug reactions, discuss the immunological mechanisms which appear to be operative, and describe some model systems of hypersensitivity where genetic controls have been indicated.

Clinical Varieties of Allergic Drug Reactions and Immunological Mechanisms

Some of the more common varieties of allergic drug reactions encountered clinically are listed in TABLE 1. Many of these reactions, although appearing to be allergic in mechanism, cannot clearly be proved to be so because of the unavailability of proper immunological assay methods. However, for penicillin, the availability of hapten conjugates, various degradation products and analytical tools have permitted some views of the immune mechanism involved.[3] Thus, immediate, anaphylactic, and various urticarial reactions to penicillin appear to be mediated by skin-sensitizing antibodies, or reagins, and involve the release of histamine (and perhaps other mediators as well) from mast cells. There is suggestive evidence that some exanthematic reactions to penicillin may be mediated by IgM antibodies (as soluble complexes with antigen). Hemolytic reactions to penicillin appear to be mediated by IgG antibodies, either through enhanced red blood cell opsonization, or cytolysis, or both mechanisms. Accordingly, in discussing "drug allergies" it is important to specify the kind of allergic reaction under consideration, as different reactions are mediated by different immunological and physiological mechanisms.

TABLE 1

SOME CLINICAL TYPES OF ALLERGIC DRUG REACTIONS

Immediate*	Accelerated†	Late‡	Unusual Late Reactions‡
Urticaria Hypotension Asthma Laryngeal edema	Urticaria Morbilliform erupjtions Laryngeal edema	Urticaria Exanthematic skin reactions Serum-sickness-like reactions Drug fever	Hemolytic anemia Thrombocytopenia Granulocytopenia Stephens-Johnson syndrome Acute renal insufficiency Lupus-like syndromes Cholestatic jaundice

* Starting 2 to 45 minutes after initiation of drug therapy.
† Starting 1 to 72 hours after initiation of drug therapy.
‡ Starting 3 days or longer after initiation of drug therapy.

The sequence of events leading to an allergic reaction to a low molecular weight chemical drug is listed below.

1. Chemical reaction of drug (or metabolite) with tissue proteins to form immunogen.
2. Induction of synthesis of antibodies of various classes, e.g., anaphylactic antibody, IgM, IgG, delayed hypersensitivity, etc.
3. Antibody-antibody binding in tissues.
4. Allergic tissue damage, most commonly through the release of pharmacological mediators, e.g., histamine.

Each of these steps consist of separate physiological events. Their possible genetic controls will be discussed separately.

Immunogenicity of Simple Chemical Drugs

It is a widely held idea among immunologists that the drug, or a trace contaminant, or a degradation or metabolic product of the drug, must bind covalently to autologous proteins in order to form the complete immunogen, i.e., the hapten-protein conjugate. This is an empirically determined view based mainly on studies of Landsteiner,[4] Eisen[5] and Gell.[6] These studies showed that of a large group of organic chemicals, only those which could react covalently with proteins or with protein model compounds (e.g. amines) could induce a strong immune response. According to this view, the simple chemical itself cannot induce an immune response, whereas the hapten-protein conjugate formed from the chemical can induce the synthesis of antibodies with immunological specificity for the hapten. A theoretical basis for this obligatory binding mechanism is not readily available. However, in accord with recent concepts on immunogenicity, it may be that hapten-protein conjugates are capable of undergoing certain metabolic processes necessary for immunogenicity, whereas the simple chemical itself cannot undergo these steps.

Where the drug itself is not chemically reactive with proteins, a metabolic product of the drug may be the reactive intermediate. For example, for aromatic drugs, especially those with nitro, hydroxy, or amino groups, a quinone may be the chemically reactive intermediate. This possibility is based on two kinds of indirect evidence:

1) Many such aromatic chemicals can be metabolized to o- or p-amino-

phenols[7] which can be readily oxidized to quinones.[8] Quinones can couple to amino or sulfhydryl residues of proteins[9] to form relatively stable hapten-protein conjugates.

2) In line with these chemical considerations, Mayer[10] and Baer, *et al.*,[11] have shown extensive allergic cross reactions among various aromatic amines and nitro compounds. These data were interpreted on the basis of a common quinone metabolite.[10,11]

If quinone structures are responsible pro-immunogens (e.g., with aspirin, procaine, etc.) then a conceivable genetic control might be through the synthesis of the enzymes which catalyze quinone-forming metabolic pathways, as well as through the synthesis of enzymes involved in alternate pathways of metabolism. Of interest in this matter are Shahidi's recent findings[12] of a patient and several members of her family who appeared to show a relatively decreased ability to metabolize phenacitin by de-ethylation. Shahidi's findings were interpreted as suggesting that in the relative absence of the usual de-ethylation pathway (pathway A, see FIGURE 1), an increased amount of phenacitin was metabolized through ortho-hydroxylation and de-acetylation (pathway C). This resulted in the formation of unusually large amounts of an ortho-hydroxy aromatic amine (Compound V). Such a compound is readily oxidized to a quinone or a quinonimine, (Compound VI) which could be expected to form immunogenic hapten-protein conjugates.

Shahidi's findings are of great interest to the clinical immunologist, as they suggest one possible kind of polymorphous genetic factor controlling hypersensitive reactions to drugs. This factor would operate by controlling the rate of metabolic formation of chemical reactive proimmunogens from the simple chemical drug.

Genetic Controls of Immune Responses

Immune responses made by individual animals to a given antigen may vary in several parameters, i.e., the molecular classes of antibodies synthesized (IgG, IgM, reaginic antibody, etc.), the serum concentration of antibodies attained, and the binding affinities of the antibodies. Each of the factors would influence the kind and intensity of hypersensitive reaction which might result from the readministration of antigen. This heterogeneous immune response is controlled by both environmental and genetic factors. Important environmental factors influencing immune responses are antigen dose, use of adjuvants, disease states, various drugs, etc. Genetic factors also have been shown to influence the immune response to a given antigen. Thus, several studies have shown a statistically significant relation between the abilities of parents and their offspring to produce high serum titers of antibody to a given immunogen.[14–16] Also, several studies have found genetically transmissible differences among rodents' abilities to respond immunologically to a given protein antigen,[17,18] or antigenic determinant.[19] Breeding experiments have shown these systems to be under complex genetic control, at least in part, because of the structural and antigenic complexity of the antigens used in these studies. More recently it has been shown that the ability of guinea pigs[20–22] or mice[23] to respond to certain structurally simple synthetic poly-amino acids is controlled by a single autosomal gene.

The essential data for the hapten-poly-L-lysine system in guinea pigs which demonstrates genetic control by a single autosomal gene are summarized below.[23]

1. Approximately 25% of random-bred Hartley can respond immunologically to H-PLL conjugates.

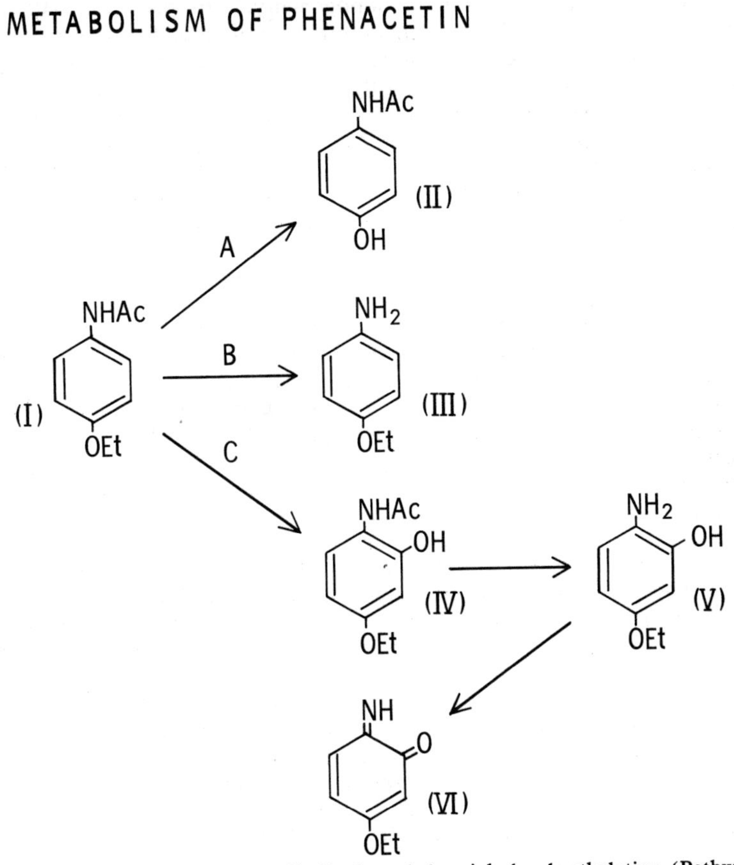

FIGURE 1. Phenacitin (I) is metabolically degraded mainly by de-ethylation (Pathway A) to form N-acetyl p-aminophenol (II) which is excreted in the urine mainly as conjugates with sulfuric or glucoronic acids.[13] A small percentage of (I) is de-acetylated to p-phenetidin (III). Shahidi's patient demonstrated in her urine after a dose of phenacitin, conjugates of 2-hydroxy-phenacitin (IV) and 2-hydroxyphenetidin (V) and considerably lower quantities of (II) than in control patients. These findings suggested a relatively high activity of Pathway C in this patient.[12] Compounds such as (V) can be readily oxidized to quinones or quinonimines (VI).

2. 100% of strain 2 and 0% of strain 13 (highly inbred strains) guinea pigs respond to H-PLL.
3. Breeding experiments:

Responder × responder ⟶ 82% responders.
Non-responder × non-responder ⟶ 0% responders.
Heterozygous responder × non-responder ⟶ 50% responders.

No evidence of sex linking.

∴ Ability to respond immunologically to H-PLL conjugates is transmitted as a unigenic, autosomal Mendelian dominant trait.

The biochemical function of this gene has not been established. It relates to the poly-L-lysine carrier, and appears to control a metabolic step performed on the carrier which is necessary for immunogenicity.[22] In the hapten-PLL system, genetic polymorphism relates to the synthetic polypeptide hapten carrier. This kind of system would probably not be of special importance in drug hypersensitivity, where the hapten carriers are autologous proteins. Of interest in this respect are the studies of McDevitt and Sela,[19] which describe a system displaying genetic polymorphism apparently based on the immune response of mice to a given antigenic determinant and not on the polypeptide backbone. However, this system is not under unigenic control. Whether genetic controls operate on the level of recognition of a foreign hapten has not yet been established.

Inheritance of Atopy in Man

Another aspect of the immune response where genetic polymorphism has been strongly suggested is the synthesis of reagins under certain conditions of immunization in man. Reagins (also called anaphylactic antibodies, or skin-sensitizing antibodies) have recently been identified as γ-E immunoglobulins.[24,25] The following lines of evidence are available to support genetic polymorphism for reagin production:

It has long been known that the atopic diseases in man are inheritable according to family studies[26–28] (see TABLES 2 and 3) as well as studies in identical twins.[28] Atopic diseases are diseases such as allergic asthma, seasonal rhinitis (hay fever) and certain cases of food and drug allergy. These diseases are grouped together because they are all mediated by reaginic antibodies, at least for certain kinds of asthma, rhinitis, etc. What appears to be heritable is not the specific allergic disease itself, but the capacity to become easily allergically sensitive (i.e., produce reagins) to an allergen with which the patient has repeated contacts. This trait, the capacity to become allergically sensitive, appears to be under complex genetic control, i.e., it appears to be neither a simple Mendelian dominant nor a recessive. Thus, with many atopic patients, neither parent is known to be atopic, and two atopic parents may have nonatopic children. However, it is difficult to make clear genetic conclusions from such family studies, since a "genotypic atopic" may not express his capacity for sensitization (i.e., develop an allergic disease) until rather late in life or not at all.

TABLE 2

RELATION OF PERSONAL VERSUS FAMILY HISTORY OF ATOPY*

Personal History		Percentage with Family History of Atopy
Atopic	(139 patients)	48%
Nonatopic	(504 patients)	12%

* From ref. #26 (Studies on patients from allergy and general medical clinics.)

TABLE 3

RELATION OF PERSONAL HISTORY OF ATOPY TO FAMILY HISTORY OF ATOPY*

Personal History		Percentage with Family History of Atopy
Atopic	(15 patients)	20% (3/15)
Nonatopic	(116 patients)	5% (6/116)

* From ref. #2 (Studies on patients from an investigation of immune responses to penicillin.)

TABLE 4

RELATION OF ATOPIC BACKGROUND TO REAGIN RESPONSE TO INTRANASAL IMMUNIZATION WITH RIBONUCLEASE*

Atopic Background		Percentage Producing Reagins
Atopic	(10 patients)	80% (8/10)
Nonatopic	(10 patients)	10% (1/10)

* From Ref. #29.

TABLE 5

RELATION OF ATOPIC BACKGROUND TO REAGIN RESPONSE TO PENICILLIN*

Atopic Background		Percentage Producing Reagins
Atopic	(15 patients)	80% (12/15)
Nonatopic	(116 patients)	30% (35/116)

* From Levine *et al.* 1966. J. Clin. Invest. **45**. 1898. The 131 patients include about 40 patients with recent allergic reactions to penicillin and 91 patients who had recent penicillin therapy without allergic reaction. Thus the frequency of reagin producers in both groups is much higher than it would be in a random population treated with penicillin (where the expected incidence of allergic reaction is about 2% and the overall frequency of reagin production is 9%).

Under certain conditions of experimental immunization with proteins,[29,30] carbohydrates,[31] or simple chemicals,[2] reaginic antibodies were produced by a significantly higher percentage of atopic patients than nonatopics (see TABLES 4, 5). It should be noted that the kind of immunization schedule used may be a crucial factor in obtaining such results. In all cases, immunization was by multiple administration of antigen, usually in low doses (in several cases by nasal insufflation). In other cases, where antigens were given subcutaneously in high dosage, there was no difference noted in the frequency of reagin response made by atopics versus nonatopics.[32–34] Utilizing these data, we should like to suggest the hypothesis that there is a genetically controlled polymorphism in man's capacity to respond to repeated small doses of certain immunogens with the production of reaginic antibody. This capacity would constitute atopy. Atopics would be then more liable than nonatopics are to those allergic reactions to drugs which are mediated by reagins, i.e., urticarial reactions as well as anaphylaxis, but not necessarily exanthematic or hemolytic reactions which are mediated by other classes of antibody. We note that Salvaggio and Leskowitz and their associates[29,31–33] have proposed that atopics may differ from nonatopics by having a greater mucosal permeability to immunogens, and that this characteristic would permit sensitization more readily to aersolized allergens. Further work is needed to clarify these questions.

Genetically Controlled Differences in Susceptibility of Guinea Pigs to Acute Anaphylaxis

Another point at which the genetic controls of hypersensitive reactions to drugs might operate is at the release of pharmacological mediators of allergic tissue damage. In studying the anaphylactic responses of Hartley and inbred Strain 2 guinea pigs to subcutaneous administration of antigen, Stone, *et al.*[35] noted that the Strain 2 animals were considerably more resistant to acute anaphylaxis. Subsequent studies[35] (summarized in TABLE 6) showed that outbred Hartley guinea

TABLE 6

GENETIC DIFFERENCES IN TOLERANCE TO ANTIGENICALLY-INDUCED ACUTE ANAPHYLAXIS IN GUINEA PIGS*

	Hartley (sensitive to acute anaphylaxis)	Inbred Str 2 (resistant to acute anaphylaxis)
Effect of i.v. histamine	Equally susceptible	
Sequestration of tagged antibody	Equally susceptible	
Histamine content of lungs	31.2 ± 15.8 μg/gm	10.5 ± 4.5 μg/gm
Histamine released from lung slices in vitro by antigen	5 to 20-fold higher in Hartley	
Bronchospasm produced by antigen in vitro	Marked	Mild to moderate

* From Ref. #35.

pigs contained in their lungs 5- to 20-fold higher amounts of histamine specifically releasable by antigen than did the inbred Strain 2 animals. These differences between inbred (Strains 2 and 13) and the outbred guinea pigs in releasable histamine, as well as the lower variability in histamine contents of the lung among members of the inbred strains, indicate genetic polymorphism. Breeding experiments have not yet been done.

Other Systems Displaying Genetic Polymorphism

Chase[36] and Jacobs, *et al.*[37] have shown genetic polymorphism in the ability of guinea pigs to become contact hypersensitive to a given simple chemical. By repeated brother-sister matings, they were able to establish guinea pig colonies whose members were either very susceptible or were resistant to sensitization with a given chemical. Genetic mechanisms were shown to be complex. The underlying biological bases for the resistant or susceptible trait have not yet been established.

West and Harris[38] found that 25% of outbred Wistar rats failed to give an "anaphylactoid" response to high molecular weight dextran injected intraperitoneally or intravenously. This reaction is manifested by edema and hyperemia of the extremities occurring within minutes after the dextran injection. The reaction appears to be nonimmunologic in mechanism, as it occurs with the first injection of dextran. Dextran apparently is capable of releasing histamine (and probably also serotonin) in the intact rat apparently on a nonimmune basis. Dextran was found to release histamine in the reactor rats, but not in the nonreactors.[38] Breeding experiments showed the reactor trait to segregate as an autosomal dominant trait. Thus, offspring of nonreactors were always nonreactors. Matings of two heterozygote parents produced 3:1 reactors: nonreactors in its offspring. F_1 (heterozygote) backcrosses to the nonreactor parent produced 50% reactors.[38] The biochemical basis for the reactor gene is not yet known, but appears related to the mechanism of mediator release by dextran.

Final Comments

Hypersensitive reactions to simple chemical drugs result from a sequence of many separate molecular events: those associated with the formation of the hapten-conjugate from the drug; the induction of antibody synthesis and the occurrence of allergic tissue damage, which in many cases involves the release of pharmacological mediators. Both environmental as well as genetic factors operate in determining the incidence and variety of hypersensitive reactions to drugs. At present, little is known about the genetic factors operating in hypersensitive reactions to drugs in man, other than the apparent role of atropy. Several hypersensitive systems where genetic factors are operative are described herein, and their possible relation to drug allergy discussed. Genetic factors of various kinds, controlling different molecular events, may have to co-exist in a given individual for a drug-hypersensitive reaction to occur. As a hypothetical example, for an anaphylactic reaction to aspirin to occur, the patient may require genetic information for the appropriate metabolism of aspirin, for the ability to produce reaginic antibodies under mild immunization, and for a high content of specifically releasable histamine (or other mediators) in the shock organ (as well as having repeated contacts with the drug). The probability of the co-existence of these genetic and environmental factors may be very low, thus accounting for the low incidence of these reactions in a random population.

References

1. Siegel, B. B. 1962. Reaginic Penicillin Sensitivity in Allergology. E. A. Brown, Ed. Pergamon Press, N. Y.
2. Levine, B. B., A. P. Redmond, M. J. Fellner, H. E. Voss & V. Levytska. 1966. J. Clin. Invest. **45:** 1895.
3. Levine, B. B. 1966. N. Eng. J. Med. **275:** 1115 and 1966. Ann. Rev. Med. **17:** 23.
4. Landsteiner, K. 1962. The Specificity of Serological Reactions. Rev'd. Edit. Dover Publ., N. Y.
5. Eisen, H. N. 1952. *In* Cellular and Humoral Aspects of the Hypersensitive States. H. S. Lawrence, Ed. P. B. Hoeber, N. Y.
6. Gell, P. G. H., C. R. Harrington & R. Michel. 1948. Brit. J. Exptl. Path. **29:** 578.
7. Fishman, W. H. 1961. Chemistry of Drug Metabolism. C. C. Thomas, Springfield, Ill.
8. Nagasawa, H. T., M. A. Morgen & H. R. Gutmann. 1958. Biochem. Biophys. Acta **28:** 665.
9. Zannone, V. G., S. E. Malawista & B. N. LaDu. 1962. Arth. and Rheum. **5:** 547.
10. Mayer, R. L. 1955. Progr. All. **4:** 79.
11. Baer, R. L., M. Leider & R. L. Mayer. 1948. Proc. Soc. Exptl. Biol. Med. **67:** 489.
12. Shahidi, N. T. 1967. Amer. J. Dis. Child. **113:** 81.
13. Brodie, B. B. & J. Axelrod. 1949. J. Pharm. Exp. Therap. **97:** 58.
14. Fjord-Scheibel, I. 1943. Acta Path. et Microbiol. Scand. **20:** 464.
15. Carlifanti, E. 1948. J. Immunol. **59:** 1.
16. Sang, J. H. & W. R. Sobey. 1954. J. Immunol. **72:** 52.
17. Arquilla, E. R. & J. Finn. 1965. J. Exptl. Med. **122:** 771.
18. Sobey, W. R., J. M. Magrath & A. H. Reisner. 1966. J. Immunol. **11:** 511.
19. McDevitt, H. O. & M. Sela 1965. J. Exptl. Med. **122:** 517.
20. Kantor, F. S., A. Ojeda & B. Benacerraf. 1963. J. Exptl. Med. **117:** 55.
21. Levine, B. B., A. Ojeda & B. Benacerraf. 1963. Nature **200:** 544.
22. Levine, B. B. & B. Benacerraf. 1965. Science **147:** 517.
23. Pinchuck, P. & P. A. Maurer. 1965. J. Exptl. Med. **122:** 673.
24. Ishizaka, K., T. Ishizaka & M. M. Hornbrook. 1966. J. Immunol. **97:** 840.
25. Stanworth, D. R., J. H. Humphrey, H. Bennich & S. G. O. Johansson. 1967. Lancet **2:** 330.
26. Cooke, R. & J. Van der Veer. 1916. J. Immunol. **1:** 201.
27. Ratner, B. & D. E. Silberman. 1953. J. All. **24:** 371.
28. Sherman, W. & W. Kessler. 1957. Allergy in Pediatric Practice. C. V. Mosby Co., St. Louis.
29. Salvaggio, J., .J Cavanaugh, F. C. Lowell & S. Leskowitz. 1964. J. All. **35:** 62.
30. Kuhns, W. J. 1964. J. Immunol. **93:** 446.
31. Salvaggio, J., J. Kayman & S. Leskowitz. 1966. J. All. **38:** 31.
32. Leskowitz, S. & F. C. Lowell. 1961. J. All. **32:** 151.
33. Salvaggio, J. & S. Leskowitz. 1965. Int. Arch. All. **26:** 264.
34. Davidson, A. G., B. Baron & M. Walzer. 1947. J. All. **18:** 359.

35. Stone, S. H., P. Liacopoulos, M. Liacopoulos-Briot, T. Neveu & B. N. Halpern. 1964. Science **146:** 1061.
36. Chase, M. W. 1941. J. Exptl. Med. **73:** 711.
37. Jacobs, J. L., J. J. Kelley & S. C. Sommers. 1942. Proc. Soc. Exptl. Biol. Med. **48:** 639.
38. West, G. B. & J. M. Harris. 1964. Ann. N. Y. Acad. Sci. **118:** 441.

TERATOLOGY AND PHARMACOGENETICS

Harold Kalter

The Children's Hospital Research Foundation and the Department of Pediatrics, College of Medicine, University of Cincinnati, Cincinnati, Ohio

Teratogenesis is one of the most widely known and most worrisome of the toxic effects of drugs, not only among professionals but among the general public as well. Reasons for this are not hard to find.

The publicity given the effects of thalidomide, and the continuing attention of the press to possible similar effects of other drugs such as meclizine and LSD, may cause fear that such dangers are common. The possibility of this danger combined with the variety and number of pills, potions, capsules, and tablets taken by us today may, in truth, be sufficient basis for anxiety. Apprehension would deepen were it better known that teratogens may do most harm during the earliest weeks of pregnancy–at a time when women seldom realize they are pregnant. Furthermore, not the least harrowing aspect of the problem is the ethical dilemma of deciding the fate of a possibly defective embryo.

To what may these fears lead? Eventually, one supposes, to demands for unimpeachably safe drugs or irreproachable procedures for testing the safety of drugs.

These ends, however, are at present beyond reasonable expectation, for the genetic polymorphism of human populations makes it unlikely that the complete absence of adverse reactions to drugs is attainable. Nevertheless, it is imperative that knowledge of the hereditary bases of unusual drug reactions be expanded, and that possible environmental modification of such reactions be explored.

Concerning teratogenesis specifically, very few environmental agents have been identified unquestionably as producing congenital malformations in human beings. And they have not been well studied from the point of view of variable responses, which is regrettable, since it is such variability that may provide clues to mitigation and prevention. Because variability of teratogenic response is not only a function of genetic differences in predisposition but also of erratic nongenetic factors such as time of exposure during pregnancy and dose consumed, it is extremely difficult to allocate responsibility for the degree or type of effect among all the influences that may have played a role.

For example, few scientists still doubt that the epidemic of limb malformations and other birth defects of several years ago was caused by ingestion of thalidomide during the first trimester of pregnancy. However, it cannot be denied that many women who took this drug during the susceptible period of pregnancy had normal children; and also that among the thousands of malformed ones the range of kinds and amounts of damage was tremendous. These qualitative and quantitative spectra were most surely the products of genetic factors as well as nongenetic ones, such as those mentioned above. But, for the most part, it has been impossible to document the first contention and the second has been partly answered for only a small proportion of cases.[1]

One of the reasons animal studies have been performed in teratology is to put these conjectures on a surer footing.

The particular facet of the subject discussed here involves hereditary differences in teratogenic response to drugs in experimental situations, and hence we are concerned with experiments in which two or more groups of teratogen-treated animals had different frequencies or kinds of malformed offspring. To facilitate the discussion and bring the analogy closer to the human situation only studies will be referred to in which different groups of the same species were used, namely, various inbred strains of mice. Quite a number of such observations have been made, and some of the teratogenic agents used are listed in TABLE 1.

As can be seen, most of the experiments were made with chemical substances such as antimetabolites, hormones, vitamins, and so on. Other experiments involved withholding of food, reduced atmospheric pressure (hypoxia), and X irradiation. Thus, the variable action of all but fasting and the physical teratogens possibly can be explained pharmacogenetically. But it would be unwise to neglect lessons that can be learned from nondrug studies, which may be of general significance, and thus we will discuss some results of X-ray studies below.

The nub of the animal teratology problem so far as pharmacogenetics is concerned is this: the action of teratogens is variable, in fact, notoriously variable. So it is common for severely and mildly abnormal offspring and even apparently unaffected offspring to occur together in the same litter from teratogen-treated females, or for the frequency and severity of defects to fluctuate greatly from litter to litter. When noninbred animals are used in these studies it is probable that such variability is the outcome of a mixture of genetic and nongenetic heterogeneities, which are tortuously intertwined and hence quite difficult to analyze.

The use of long-inbred, and thus genetically highly uniform, strains of mice, while it apparently does not greatly reduce the amount of variability occurring in teratogenic experiments, does permit apportioning the sources of this variability into their genetic and environmental components and facilitates further probing of each of them. Where such probings have been made, a complex, multifactorial picture has emerged.

A malformation that has been studied from various points of view and which well exemplifies the problems and achievements of experimental mammalian teratology is the cleft palate induced in mice by glucocorticosteroids.[2–4] It is a convenient defect to study because it is diagnosed easily and because it is an all-or-none abnormality, and hence questions of degree of severity do not obtrude. It is induced in mice (but not rats) and its frequency varies greatly from strain to strain. Furthermore, it is subject to marked environmental modification.[4] Concerning its genetics, although not thoroughly analyzed, susceptibility to cortisone-

TABLE 1

TERATOGENS USED IN STUDIES IN WHICH DIFFERENCES BETWEEN INBRED STRAINS OF MICE OCCURRED

Teratogen	References
Cortisone acetate	2, 3, 4
Galactoflavin	5, 6
Hypervitaminosis A	7
5-Fluorouracil	8
ACTH	9
Insulin	10
Tolbutamide	10
6-Aminonicotinamide	11
6-Azauridine	12
Fasting	13
Hypoxia	14
X irradiation	15, 16

induced cleft palate appears to be a quantitative trait governed by several gene loci. Furthermore, the response is controlled by an interaction of both the maternal and fetal genotypes.[3]

A recent study by Dagg, *et al.*[17] of the genetics of the teratogenic response to 5-fluorouracil also revealed a complex mode of inheritance with some environmental factors operative as well.

We ask now—what is the mechanism through which teratogens act and how do genes regulate these activities? A means of gaining insights into these problems lies in exploring the basis of strain differences. Interesting facts have been emerging from studies of these phenomena concerning embryonic growth patterns.

For example, embryological studies[18] of cortisone-induced cleft palate showed the fetal palate was, on the average, more developmentally advanced at given chronological ages in resistant-strain mice than in a susceptible strain. Another study suggesting growth factors as an explanation was one in which x-irradiation was used.[16] It was found that early in gestation embryos of the more susceptible strain were smaller than resistant-strain embryos. When they were x-rayed at those times when they were approximately the same size, the strains responded quite similarly, Thus, in these instances the effects of teratogens may have depended on the embryonic growth attained at given times during pregnancy.

Other growth factors can also be postulated. Teratogens may have different consequences according to the amount of destruction or retardation they cause, or the amount of recovery that takes place afterward. These things too may be subject to gene control and hence vary from strain to strain. Finally, especially for this monograph, the possibility must be considered that strain differences may be based on differences in the speed and type of distribution and transformation of teratogenic substances. Ultimately, of course, all effects on embryonic development must be referrable to initial chemical or molecular changes, whether in structure or function. And, thus, it is possible that strain differences may be the outcome of variable gene-controlled responses at this primary level, which in the broadest sense is pharmacogenetic.

It should not be imagined, however, that such possible pharmocogenetic phenomena are of the same order as those that largely have been the concern of this monograph. For there is no evidence whatsoever that experimentally produced defects are associated with any such simple situation as the presence or absence of alleles at single loci determining the level or type of enzymes. Presumably the same can be said for the majority of human congenital malformations, since they have no neat genetic, or any other, explanation.

Indeed it would be unrealistic to expect analogies in this respect between pre- and postnatal life. Embryos are the most vulnerable of creatures to death and disruption. The control of their complex and delicate processes is imperfect. Their most pressing need is to maintain a plasticity that will enable them to adapt to environmental fluctuations. This could not be done if their existence or well-being were imperiled by harmful situations of single gene origin. The only means of minimizing the dangers of environmental impacts lie in multigenically controlled hemeostases.

References

1. Nowack, E. 1965. Die sensible Phase bei der Thalidomide-Embryopathie. Humangenetik **1:** 516–536.
2. Fraser, F. C. & T. D. Fainstat. 1951. Production of congenital defects in the offspring of pregnant mice treated with cortisone. Pediatrics **8:** 527–533.
3. Kalter, H. 1954. The inheritance of susceptibility to the teratogenic action of cortisone in mice. Genetics **39:** 185–196.

4. KALTER, H. 1965. Interplay of intrinsic and extrinsic factors. *In* Teratology: Principles and Techniques. J. G. Wilson & J. Warkany, Eds. : 57–80. Univ. Chicago Press, Chicago.
5. KALTER, H. & J. WARKANY. 1957. Congenital malformations in inbred strains of mice induced by riboflavin-deficient, galactoflavin-containing diets. J. Exp. Zool. **136:** 531–566.
6. WALKER, B. E. & B. CRAIN, JR. 1961. Abnormal palate morphogenesis in mouse embryos induced by riboflavin deficiency. Proc. Soc. Exp. Biol. Med. **107:** 404–406.
7. WALKER, B. E. & B. CRAIN, JR. 1960. Effects of hypervitaminosis A on palate development in two strains of mice. Am. J. Anat. **107:** 49–58.
8. DAGG, C. P. 1960. Sensitive stages for the production of developmental abnormalities in mice with 5-fluorouracil. Am. J. Anat. **106:** 89–96.
9. KALTER, H. 1962. ACTH, congenital malformations and "stress." Am. Zool. **2:** 419. (Abst.)
10. SMITHBERG, M. & M. N. RUNNER. 1963. Teratogenic effects of hypoglycemic treatments in inbred strains of mice. Am. J. Anat. **113:** 479–489.
11. GOLDSTEIN, M., M. F. PINSKY & F. C. FRASER. 1963. Genetically determined organ specific responses to the teratogenic action of 6-aminonicotinamide in the mouse. Genet. Res. **4:** 258–265.
12. YOSHIHARA, H. & C. P. DAGG. 1967. Teratogenicity of 6-azauridine in inbred mice. Anat. Rec. **157:** 345. (Abst.)
13. MILLER, J. R. 1962. A strain difference in response to the teratogenic effect of maternal fasting in the house mouse. Can. J. Genet. Cytol. **4:** 69–78.
14. INGALLS, T. H., F. R. AVIS, F. J. CURLEY & H. M. TEMIN. 1963. Genetic determinants of hypoxia-induced congenital anomalies. J. Hered. **44:** 185–194.
15. CALLAS, G. & B. E. WALKER. 1963. Palate morphogenesis in mouse embryos after X-irradiation. Anat. Rec. **145:** 61–72.
16. DAGG, C. P. 1964. Some effects of X-irradiation on the development of inbred and hybrid mouse embryos. *In* Effects of Ionizing Radiation on the Reproductive System. W. D. Carlson & F. X. Gassner, Eds. : 91–102. Macmillan, N. Y.
17. DAGG, C. P., G. SCHLAGER & A. DOERR. 1966. Polygenic control of the teratogenicity of 5-fluorouracil in mice. Genetics **53:** 1101–1117.
18. WALKER, B. E. & F. C. FRASER. 1957. The embryology of cortisone-induced cleft palate. J. Embryol. Exp. Morph. **5:** 201–209.

CONCLUDING REMARKS

Werner Kalow
University of Toronto, Toronto, Canada

On the pages of this monograph many interesting ideas have been presented. Obviously I cannot allude to everything that was said. Some of the topics like primaquine sensitivity, prolonged action of succinylcholine and slow inactivation of isoniazid have been godfathers to the field of pharmacogenetics. Sufficient progress has been made in these areas of research to warrant several papers on each of them to properly present the subject. Also, many of the other older topics have been expanded, in some cases with the introduction of completely new concepts. For example, Dr. Tschudy in his report on hepatic porphyria presented evidence for the importance of disordered hormonal function. The study of familial dysautonomia has opened new vistas onto the function of autonomic transmitters. Malignant hyperpyrexia has been sufficiently defined to permit a rational study.

Some topics have not been presented before in the context of pharmacogenetics. Examples are the papers on acetophenetidin, on diabetes insipidus, and on atypical alcohol dehydrogenase. I feel I would commit a serious omission by not pointing here to Dr. Levine's critical review on genetics and allergic drug sensitivities, and to Dr. Hirschhorn's study of chromosomal breaks due to LSD and other agents.

Ideally, all clinically important topics should have been presented in this monograph, but it is clear that not all have been covered. The whole group of agents that have particular odors or tastes has not been mentioned. For the student of human genes, hereditary deficiencies in the perception of these agents are as important as the biochemically defined metabolic defects. The striking person-to-person differences in response to some tranquillizers, stimulants and particularly hallucinogenic agents have been omitted from presentation mostly because the genetic background has not been established. One may hope that appropriate data will be ready in the not too distant future.

Some of the papers presented showed important progress in studies involving animals. The report by Dr. Vesell represents fundamental investigations with wide implications for bioassay and deserves special mention.

The great majority of papers have been presented by investigators who are defacto clinical pharmacologists. We may take this as an indication that in the field of clinical pharmacology particularly, pharmacogenetics will be able to assist medical advance. Vice versa the more clinical pharmacologists there are, the more rapidly is pharmacogenetics likely to advance.

In concluding, I wish to state my appreciation to the National Institute of General Medical Sciences for the financial support that made the conference and this monograph possible. I am sure I express the sentiments of all participants by saying thanks to Admiral Schanze and the Academy staff for their organizational arrangements which made it a pleasure to attend the Conference.

Printed in the United States of America